Beryl Crane is the founder and director of the Crane School of Reflexology, which holds the prestigious James Accreditation Award from the International Therapy Examination Council, a leading examining body in complementary therapies. Beryl became a Fellow of the Reflexologists' Society in 1989. She has been their Publicity Officer since that time. Since 1995, when she was nominated, she has been their Chairperson. Beryl also teaches and lectures internationally and was asked to present and help with advanced courses with the China Reflexology Association in 1995, after which they made her a Full Honourable Member. Beryl is also Reflexology Advisor for the Institute for Complementary Medicine (Reflexology Division), Guild of Complementary Practitioners, and she is one of the Directors of the International Council of Reflexologists in the USA. She is also a member of the British Complementary Medicine Association (BCMA), The National Back Pain Association, St John's Ambulance, the All Party Parliamentary Group on Skin and The Institute for Optimum Nutrition.

I would like to dedicate this book to my husband of 43 years, who I love dearly for his patience, understanding and love, which were sorely tested throughout the time that this book was in the making.

Reflexology

THE DEFINITIVE PRACTITIONER'S MANUAL

*Recommended by the
International Therapy Examination Council
for Students and Practitioners*

BERYL CRANE

E L E M E N T
Shaftesbury, Dorset ● Rockport, Massachusetts
Melbourne, Victoria

© Element Books Limited 1997
Text, illustrations and charts © Beryl Crane 1997

First published in Great Britain in 1997 by
Element Books Limited
Shaftesbury, Dorset SP7 8BP

Published in the USA in 1997 by
Element Books, Inc.
PO Box 830, Rockport, MA 01966

Published in Australia in 1997 by
Element Books
and distributed
by Penguin Books Australia Limited
487 Maroondah Highway, Ringwood,
Victoria 3134

Illustrations by Paul Girling, Greystoke Graphics, Banham, Norfolk
Additional illustrations by David Gifford
Photographs by Malcolm Tinn, Tangles Photographic, Harlow, Essex
Design by Page
Typeset by Footnote Graphics, Warminster, Wilts.
Printed and bound in Great Britain by Butler & Tanner, Frome, Somerset

British Library Cataloguing in Publication
data available

Library of Congress Cataloging in Publication
data

Crane, Beryl.
    Reflexology : the definitive practitioners manual / Beryl Crane.
        p.   cm.
    "Recommended by the International Therapy Examination Council for students and practitioners."
    Includes bibliographical references and index.
    ISBN 1–86204–125–3 (hardbound)
    1. Reflexology (Therapy)—Handbooks, manuals, etc.   I. Title.
RM723.R43C73   1997
615.8'22—dc21   97–29169
                                                          CIP

ISBN 1 86204 336 1

Contents

Acknowledgements

Many thanks to my models: my daughter Alex for the use of her feet and hands, my daughter-in-law Susan for her help in the plate section, and my granddaughter Sarah for the use of her ear. A big thank-you to baby Isaac Verral, who smiled throughout whenever his feet, hands or ears were touched, no matter how long the photographic session took. I would also like to thank my many students and the practitioners who wrote to me encouraging me to write this manual.

Acknowledgements are due to Health Research, Mokelumne Hill, California for continuing to produce facsimiles of the early writings of Fitzgerald, Bowers, White and Shelby-Riley.

I would also like to acknowledge the following works which I have consulted in the course of writing:
The Anatomical Atlas of Chinese Acupuncture Points, Shandong Science and Technology Press, 1982; *Black's Medical Dictionary*, A & C Black, 38th edition, 1995; *Churchill Livingstone Medical Dictionary*, Churchill Livingstone, 14th edition, 1987; *Gray's Anatomy*, Jarrold & Son Publishers, 35th edition, 1973; Badawy, *The Tomb of Nyhetep-Ptah and the Tomb of Ankhm'ahor at Saqqara*, University of California Occasional Papers © 1978.

Foreword

The author has been known to me for many years and I have great respect, not only for her expertise in the field of reflexology, but for her very wide knowledge of the subject.

As a complementary therapy, reflexology is daily gaining the approbation of patients and other professionals including general practitioners and hospital doctors. This is due to the work and dedication of reflexologists, of whom Beryl Crane is an outstanding example.

It gives me the greatest of pleasure to recommend this excellent and well researched book to all serious students of this therapy.

Dr William Arnold-Taylor MSc, PhD
Member Clinical Forensic Medicine;
Fellow of the Royal Society of Medicine;
Chairman of the International Therapy Examination Council Limited

Preface

What is reflexology?

Reflexology is a science based on the principle that reflexes, or areas, in the feet, hands and other parts of the body relate to the internal organs and other structures of the body.

There are several definitions of the word 'reflex', all of which are relevant here:

- 'an involuntary unconscious response to stimuli'
- 'a mirror image'
- 'to turn or be directed back'.

The definition of 'ology' is the study of that branch of science. The term 'microcosm' is also relevant: this is defined as 'a small system regarded as a little self-contained world that represents all the qualities or activities of something much larger'. In reflexology the feet, hands and ears are seen as a perfect microcosm of the body, with a somatic replication of all organs, glands and muscles of the body on to an area or a reflex point. Palpation or pressure on such points helps to achieve balance in the body by normalizing the function of internal organs through a system of zones that link particular reflexes with particular organs. This treatment by pressure helps to stimulate the body's healing process and to allow the person to achieve physical and emotional well-being. There are many ways to apply pressure. Even wringing the hands or rubbing them together can be quite beneficial, while putting the fingertips together helps to stimulate the brain, and squeezing the fingers can relieve a headache or toothache. The points to which pressure is applied are located by reference to both Traditional Chinese Medicine (TCM) and the zone theory. The area just behind the ball of the foot is known as 'Bubbling Spring' (or 'Well') point, a vital point in the Chinese meridian theory; this is the same point where the solar plexus is represented on the feet in the reflexology theory. It is on these minute reflex areas that the reflexologist will apply precise alternating pressure techniques, thus bringing about a therapeutic effect on the corresponding area of the body.

Reflexology is truly a holistic non-invasive therapy, where the practitioner sees the patient as a whole; it is most important that the practitioner is aware of this concept from the onset of treatment, as it is this approach and perspective that is so advantageous. Patients' problems should not be viewed as just a bad shoulder or stiff neck and so forth. The body does not function as an individual part but as an interaction of many structures and systems (*see* chapter 2).

Reflexology is a must for the 21st century. We need to make this age-old therapy an essential part of everyday life for all, young and old alike. Reflexology treatment has many benefits. It leads to a better functioning of the circulatory system, as blood flow is improved, taking all the nutrients to the appropriate parts more efficiently. Blood and nerve supply to muscles improves, aiding and relaxing muscle spasm and tension. The treatment also promotes good muscle tone through nerve stimulation, so reflexology helps compensate for lack of exercise in cases of illness or old age. It also promotes a more active peripheral vascular return. This is especially helpful in people who have a sedentary lifestyle, whose skeletal muscles often lack the ability of squeezing the veins to increase the venous blood pressure; as a result of the therapy their hearts do not have to work quite so hard to bring about the venous return. The person often finds the therapy warming and exhilarating, as it calms the nervous system. Since stress-related problems do not seem to have the same adverse effects the person is better able to cope. Reflexology can in fact be both sedative and stimulating to the nervous system; this is why it benefits and relieves pain in many nervous and autoimmune disorders. Also, the processes of elimination work more efficiently, so that there is no accumulation of excess waste within the system, which many therapists consider the primary cause of disease. Stimulating the circulation helps the elimination of excess waste products and contributes to increase of excretion of fluids. The treatment generally also lessens inflammation, pain, swelling, heat and redness, which may occur as reactions of the body's tissues to injury. In cases of injury, in reflexology there is no need to touch the impaired part itself. Stimulation to the lymphatics helps the oedema that is often the body's reaction to injury, and the accumulation of fluids that could also be the result of a defective kidney or a circulatory disorder.

Research on its physiological effects is still in its very early stages; many studies of treatment outcomes have been published but more in-depth clinical trials are needed to verify the many noted outcomes and to test some of the hypotheses so that the possible theories of action can be elucidated. Reflexologists world-wide are communicating with each other to further research that is not just anecdotal evidence, but demonstrates comprehensive outcomes showing the benefits of treatment; however, more advanced study of how and why reflexology works is still needed. This will be achieved only when research moves in the direction of standardized, randomized, controlled studies of the reflexology treatment. Studies to date have shown how reflexology has a sedative or stimulating effect on the nervous system depending on the type (firm or gentle pressure) and length of treatment. There is also the question of whether it is stimulating or sedating nerve pathways (for a full discussion of the nervous system and reflexology see chapter 2). The tradition of pressure for relieving pain has been under much discussion since the late 1800s. Many great medical men have been involved in studies of reflexes and how nerve signals are transmitted, and have shown how such pressure affects the autonomic nervous system, which in turn improves the function of all the organs and structures of the body. Studies of nerve innervation have demonstrated that such pressure either increases or decreases the rate and strength of the heartbeat, depending on whether the sympathetic or parasympathetic nervous system is stimulated. Analysis of the sensory stimulus to the nerve endings by touch shows how reflexology enables the body to provide better functioning of all the structures and organs within it. There is a hypothesis that reflexology treatment may also encourage the process of cell renewal, acting at cellular level to provide better intercellular communication. Studies on outcomes of treatment show that the sensory stimuli to all the reflexes aids the body in repairing itself. Theories of its effect include activation of the sebaceous glands and sweat glands, which help in moisturizing and lubricating the skin. Other glands and organs would also benefit by stimulation of the blood circulation, because this is like a transport system, and through the continuous flow of blood around the body nutrients from the alimentary tract are distributed to all tissues of the body. So more oxygen from the lungs reaches all the tissues, and waste material (including carbon dioxide) is transported to the excretory surfaces. Hormones are transported from endocrine glands to other organs and tissues. In the immune system the lymphocytes, which have a defensive action in removing waste, germs and dead cells, are activated. The leucocytes, or white blood cells, are transported to the site of infection quicker, helping to reduce pain and stiffness of joints, improving mobility, and helping in antibody production.

Reflexology is the subject of many research programmes, each organization conducting its own investigation. The many societies and associations, together with the present-day umbrella bodies within the UK, are all recording outcomes of treatment. We also have a research Council for Complementary and Alternative Medicine. The International Council of Reflexologists in America is made up from many leading health care practitioners from around the world, all with the same aims and goals. This organization openly encourages research and is also promoting critical thinking skills amongst its members. The latest news from the research committee of the federation of Danish reflexologists, the Forenede Danske Zoneterapeuter (FDZ) (summarized from an article in their newsletter), is as follows: In 1995 the National Board of Health Council for Alternative Treatment published the results of a country-wide study entitled 'Headaches and reflexological treatment' in which 220 patients were treated by 78 reflexologists throughout the country; they were monitored from the time they decided to begin reflexology treatment until they finished the course, and again 3 months after the final treatment. Seventy-eight per cent of patients reported that they had been either cured (23 per cent) or helped (55 per cent). These results are reported with the permission of Christine Issel (*see* Useful addresses, page 431).

Today there is no concise explanation of the rationale of how and why reflexology works, that is accepted by the medical fraternity. Just like any other therapy, however, so much depends on the practitioner in the art of using this technique. It is often said that a poorly trained reflexology practitioner will not necessarily harm you; however, the benefits of receiving treatment from a competently trained practitioner are astounding and it can work wonders if applied correctly.

We should not need to postulate about the benefits of reflexology treatment, because any recipient can attest whether they are in pain prior to treatment. There are comparatively few that leave with the same degree of pain and discomfort. While this relief may not last until the next session, on subsequent visits the problem will often right itself. Most reflexologists will also substantiate that since they have been practising reflexology they often themselves feel better; this may indicate that the stimulation of their own fingers is affecting their nervous systems and benefiting them in some way.

The following chapters explain the history and theory of reflexology by reference to the concepts of zones, reflexes, meridians and nerve pathways. It is to be hoped that by the end of this book, readers will agree that it does not matter whether one is working on a meridian, or a reflex, or a nerve pathway, or an energy line. They may decide just to accept the zone theory. Whatever is transmitted by the technique is powerful and potent to the body. Reflexology achieves homeostasis of all the systems of the body, through the reduction of the effects of stress, and by giving complete relaxation to the recipient.

Aims of this book and how to use it

The aims and objectives of this text are to give clear guidelines for the student or practitioner of reflexology to follow. Each chapter is clearly defined with its contents, so that the reader may obtain a brief outline of the facts and information within each section. This will enable the reader to cross-reference against any previous data.

This manual also undertakes to raise the standards and levels of competency of the student or practitioner. It is not a book on anatomy and physiology, but looks at the wider understanding that is needed in this totally holistic, natural therapy. The reader is made aware of the cellular make-up of the body, and of how each cell has one particular job to do, and even though it has its own in-built chemistry to carry out a particular function it does not accomplish all the activities that are necessary for its existence. This is all brought together by the co-ordination of the different mechanisms of the body to achieve balance and unity.

Material is presented to enable students to understand the different levels of understanding required for reflexology, and various ideas and theories are discussed. Readers should acquire a knowledge of how deeply relaxing reflexology is and how this benefits a wide range of disorders, whether related to stress, emotional or mental, or even more deep-rooted tensions leading to manifestation of physical problems. The expertise and enlightenment gained from this manual will enable the reader to conduct a therapeutic healing session for all ages, from the very young to the more elderly person, to the sick and infirm.

This practitioner's manual enriches your knowledge and understanding of how reflexology works and how it is beneficial to those who are extremely fragile in health and how reflexology works safely by gently removing congestion or blockages, restoring balance and improving energy generally throughout the body. It explains how our feet are the very foundation of our body, and how any deviation from normal structure or function can be reflected back into the body, often resulting in stress and imbalances to organs and a burden on the skeletal function. All these observations are helpful in diagnostic techniques and foot analysis.

The text also explains how to use reflexology without risk, as with the correct treatment there is no great shock to the system, and each session is balanced according to each individual's needs, thus allowing the body to adapt to the necessary changes that take place over a period of a few weeks, with more chronic problems often needing a little more time before they respond.

The book utilizes the concepts of zones and meridians throughout, and these are detailed in chapter 2. These channels are systematically mapped out showing the reflex point and acupuncture (acu) points that are linked to specific organs and functions of the body. This manual also takes you through the history of reflexology, from the very early beginnings of the discovery that pressure on specific areas of the skin brought about a therapeutic action on the functioning of different body organs, to the present-day standard and refinement of this therapy.

The text also outlines how reflexology has currently been lifted to new heights with in-depth training now covering a period of an academic year, setting high standards in professional practice. Values and ethics also are an integral part of the reflexologist's work. Good and safe practice is explained throughout this manual, while professional standards are detailed and encouraged. Advice on setting up and running a reflexology practice is also included.

In conclusion, this work has the following aims:

- to give a knowledge of the history and theory of reflexology from its early methods and aims through to present-day evidence of the art and skill, and current techniques used throughout the world in clinical reflexology
- to develop the student or practitioner's understanding and appreciation of the principles of reflexology and the holistic concept
- to create opportunities for the student or practitioner to learn how to assess the state of a person's health and be able to identify where there may be an imbalance within the body by: observation – of the patient or client and of the hands, feet and ears; a knowledge of hand, foot, and nail conditions that may relate to a patient's health; use of correct consultation procedures, including listening skills; palpation of specific reflex points, and understanding of the basis of reflex stimulation to analyse imbalances and to boost the body's own healing process
- to explore promotion and maintenance of each individual's health and emotional well-being through palpation of specific reflex points, and how these relate to the zone theory and the meridian theory
- to develop a student's or practitioner's competence and improve

their practice, by making them aware of research and investigative procedures in relation to complementary medicine
- to enable students and practitioners to develop an understanding of general practice management.

By the end of the manual the student or practitioner will be able to:

- make a diagnostic assessment of a client before treatment, taking into account the previous medical history and contraindications if any, and evaluate all other relevant factors that may cause them an imbalance
- be aware of their own abilities and when it is necessary to refer a patient to other health care professionals if so required
- complete a full and thorough competent treatment procedure employing all the clinical skills acquired throughout their course of study, including knowledge of the zone and meridian theories, and be able to adapt treatment accordingly in respect of specific areas to treat, amount of pressure and length of treatment
- evaluate treatment sessions through practice and experience throughout the course, and develop both skills and practice using the cyclical learning process, that is, assessing, planning, carrying out procedures, evaluating when needed, and improving if possible
- promote and implement values of good and safe practice in reviewing future treatments with patients, and discuss with them any factors that could affect their health, such as behaviour patterns, lifestyle, nutrition and diet
- analyse and discuss all relevant articles and contemporary research regarding the practice of reflexology, both hypothetical or speculative and established theories and facts, and take account of other therapies that would be an adjunct to it.

1   A brief history of reflexology

Healing by touch is as old as mankind. It requires insight, intuition and the use of specialized skills and techniques.

The word 'massage' comes from the ancient Arabic word *'mass'*, meaning 'to touch or palpate'. Touch or massage has historically been used as a restorative to bring back health and strength. Many of the touch therapies are based on the theory that for good health the body's energy must flow unimpeded, or that a holistic and integrated approach to maintain health should be followed. For instance, Hippocrates (460–375 BC) advocated a system of treatment that incorporated diet, fresh air and exercise (or gymnastics, as they were known then) and advised massage, or rubbing an area of the body, as a therapeutic relaxation.

This chapter examines the ancient and recent origins of reflexology, both in the West and in the Orient, and the recent development of the zone concept.

Egyptian origins

The Egyptian origins of reflexology can be seen in a frieze at the tomb of Ankhm'ahor that is thought to illustrate a reflexology treatment taking place (figures 1.1 and 1.2). This tomb in Saqqara is known as the 'physician's tomb' owing to the marvellous portrayal of many medical scenes found on its walls. The tomb was discovered by V Loret in Egypt in 1897. Saqqara is one of the richest archaeological sites in Egypt, containing monuments constructed over a span of more than 3,000 years, the earliest being the Mastabas, the earlier name for a tomb. Saqqara is the largest necropolis found (a large burial ground of the ancient city). Activity was extremely intense in this area during the Old Kingdom.

The Old Kingdom encompassed the period from the 1st to the 6th Dynasty when all the great pyramids were built in Giza and in Saqqara this period lasted from 3000 to 2250 BC when it came abruptly to an end, owing to a civil war breaking out, and

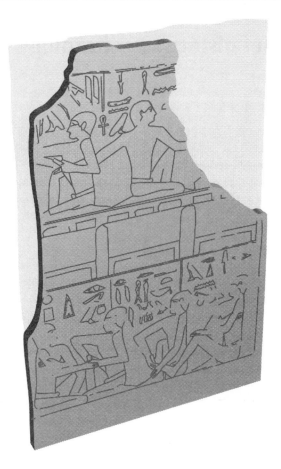

Figure 1.1 Illustration of patients having hands and toes treated (lower picture) and a patient having hand treatment (top picture), from the tomb of Ankhm'ahor.

the whole empire collapsed. To the Ancient Egyptians the afterlife was just as important as the earthly life, hence the reason they surrounded themselves with many murals and pictures on the walls of their many tombs; these portray agricultural scenes and abundant harvests as well as hunting, fishing and dancing scenes and many games. All of these were of an afterlife modelled on a visionary earthly life. Ankhm'ahor was an able master-builder and was considered an expert because he controlled the work of the many sculptors at the tomb. This project disclosed his keen interest in medicine as he displayed recurrent images of medical themes and surgical operations taking place on the walls. His interest in pathology was attributed to his admiration of another architect named Imhotep, who was made an object of worship and was later known as Imuthes, God of Medicine. (Imhotep built the first step pyramid for King Zoser the Pharaoh of the 3rd Dynasty in 2686 BC when Zoser was the King of Upper and Lower Egypt.)

In the Masataba of 'Ankhm'ahor' on the west door entrance are

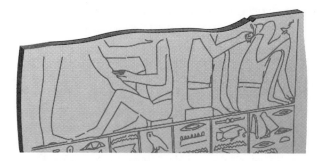

Figure 1.2 Patients having massage or manipulation of the foot or leg and shoulder, from the tomb of Ankhm'ahor.

two registers representing the treatment of hands and feet. These are referred to as a manicure and pedicure by Alexander Badawy in his book *The Tomb of Ankhm'ahor at Saqqara* in which he gives a very fine detailed translation of the wall scenes. In one scene on the wall the right hand of one person is being treated and the other person is having a toe on the left foot treated. The text reads: (patient) 'Make these give strength.' The operator responds, 'I will do to thy pleasure sovereign!' (This answer is between the two operators, so it could be valid for both.) The patient who is having his toe treated is begging, 'Do not cause pain to these.' There also appears to be a probe in the operator's hand (see figure 1.1) (although this is not shown in the many reproduced copies that are included in many reflexology books). An upper fragment on the same wall shows a patient having both hands treated; however, the inscription was badly defaced (see figure 1.1).

Another relief shows massage or manipulation to the foot or leg and shoulder (figure 1.2), which could indicate some form of pressure therapy. As massage was often mentioned in many of the texts and old medical papyri it is quite reasonable to believe that this could be a form of reflexology treatment taking place on the hands and feet with massage or manipulation to the legs and back.

Ankhm'ahor himself is represented on two door-jambs in identical striding attitude. The inscriptions indicate the many titles he held; these include 'Hereditary Prince', 'Count', 'Chief Justice', 'Vizier' and 'Court Physician'.

Chinese origins

Ancient Chinese writings described a pressure therapy using the fingers and thumbs. Acupressure is an old Oriental therapy, 'acu' meaning 'needle point'; however, finger pressure was used long before needles. There are different types of acupressure, from the very gentle to deep digital and thumb pressure. There were many early books written on massage or 'examining foot method' as it was then called. In reflexology, the varying pressures are used according to each individual's requirements and the diagnostic techniques are very similar to those used in Chinese acupressure.

In the Sung Dynasty (AD 960–1280) a paper that first appeared in *Essentials of Preserving Life* showed some exercise routines, which, when repeated, were supposed to be excellent for health. One of these routines was to stretch the hands forward and clench firmly the balls of the extended feet and lower the head as if paying homage; this was repeated 12 times, after which you then returned to the crossed leg position and placed your clenched hands back into your lap. Many ancient diagrams survived of these early 'Dao Yin' exercises that were the earliest forms of Chi Kung (Qigong); these were traditionally considered representations from the Chinese ancients of longevity each of whom had their own special method of healing diseases. One in particular is an acupressure cure for lumbago or any low back pain; it shows the person facing the wall, pressing the palm of the right hand against the wall, letting the left hand drop naturally; the right foot is also placed against the wall, and the person then proceeds to exhale very slowly 18 times. This is then repeated with the left hand and foot. This exercise is claimed to heal strain of the lumbar muscles, and relieve lower back pain and lumbago. These actions indicate how important the hands and feet are considered to be in maintaining good health in TCM.

Acupuncture itself developed throughout the early Shang Dynasty in the 16th to 11th centuries BC. It became a method of treating disease and pain by the insertion of many different types and sizes of needles into specific areas of the body. These areas, or acupuncture points (acupoints), were thought to lie on lines or channels known as meridians (*see* chapter 2 for a full description). Acupressure and acupuncture were, however, only a small part of the treatment of TCM. The system also included a vast herbal tradition and dietary practices.

Buddhism was a religion of East and Central Asia that grew from the teachings of Gautama Buddha. His philosophy was that pureness of spirit was the answer to all suffering. Buddhism spread to China around the time of the Han Dynasty (about 206 BC). There is evidence from this period that in ancient times the feet symbolized many things. A Buddha's footprints carved in the rock at Kusinara, China, shows signs on the second, third, fourth and fifth toes depicting the Sun, in ancient times possibly symbolizing the Qi energy within the toes (*see* figure 1.3).

Yin, Yang and Qi

The terms 'Yin' and 'Yang' are widely used in Traditional Chinese Medicine. They describe, for instance, the quality of the Qi (Chi) energy, which flows through channels called meridians. Illness is caused by an imbalance of Yin and Yang in the body. The idea of Yin and Yang polarities appears continually throughout Chinese thought. Yin is conceived as the soft, inactive female principle or polarity in the body and in the universe generally, while Yang is the active, male principle or polarity. Although opposites, they are also interrelated, and to keep healthy these two opposing but complementary energies must always be balanced.

One energy ascends in the body; the other descends. TCM theory states that if the blood and the energy are not in equilibrium, there is disharmony between the Yin and Yang qualities, and illness will soon follow. A blockage or malfunction is considered to indicate a deficiency or excess of energy of one or the other within the body, manifesting as a functional disturbance, or an imbalance in the way in which an organ or body system functions; from this, physical ill-health can develop. A saying that describes this idea is 'If there is a kink in the life force disease will manifest'. In disease these terms also refer to Yang being all acute problems, in which the patient feels hot and may have a temperature, and is restless. Yin indicates a more chronic problem,

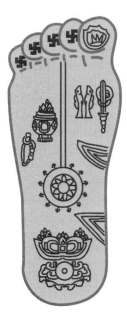

Figure 1.3 Buddha's foot, showing the Sun sign on the toes, possibly indicating Qi.

in which the patient is weak and often cold and has no wish to move about.

Good health depends on the correct balance between these two opposites, the negative and positive. To follow the general principles of Yin and Yang one needs also to be aware of the environment and the changes of the season; all of the above had to be taken into consideration to preserve life. Today China is known for its many centenarians, and longevity is something all Chinese people cherish; many feel that it can be attained through correct living and the use of TCM principles.

The Zangfu organs and the meridians

TCM theory divides the body into 12 organ systems, 6 of which are Yang (Fu or hollow organs): Stomach, Small Intestine, Large Intestine, Bladder, Gall Bladder and Triple Burner (or Triple Heater or Triple Energizer), and 6 of which are Yin (Zang or solid organs): Heart, Liver, Spleen (and Pancreas), Lungs, Kidneys and Pericardium. Together they are called the Zangfu.

Each of the Zang organs is related to one of the Fu organs. So there are six pairs. Often when treating a patient, these Yin and Yang organs can be coupled together because they are so closely related, and treatment of one will often affect the other. The pairs are: the Liver and Gall Bladder, the Spleen and Stomach, the Lungs and Large Intestine, the Kidneys and Bladder, the Heart and Small Intestine, and the Pericardium and Triple Burner. The Triple Burner (Sanjiao) regulates the functioning of all the Zangfu organs; it also acts as a passageway for the movement of all fluids.

The organs are also designated according to the Five Elements theory. According to ancient Chinese traditions, the elements comprise Wood, Fire, Earth, Metal and Water. These elements are thought to influence each other, in a cyclical manner.

The balance of Yin and Yang within each of the above organ systems is regulated and influenced by the Yin–Yang balance of the Qi flowing through the meridians connected with them. This Qi is particularly easy to influence for the purposes of treatment at particular points called acupuncture points (or acupoints). Acupoints at the extremities (hands and feet) are thought to be the most powerful to use (*see* figure 1.9).

There are 12 major meridians in the body and limbs, each connected to one organ system; 6 connect the hands with the face or chest, and 6 connect the feet with the face or chest. These meridians are often classified in three ways:

1 According to their cycle of energy. This is as follows: Lungs, Large Intestine, Stomach, Spleen, Heart, Small Intestine, Bladder, Kidneys, Pericardium, Triple Burner, Gall Bladder, Liver. The cycle of energy goes: hands–hands, feet–feet, hands–hands, feet–feet, hands–hands, feet–feet; we can balance the energy by working on this theory.

2 According to the division of the two groups into Yin and Yang:
the Yin meridians of the feet and legs are: the Liver, Spleen and Kidneys – these ascend from the feet to the breast (figure 1.4)
the Yin meridians of the hands and arms are: Lungs, Heart, Pericardium – these descend from the breast to terminate in the fingers (figure 1.5)
the Yang meridians of the hands and arms are: Large Intestine, Small Intestine and Triple Burner – these ascend from the fingers to the face (figure 1.6)
the Yang meridians of the feet and legs are: the Stomach, Bladder, Gall Bladder – these descend from the face to the toes (figure 1.7).

3 According to where they are located: the six meridians on the hands and arms include the Lungs, Large Intestine, Triple Burner, Pericardium, Heart and Small Intestine. The six meridians on the feet and legs are the Kidneys, Spleen, Liver, Stomach, Gall Bladder and Bladder.

There is an involved association between an organ and a meridian. They are often paired together because of the anatomical closeness of the corresponding meridian, which links the Yin and the Yang organ. In reflexology this opposite point becomes an area of assistance to work.

We begin to see a combination between the groups as follows:

- The three Yin meridians descend from the breast area to the hands (*see* figure 1.5); that is the Lungs, Heart and Pericardium, (for details of each meridian pathway *see* figures 2.8–2.20, pages 51–64).
- The three Yang meridians of the hands ascend from the hand to the face (*see* figure 1.6) that is the Large Intestine, Small Intestine and Triple Burner.
- The three Yin meridians of the feet ascend from the feet to breast area (*see* figure 1.4); that is the Spleen, Kidneys and Liver.
- The three Yang meridians of the feet descend from the face to the feet (*see* figure 1.7); that is the Stomach, Bladder and Gall Bladder.

There are many interactions between the organs and meridians, and they are paired in many ways. Some old doctrines link the

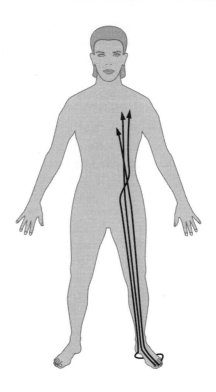

Figure 1.4 The three ascending Yin meridians of the feet (Spleen, Liver and Kidneys)

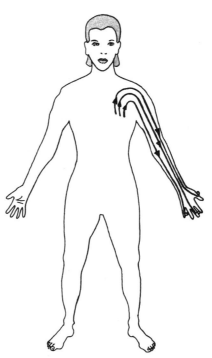

Figure 1.5 The three descending Yin meridians of the hands (Lungs, Heart and Pericardium)

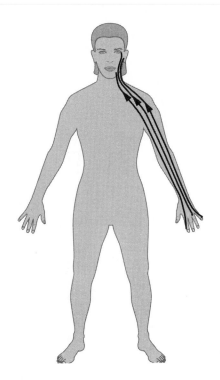

Figure 1.6 The three ascending Yang meridians of the hands (Large Intestine, Triple Burner and Small Intestine)

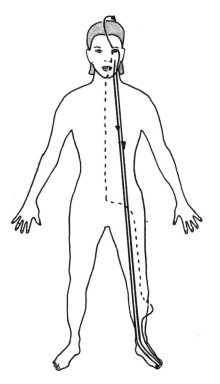

Figure 1.7 The three descending Yang meridians of the feet (Stomach, Bladder and Gall Bladder)

(a)

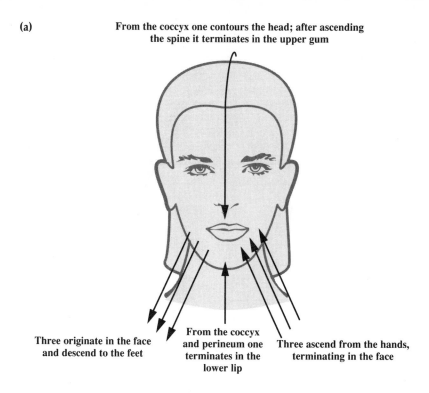

From the coccyx one contours the head; after ascending the spine it terminates in the upper gum

Three originate in the face and descend to the feet

From the coccyx and perineum one terminates in the lower lip

Three ascend from the hands, terminating in the face

(b)

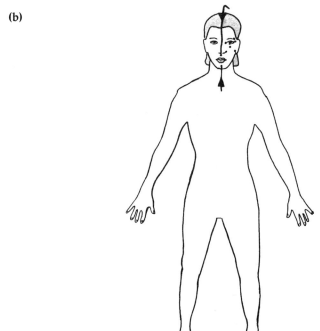

Figure 1.8 (a) Eight major meridians converge on the face. (b) The face has three originating points, three terminating points, and two terminating points from the vessels.

Yin organs in a cycle, and then the Yang organs, in a theory that attempts to describe the movement of Qi energy. One idea is that there is an area of the body where Qi undergoes a fundamental change in polarity, where Yin is converted into Yang or vice versa (figure 1.9). One speculation is that at such an area or point the therapist gets a much more positive result, because the energy is unstable and nearer to the surface here. However, there are areas which contain the points where the ascending Yang meridians terminate on the face and where the descending Yang meridians originate from prior to descending to the feet: these are thought to be more stable yet not so potent. Yet if this is so, why is it that these facial distal points are so powerful? It is imortant to note that there are eight major meridians converging on the facial area (*see* figures 18a and 18b, and chapter 7). Is this why the ears, head and facial points are so effective? This interchange of energies takes place on the fingers of the upper limbs as the Yin energy is near its end, and the Yang energy is about to commence; this fluctuation extends from the fingers to the elbow. So we see the three Yin meridians conveying their energy to the three Yang meridians, anywhere in this area. This leads to the traditional pairing of these organs on the hand:

- Lungs (Yin) paired with Large Intestine (Yang)
- Heart (Yin) paired with Small Intestine (Yang)
- Pericardium (Yin) paired with Triple Burner (Yang).

The same metamorphosis takes place on the feet, with the area from the tips of the toes to the knee being the most advantageous area to work, and around the ankles being very potent. Again, a pairing of the Yin and Yang meridians takes place:

- Stomach (Yang) paired with Spleen (Yin)
- Bladder (Yang) paired with Kidneys (Yin)
- Gall Bladder (Yang) paired with Liver (Yin).

It is important when treating always to balance these points, incorporating pressure points of both upper and lower limbs. This stabilizes the energy from the upper part of the body with that of the lower part of the body. The combination of such points is very forceful and effective, so working upper pressure points with lower pressure points or working on the paired organ becomes a powerful therapy.

The Chinese often utilize these combination points according to their forceful action or their compatibility. The meridian channels form a complete circuit and TCM principles state that these energies within each meridian are balanced; hence, on that account they have always been used in treatment. The points on the extremities are referred to as the fountain head or well points (figure 1.9), for instance those at the tips of the fingers and the tips of the toes, and KI-1 located at the centre of the ball of the foot. These are considered to be extremely powerful as they are barely skin deep at this terminal or starting point, so they are easy to stimulate by palpation as is done in reflexology. The spring points are extremely potent and forceful; these are found around the wrist and the ankles, with the feet points being more dynamic than those of the hands. At the sea points, which lie at the elbows or knees, the energy is more general and less active, achieving a slower response.

Recent history

When the People's Republic of China was formed in 1949 TCM came under threat because of superstitions and ancient theories and was almost lost. It was Chairman Mao who came to the rescue. The story goes that he became very ill and orthodox medicine did not

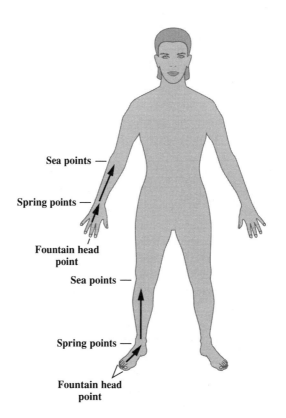

Figure 1.9 The most potent areas to work

help him, so he turned to the traditional folk medicine, which saved him. Following this, he declared 'Traditional Chinese Medicine is of immense value, it needs to be constantly explored and further developed'. Because of this, since 1950 work was encouraged on research and tests on TCM, and Western medicine and TCM were practised side by side. Research on TCM has continued in China and has been maintained over the last 40 years and more recently they have also researched treatment by reflexology. To date the China Reflexology Association have accumulated over 10,000 case histories on reflexology treatments. There are 31 provinces in China, half of which have set up a reflexology branch. Among 7,000 members of the national and the local associations, there are now over 1,500 medical doctors in China who practise reflexology in their hospitals, or clinics, sanatoriums, and other centres.

The history of the zone concept

The founder of zone therapy

Zone therapy is a system discovered many years ago by an eminent American physician, William H Fitzgerald, who was born in 1872 and who died in Stamford, Connecticut on 21 October 1942. He was an MD in Hartford, Connecticut. Dr Fitzgerald graduated from the University of Vermont in 1895 and worked his first 2½ years at the Boston City Hospital; he then went on to serve a further 2 years at the Central London Ear, Nose and Throat (ENT) Hospital in England (1902). This was followed by a further 2 years in Vienna's ENT Hospital under Professor Politzer and Professor Otto Chiari, who were well known in the medical world at that time. All of this gives some indication of Dr Fitzgerald's qualities as a doctor and surgeon. Dr Fitzgerald was senior nose and throat surgeon at St Francis Hospital, Hartford, Connecticut for several years. It was during that period that he made his findings of zone therapy, as it was called at this time, known to the medical world.

He developed this therapy because he observed, while working, that when applying pressure over certain points of the toes and hands, and other parts of the body, if the pressure was firm enough it caused a type of anaesthesia in a limited area. This enabled him to perform minor operations on the nose and throat without using cocaine and other local analgesics while the patient could be treated without pain. Fitzgerald stated in his book that pressure over any bony eminence, or upon the zones corresponding to the location of the injury, would tend to relieve pain, and that not only would it relieve pain but if pressures were firm enough it would produce an anaesthetic effect, often removing the cause of the pain.

Dr Fitzgerald published his first book in 1917 with Dr Edwin Bowers. The title read '*Zone Therapy, or Relieving Pain at Home*'. In this he related all his important findings on zone therapy. A zone is an area or part that is marked off, with stated qualities. Fitzgerald diagrammatically depicted this in his early drawings by dividing the human body into zones both anterior and posterior (figure 1.10) and he speculated that the body could be divided into ten such longitudinal (meaning vertical) zones, five each side of the median or middle line. The first ran from the medial edge of the great toe through the centre of the nose to the brain, and then out to the thumb or vice versa. He spoke of these zones as numbering one to five on the right side of the body and the same on the left side. He called them 'ten invisible currents of energy through the body' in line with the fingers and toes. (Note that the zones extended from the toe to the brain and out to the thumb or fingers or vice versa, not from the brain to the toe and brain to fingers, as stated in some books.) Fitzgerald also said that his five lines marked out and represented the *centre* of the respective zones. (Many books do not show this but instead depict four lines coming from each of the webs of the toes, showing the digits as the ten zones.) He then demonstrated the correlation between areas in distant parts of the body and how pressure of between 2 and 10 pounds on given fingers or toes would alleviate pain anywhere in a particular zone. He also stated that the upper and lower surfaces of the joint and side areas must all be pressed for good results (figure 1.11). Each zone could be worked on either hands or feet because the zones ran either way. The distance between the area treated and the organ was of no importance as the whole zone would be treated.

Fitzgerald outlined how pressure over the great toe or on the corresponding thumb helped the entire first zone; this first zone included the incisors and cuspid teeth, and an analgesic effect would often be felt throughout the zone. The second zone included the bicuspid and the third zone the two molars (knowing the zonal pathway enables you to work on the corresponding area for teeth problems). He stated that zones 4 and 5 usually merged in the head. The shoulder and axilla were in all five zones. Also he considered that in zone 4 was the middle ear. (My opinion is that the eustachian tube and middle ear combined are in zones 3 and 4.)

(a)

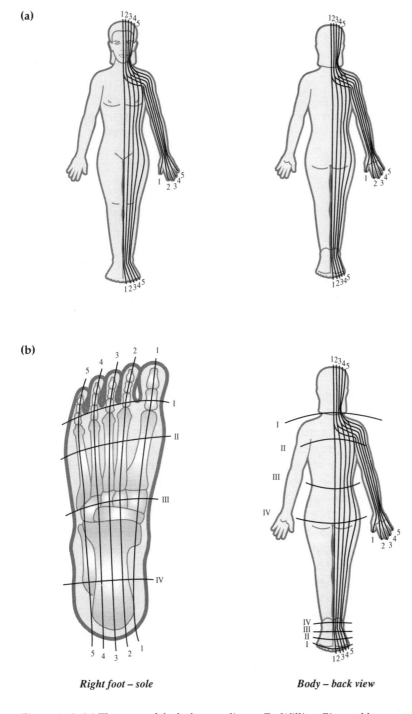

(b)

Right foot – sole   *Body – back view*

*Figure 1.10 (a) The zones of the body according to Dr William Fitzgerald.
(b) Corresponding longitudinal and lateral zones in the body and the foot.*

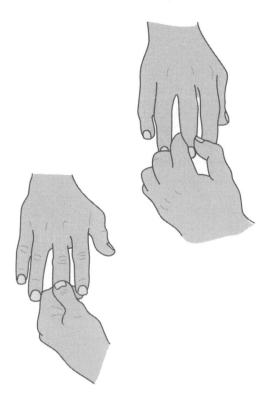

Figure 1.11 Applying pressure to all surfaces of the finger

Zone therapy demonstrates the correlation and interdependence of all parts of the body. In his chapter 'Zone therapy – for doctors only', Fitzgerald commented: 'six years ago I accidentally discovered that pressure with a cotton-tipped probe in the mucocutaneous margin of the nose gave an anaesthetic result'. He also went on to explain about how pressure on hands and feet and over joints reproduced the same characteristic results in pain relief. He stated that, when the pain was relieved, the condition that produced the pain was most generally relieved also, and that this led to the 'mapping out' of these various areas and associated connections and also to the conditions influenced through them.

He wrote that clasping the hands firmly was effective for many conditions including nervousness, anxiety, insomnia. Also clasping them for 10 minutes would help all pulmonary problems and even the common cold, while changing the clasp position from one hand to the other for 10 minutes each time would help to relieve many minor symptoms and in some cases even more involved problems.

He stated that neck and thyroid problems could be relieved by using distal pressures on the base of the first phalanx of the great toe or thumb and second and third digits respectively. (This was clearly stated so that errors in later books should not arise.) For lumbago one should work on the edge of the palm in line with the ring and little finger, but the most rapid relief for sciatica was secured by attacking the soles of the feet. Fitzgerald often spoke of curing lumbago with a comb; his instructions were to press the teeth into the palmar surface of the thumb first and then the second and third fingers and occasionally work on the webs, especially between thumb and first finger, and to work even the very tops of fingers and right up to wrists as this would help the entire zone. The palmar surface of the hands was to be attacked for pains in the back of the body and the dorsal or top surfaces of hands and fingers for any problems in the anterior (front) surface of body.

He added that, for eye problems, pressure could be applied to the index finger and sometimes middle finger if the eyes were set far apart. He spoke of squeezing the big finger or corresponding toe for ear problems. Pictures showed the distal phalange being squeezed by thumb and forefinger, or tight elastic bands being placed around them; one of the most effective methods for ear problems was placing a clothes peg to the tip of the ring finger or the fingers on either side, or raising the nail of the fourth finger for tinnitus. This point is a known acupuncture point (*see* figure 6.8b).

Pressure was often applied using aluminium combs, pointed instruments, tight elastic bands, clothes pegs or clamps on the fingers or toes (figure 1.12). Fitzgerald also spoke of how to use pressure with fingers and thumbs from anything between 1 and 4 minutes. The use of the many non-electrical applications such as surgical clamps, aluminium combs, elastic bands, pegs and percussion motors never really caught on because they were so invasive. Fitzgerald also had 'therapy bites' and 'therapy grips'; these were saw-edged articles or sometimes just metal combs. He even used rubber erasers. However, hands and the precise techniques of the correct pressure were all that was really needed.

He stated how all the zones must be free from irritation and obstructions to get the best results. His writings spoke of how important teeth were and how they should be preserved, also how offending corns, warts, calluses, etc. created an inflammatory process, which could cause a problem in a corresponding part of the body, how fingernails and toenails should be kept trimmed and how too much pressure from shoes could be detrimental to health within that zone.

Fitzgerald gave four different reasons in his book for how zone therapy worked (this is also outlined in the book *Reflexology: Art, Science and History* by Christine Issel). He stated:

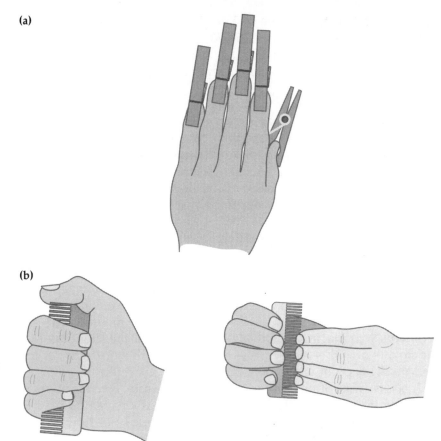

(a)

(b)

Figure 1.12 (a) A method of treating earache, toothache and any pain. (b) Combs applied to the fingers to treat complications of the midthoracic and lower back, and other deep-seated problems.

while we know the fact of pain relief, through the laying on of the hands, or by kindred measures, we only know part of its reason for operation. There are several of these. They are:

1 Through the soothing influence of animal magnetism

2 The manipulation of the hand over the injured place tends to prevent a condition of venous stasis

3 Pressure over the seat of injury produced 'blocked shock' or 'nerve block' which meant that by pressing on the nerves running from the injured part to the brain area we inhibit or prevent the transmission to the brain of the knowledge of the injury

4 Pressure over any bony eminence injured, or pressure applied upon the zones corresponding to the location of the injury will tend to relieve pain. Not only will it relieve pain but if the pressure is strong enough and long enough and in the right place it will frequently produce analgesia, or insensibility to pain.

These are some of the many ailments that Fitzgerald said he treated:

Abdominal pains
Abortion (prevention of)
Angina pectoris
Arm problems
Asthma
Backache
Bladder problems
Blood pressure disorders
Brachial neuritis
Breast problems
Bronchitis
Cancer (he never claimed to cure)
Colds
Conjunctivitis
Constipation
Coughs
Deafness
Diarrhoea
Epilepsy
Eustachian tube problems

Eye problems
Falling hair
Foot problems
Gall bladder problems
Goitre
Haemorrhoids
Hay fever
Headache
Heart problems
Hiccough
Hysteria
Insomnia
Intestinal problems
Labour pain
Laryngitis
Liver problems
Locomotor ataxia
Loss of voice
Lumbago
Lung problems
Menses
Migraine
Morning sickness

Mumps
Nasal catarrh
Nervousness
Neuralgia
Ovarian problems
Paralysis
Pneumonia
Prostate
Quinsy
Rheumatism
Sciatica
Sea sickness
Sneezing
Sore throat
Testes problems
Throat problems
Tinnitus
Toothache
Torticollis
Tuberculosis
Tumours
Uterine problems
Whooping cough

Zone therapy and acupuncture points

Fitzgerald never clarified where he became acquainted with the theory of zone therapy. He only spoke about how he stumbled upon the concept of zone therapy, and never ever mentioned whether there was any Oriental connection. Many of his reflex areas do correlate with acupuncture points, however.

For example, he spoke of Signor Umberto Sorrentino, a noted tenor, relieving his tight throat by squeezing the lateral aspect of the forefinger and thumb; these are acupoints governing the vocal chords. He also spoke of digging the fingernails into the inner side of the thumb. There is another well-known acupoint at the base of the thumbnail known as Lung 11 (abbreviated to LU-11) and it is effective for any throat problems or shortness of breath.

Fitzgerald also stated that scratching stimulates, deep pressure relaxes and that this knowledge should help many stomach problems. Morning sickness in pregnancy responded to deep pressure on backs of hands or the palmar surface of wrist and forearms. There is an acupoint on the inner forearm just below the wrist, Pericardium 6 (PE-6), used for nausea including motion sickness (utilized commercially in 'Sea-Band' wristbands).

In his chapter on painless childbirth, Fitzgerald spoke of pressures applied to the foot to alleviate pain and to enhance advancement of labour. He related how when contractions began and the mother started to feel discomfort, he would press on the foot with the thumbs of both hands at the metatarsal phalangeal joint for 3 minutes each time, and this greatly relieved the pain for the mother-to-be. On the great toe on the medial edge at the base of the nail bed there is a well-used acupoint, Spleen 1 (SP-1); this point relieves spasm in the uterus. On the lateral edge there are two points, Liver 1 (LIV-1) at the base of the nail bed and Liver 2 (LIV-2) on the metatarsal phalangeal joint; both points are helpful for problems of the genitourinary tract. (All of these points can be located by reference to figures 5.41 on page 180 and 6.8a and b on pages 209 and 211.)

For any pain in the head Fitzgerald suggested using pressure on the middle or tips of the fingers and toes, holding this pressure for up to 3 minutes. On the toes and fingers are several acupoints that help the head area. The tips of the toes are known as 'Qiduan'; the tips of the fingers are known as 'Shixuan', and both benefit the whole nervous system. On the dorsal surface of the foot are the following acupoints: SP-1, the first point on the great toe, and LIV-1, on the lateral edge of the great toe, both help to calm the mind; Gall Bladder 44 (GB-44), on the lateral edge of the fourth toe, relieves headaches and also helps eyes and ears; Bladder 67 (BL-67) alleviates headaches. On the hands, starting from the index finger, all meridians arise on the dorsal surface at the base of the nail. First Large Intestine 1 (LI-1), on the medial edge of the index finger, calms the mind, is for any anxiety, and will also restore consciousness; Pericardium 9 (PE-9), on the medial edge of the middle finger, helps calm the mind when anxious; Triple Burner 1 (TB-1) on the lateral edge of the ring finger, aids all ear problems and painful stiff shoulders; Heart 9 (HE-9), on the medial edge of the little finger, is a marvellous point for headaches; the Small Intestine (ST-1) meridian also arises on the little finger, but on the lateral edge, and points on this benefit headaches and stiff neck. For detailed maps of the meridian pathways *see* figures 2.8–2.20 on pages 51–64.) Did Fitzgerald know of the existence of these acupoints, or was his knowledge obtained solely from observations? It is interesting that all the three Yang meridians of the upper body run to the face and pass their energy to the descending three Yang meridians of the lower body. These Yang meridians could be seen as three continuous channels, from hands to face, face to foot, or vice versa. The three Yin meridians could also be seen as three continuous channels from foot to breast, breast to hands or hands to breast, and breast to foot. According to the philosophy of the meridians, these are accessible on both sides of the body, so we would see six channels almost running longitudinally, being accessible on either the feet or the hands (figure 1.13). Fitzgerald possibly saw this connection as the meridians merging in the body, and this encouraged him to experiment with his zonal theory. (Remember his comment: 'Five lines there marked out. I have designed these figures in this manner purposely to avoid making six lines, which would be confusing to the student.') This seems to be a simplified version incorporating all the meridians. So regardless of how he gained his insight he did produce a simplified version of the meridian theory.

We can also compare the practices derived from the meridian theory with those of the reflexology theory. For instance, in the latter in many cases the feet are found to be far more energetic and forceful in the outcome of treatment, while the hands still being potent but with less chance of creating too much movement of

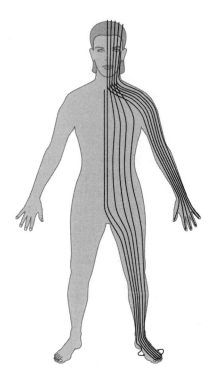

Figure 1.13 Merging of the meridians, making six lines of energy either side of the medial line

energy within the body; hence they must always be the first area to work on in anyone who is seriously ill, or the very young or elderly. This is understandable by reference to the interchange of Yin and Yang energy believed to occur on the hands and feet.

The statements by Fitzgerald that all zones must be free from irritation and obstruction, and that pressure could be given with rubber bands, pegs or clamps on any bony prominence, are of interest. The meridians in TCM are believed to lie alongside the bones, often following neural pathways. Fitzgerald expounded that pressure stimulated certain control centres in the medulla oblongata, or even functions carried out by the pituitary body and its many nerve pathways. The connection between nerve function, reflexology and acupuncture is discussed in detail in chapter 2.

Reflexology after Dr Fitzgerald

Dr William H Fitzgerald (1872–1942) was one of the most forward-thinking of medical men who became a natural healer through the art of using a pressure therapy to benefit and heal the human body. Many colleagues who assisted him throughout those early years of discovering the art of zone therapy went on to elaborate these techniques. This was based on the idea that the body was marked off with imaginary lines running from digits on the feet to the digits on the hands, each line passing through an organ. Pressure was applied on a given point and caused a reflex action; this led to normalization of muscle fibres in the corresponding organ within that zone, or stimulated the interrelated muscle to relax. The theory was based on observations over a period of people who were in discomfort; if they hurt themselves they rubbed the offending part. If they expected pain they would clench their fists or hold on tight to a chair. The hypothesis was developed that if the correct action were adopted then relief from pain would ensue and discomfort could be eased. The pressure was not just a nerve block with an analgesic effect or loss of sensation in that zone, rather that if the right pressures were used on the correct points the problem or disorder the person was suffering from could be alleviated.

From 1913 to about 1920 most work on zone therapy was being developed by two other medical physicians, Doctors Bowers and White. Edwin F Bowers MD, a well-known medical critic and writer, wrote an article on Dr Fitzgerald's work. The method was unnamed at the time so he christened it 'zone therapy'. He further elaborated that 'Man was admittedly of chemical formation controlled by electrical energy, or electronic vibration' introducing the concept of energy to the system. Dr Fitzgerald also taught George Starr White MD, who acknowledged in his writings *A Lecture Course to Physicians* (seventh edition revised) that credit must be given to Dr Fitzgerald for the discovery of mapping out the body into five zones each side of the medial line. He also stated that others had used a form of pressure for the relief of pain but prior to this there was no system regarding its use. He also said '"Zone Therapy" must be classed with the best and most original procedure in medicine today.' Further, he quoted Dr Fitzgerald's statement that, 'Zone therapy is not a cure-all, but it is a valuable adjunct in therapy.'

It was during this time that William Fitzgerald lectured to Dr Joe Shelby-Riley and his wife Elizabeth Ann Riley. They had a school of chiropractic in Washington DC. Fitzgerald found that naturopaths, chiropractors and osteopaths were willing converts as they were interested in any drugless therapy. Dr Shelby-Riley became more than just interested in zone therapy during his lifetime; he also wrote 12 books, his first *Zone Therapy Simplified* (written in 1919) was mentioned in his later work *Science and Practice of Chiropractic with Allied Sciences* (1925). A later book was just entitled *Zone Reflex*; the 12th edition was copyrighted in 1942. By then the Rileys had elaborated and greatly broadened their instructions and introduced a technique called hookwork in which the fingers are hooked under bones (eg the scapula) in connection with zone therapy. Elizabeth Ann Riley was a remarkable teacher of zone therapy.

In 1919 a young man named Harry Bond Bressler graduated from the Shelby-Rileys' chiropractic school, receiving a Degree of Chiropractic, and joined Dr Shelby-Riley in his practice in 1920. He wrote a book in 1955, confirming everything that had previously been written by Fitzgerald. Bressler considered that Fitzgerald had become acquainted with the art of pressure therapy in Vienna, which was very possible because many doctors and naturopaths visited the continent for seminars and meetings. Note that both in this book and in subsequent books written, some anomalies regarding reflexology points arose. Bressler made an issue of the terminology to be used when referring to the digits, because he felt that some people were confused. He called the first phalanx or finger joint the proximal phalanx (nearest the palm), the next was the middle or second phalanx, and the one nearest the end of the finger was the distal or third phalanx (with exception of the thumb and great toe, which have only two phalanges, a proximal and a distal). He clearly stated that the eyes related to the tips of the index finger and second toe, being the third or end joint (he said to try the third or middle digits). For the ears he said he used the fourth finger, the ring finger (note that the ring finger is actually the *third* finger); the third finger in TCM contains the Triple Burner meridian and is always used for ear problems. Fitzgerald had specified raising the nail on the *third* finger for tinnitus of the ear; however, Bressler wrote that he had confirmed Fitzgerald's work of raising the lateral edge of the nail of the *fourth* finger for ear noises for 2–5 minutes, three or four times each day. Harry Bond Bressler also linked ear problems to the liver; I think this was because the Gall Bladder channel commences on the face and contours the ear to terminate in the fourth toe. The toe terminal point is also used for ear problems, as because many of the disorders linked to the Gall Bladder meridian are often high congested states the liver would definitely also be out of balance. In his chapter on ears he also included ear massage, but his points do not relate to the known acupoints.

Reading through Fitzgerald's book you are made aware that, even though he worked on the actual organ involved, often he was also looking for other organs that might be contributing to the condition. That is, he was looking for 'areas of assistance' or associated areas, one of the basic concepts of reflexology today. For instance, not only did he refer to ingrowing toenails contributing to headaches but he stated that this would affect the entire zone and could be the contributing factor for a discordant condition expressed in a distant organ within that area. Undue pressures would cause a problem within any part of that zone.

Bressler's one main deviation appeared in his depiction of the zones. Fitzgerald's early work had always depicted the zones as ten lines of energy, five each side of the medial line, and his diagrams clearly show this (*see* figure 1.10). The five lines are quite clearly marked out, and each line represents the centre of that respective zone. Fitzgerald clearly stated that he designed these figures in this way to avoid confusion. However, Harry Bond Bressler states that the zones commence in the web of the first phalange; this results in only four lines either side of the median line, which is not as Fitzgerald's original concept. It is important to be aware of this alteration.

Eunice Ingham, another author, was also a student of the Riley chiropractic school. In her book she stated that Dr Fitzgerald, in his work *Zone Therapy*, blazed the path for further developments, as he 'brings to light for our consideration his discovery of the ten various zones of the body and location of each organ in the body in one or more of these zones'. If the feet and the hands are supposed to represent the physical body with all organs laid out in a similar arrangement, every book or chart should be the same, with variations only being in the format. However, in Ingham's books the eye and ear reflexes are clearly depicted at the base of toes two, three and four and this arrangement has been followed in many later books. Was this due to the fact that the acupoint just before the terminal point on the Stomach meridian (*see* figure 5.41, page 180) is at the metatarsal phalange at the base of the second toe, a point that is used for all facial problems? Similarly, on the fourth toe the last but one point on the Gall Bladder meridian (GB-43) is for all ear and eye problems (*see* figure 5.41). Ingham also shows the Heart area covering the same area as that of the Lungs, and suggests working on the shoulder reflex under the fourth and fifth toes, which correspond to the fourth and fifth zones. In TCM the Heart meridian is on the fifth finger, so we should be able to access the heart through the zone. Ingham states 'take any of the internal organs of the body and determine what zone line passes through them'. This system will guide you in reflexology as we know it today. Ingham stated that the zone concept had become a powerful and important tool in the relief of many disorders and that zone therapy had the ability to stimulate the body's own natural healing process and allow it to balance its own natural energies. A balanced energy flow should have no blockages.

Doreen E Bayly was trained by Eunice Ingham in America and was responsible for bringing the therapy to Great Britain in 1966. Her book *Healing through the Feet* was published in 1978.

In the 1960s a young Yorkshire man named Joseph Corvo was taught the zone principle by one of Dr William Fitzgerald's believers. Today he practises and teaches zone therapy, but does not link it with reflexology. He claimed the system is as old as the human race, that it is a natural instinct to put your hand on a painful part and press it, and that it not only relieves the effect but also removes the cause. He also maintained that you could not harm yourself in any way using the 'zonery system' and that it was absolutely safe. To date Joseph Corvo must be listed amongst the great masters for the vast amount of treatment that he has given to help so many and the many books that he has also written.

Regardless of what name we call this therapy by – the zonery system, zone therapy, reflex zones of the feet and hands, or just simply reflexology – there is no doubt it is an ever-expanding activity. As more details are discussed, explanations sought and more research is undertaken our knowledge will expand greatly. If William Fitzgerald was known as the 'grandfather' of the zone theory then Eunice Ingham is known as the 'mother' of contemporary reflexology. Regardless of how these forward-thinking people developed their theories, even if we do not exactly agree with them let us explore them all. Daily new theories and techniques are being developed world-wide but many of Fitzgerald's and Ingham's basic methods and procedures are still taught today.

Through the years we have also had many great naturopaths who believed in the wonderful art of natural self-healing for treating illness; their methods included changing the food that people eat and utilizing the forces of nature such as fresh clean air, light, heat, cold and water (which has been used therapeutically for thousands of years). These drugless methods also incorporated physical exercises and massage.

Important events in the development of reflexology

This calendar in Box 1.1 outlines some important medical events from ancient history to the present day, showing how it may appertain to the whole theory of reflexology, and how the West and the East have something in common with this incredible therapy.

Box 1.1 Important Events in the Development of Reflexology

c2500 BC   China   Beginnings of acupuncture in China
c2330 BC   Egypt   Tomb of Ankhm'ahor built depicting representations of surgical operations, or treatment of hands and feet
c1558 BC   China   Acupuncture in China became more refined
c500 BC   Japan   Acupuncture reached Japan
AD 420   China   A bronze statue was cast showing the location of all the points of acupuncture
1582   Europe   First book of zone therapy published by Doctors Adamus and A'tatis
1776   Per Henrick Ling was noted for his gymnastics; lingism, as it was later known, was the treatment of disease with both active and passive moves
1800s   Britain   Treatment by acupuncture was introduced into Britain and the term 'reflex' used by many medical men
Early 1800s   Japan   Reiki, an ancient energy healing system based on very old Tibetan texts, arose from the teachings of Dr Mikao Usui; its theory was that the universal life energy was channelled through to the practitioner, who in turn conveyed it through the fingertips to those who needed it
1823   Britain   First issue of the *Lancet* was printed. A case of acupuncture treatment was reported. Successful treatment was carried out by a Dr Tweedale of Lyme Regis
1827   Britain   Acupuncture was used in the Royal Infirmary, Edinburgh and St Thomas's Hospital, London
Early 1800s   Italy   Filippo Pacini (1812–83), an anatomist, discovered Pacinian corpuscles: sensory receptors in the skin particularly sensitive to changes of pressure, also found in joints and tendons. Angelo Ruffini (1864–1929), an anatomist, discovered Ruffini corpuscles, which record dermal distortions; they are cylindrical sensory organs that respond to pressure and warmth, found in finger pads, joints, tendons and tendon sheaths

Early 1800s   Germany   Johannes Peter Müller (1801–58), a physiologist, proposed the principle of the law of specific irritability, the principle that each nerve is excited via sense organs responsive to a specific form of energy, and its excitation, because of its connections, can give rise to only one modality of sensation, regardless of whether the nerve is electrically or mechanically excited. Karl Ludwig Merkel (1812–76), an anatomist, discovered Merkel's discs, tactile end-organs; these are slow-acting mechanoreceptors, responding when the tissue is stretched. George Meissner (1829–1905), a histologist, discovered Meissner's plexus, a fine network of nerves in the wall of the alimentary canal, also Meissner's corpuscles, found in the fingertips and lips

1880   Europe   Acupuncture was used in Europe. The connection could be the French Consul in China, Soulie de Morant, who became closely associated with Chinese philosophy. He studied the Chinese language and many ancient treatises on the subject. Many of them were thousands of years old and he translated them into French

Late 1800s   Europe   From the latter part of the 1800s great strides were made by the medical profession in the study of reflexes. Many devices were used to deliver electrical stimuli to parts of the body. These were to establish the identity of nerves, such as whether they were sensory or motor. They also established, by the response raised, if a nerve or tract was damaged or absent. As these responsive actions indicate externally what is taking place within the body, it is my belief that we can send a message in on the same pathway

Late 1800s   Germany   Mendel–Bekhterev reflex abnormal response was found showing dysfunction in the corticospinal tract; Kurt Mendel (1874–1946) was a neurologist. Hermann Oppenheim (1858–1936), a neurologist, found that when pressure is applied on the tibial crest there is a fanning of all the toes and an extension of the great toe. This is indicative of lesions within the pyramidal tract

Late 1800s   USA   Charles Gilbert Chaddock (1861–1936), a neurologist, found that reflex extension of the great toe was induced by percussion on the external malleolar region and this was indicative of pyramidal tract lesion. Alfred Gordon (1874–1953), a neurologist, found the knee jerk reflex and extensor plantar response evident in pyramidal tract disease; this was produced when squeezing the calf muscles

1886   Russia   Vladimir Michailovitch Bekhterev (1857–1927), led historical development in experimental methods of reflexology on animals and then the study of human behaviour

1886–7   Russia   Ivan Petrovitch Pavlov (1849–1936), a physiologist, studied conditioned reflex activity in dogs and received the Nobel Prize in 1904 by proving that there was a direct association between a stimulus and a response reflex action (*see* chapter 2)

Late 1800s   Russia   Lyudvig Martinovitch Puussepp (1875–1942), a neurosurgeon, discovered that there is a slow abduction of the little toe in response to stroking the outer aspect of the foot, which is indicative of upper motor neurone disease. These abnormal reflexes are not present in healthy individuals

1892   France   Dr Joseph François Felix Babinski (1857–1932), a neurologist, ascertained the plantar reflex (*see* chapter 2, page 46)

1893   England   Sir Henry Head (1861–1940), a neurologist, published research proving a direct relationship between pressure applied to the skin and its effect on internal organs. This was later clarified to be the effects of dermatomes (*see* chapter 2, page 43)

1895   United States   Dr William Fitzgerald (1872–1942) qualified at the University of Vermont, and was the originator of the theory of zone therapy (died 21 October 1942 in Stamford, Connecticut)

1897 Egypt Tomb of Ankhm'ahor at Saqqara discovered by V Loret depicting treatment of feet, hands and legs

1902 Vienna Fitzgerald studied and taught in Vienna

1906 England Sir Charles Scott Sherrington (1859–1952), an Oxford physiologist, proved that the whole nervous system responded to stimuli from proprioceptors, specialized sensory nerve endings that monitored internal changes in the body. He published his findings in *The Integrative Action of the Nervous System*

1907 Russia Bekhterev formed the Psychoneurological Institute, and later became the Director of the State Reflexological Institute for the study of the brain in Leningrad

1913–20 Washington Fitzgerald went to Washington to teach and lecture to Shelby-Riley students

1915 United States Edwin Bowers article published 'To stop that toothache squeeze your toe'

1917 United States Edwin Bowers MD and William Fitzgerald MD published *Zone Therapy*. Many other books were published during this period

1919 United States Dr Joe Shelby-Riley published first of 12 books about zone therapy, the last being published in 1942

1928 Russia Bekhterev had his work translated into English

1938 United States Eunice Ingham (24 February 1889–10 December 1974) published *Stories the Feet Can Tell*

1945 United States Eunice Ingham published *Stories the Feet Have Told*

1949 United States Dr Roy S Ashton published *The Fundamental System Bad Feet–Bad Spine* showing the connection between foot abnormalities and the spine

1955 United States Harry Bond Bressler published his book *Zone Therapy* confirming all of Dr William Fitzgerald's work

1966 England Doreen Bayly returned from America after training with Eunice Ingham and introduced reflexology to Britain; she published her first foot chart in black and white in 1966 entitled 'The Eunice Ingham method chart produced by Doreen Bayly'

1974 Germany Hanne Marquardt studied with Ingham in 1970; then she published *Reflex Zone Therapy of the Feet*

1978 England *Reflexology Today. The Stimulation of The Body's Healing Forces Through Foot Massage* was published by Doreen Bayly. Her earlier chart was reproduced in colour in 1970

1978 Taiwan Father Joseph Eugster began his dedicated work, teaching reflexology

1980s England Complementary medicine and reflexology specifically became a growth area; by this time over 80 books had now been written, and many articles, some with conflicting points but many stating a similar theme. Societies and associations were formed from 1983 onwards around the world. Schools were set up with many offering short training programmes leading to a certificate to practise

1990s England Directories were set up but are not conclusive, as many people do not choose to advertise this way. The Institute for Complementary Medicine formed a British Register of Complementary Practitioners (BRCP). The British Council of Complementary Medicine is a registered charity, which was formed to establish national standards in all developing areas of complementary medicine. It works in tandem with the BRCP. The British Complementary Medicine Association (BCMA) was formed in 1992 to assist therapists in the setting of standards of practice and to encourage them to join together in self-regulatory bodies. The BCMA is a leading member of the Independent Care Organisations (ICO) – the body charged with setting standards in private health care.

Research programmes are being initiated. The years ahead look promising.

2   A holistic approach to medicine

The concept of holistic medicine

Holistic medicine is an approach to health care in general; it is based upon the idea that health is the result of harmony between the body, mind and spirit and any extreme stress of any kind, which includes physical, psychological, social and environmental pressure, is inimical to good health.

Natural healing takes place every day. When you cut yourself, the body's innate power draws and knits together tissue and heals the wound. If we fracture a bone, many parts of the body perform different tasks for healing to occur; a team effort is needed, as no single body part works alone. The body is like a machine with many component parts that perform daily chores in maintaining blood circulation, and ensuring the correct level of fluids and enzymes to keep it in good running order. These functions would not be able to take place without energy. Food is the fuel that provides the energy the body needs for its cells to perform their intricate tasks. Every part of the body is involved with a complex nerve network, with the brain as the control centre, monitoring and co-ordinating every function. All the component parts need to be in balance.

Reflexology provides the means whereby the body can be synchronized to balance the timing of its engine. Reflexology is a fascinating study of the links between reflex points of the feet and hands and longitudinal (vertical) pathways or zones. As we work on the feet, we thus form a picture of the entire body. In this way the feet or hands are considered a microcosm of the body, with all organs, glands, and so on laid out in the same arrangement (for details of the reflex areas, *see* plates 1–4).

As mentioned above, all processes that take place in the cells of the body need energy. The energy transfer that is central to reflexology and other healing systems such as shiatsu, acupuncture and acupressure allows the body's integrated systems to achieve homeostasis. We often hear in traditional medical systems terms such as 'Chi', frequently translated as 'life energy' or 'life force', or

'Prana', meaning breath of life. Energy is indeed constantly circulating through the body and is the very foundation of life. At a cellular level, we need energy to survive, we draw energy from the food we eat and this powers every cell within the body, which in turn needs its own energy to function. It is this much deeper level of biotic energy, the innate energy at cellular level, which maintains the metabolic processes that we work on.

At the neurological level, every machine needs a control system, and the complex brain is the control and computer system of the body. The brain, which is the source of conscious awareness of each and every thought process, is also a motor centre initiating and co-ordinating the voluntary movements of the body, and interpreting all the fast incoming information received from the sense organs. It monitors and discharges the necessary signals to muscles, glands or other parts of the nervous system to respond appropriately. It is a vast network, and is the body's greatest user of energy, to power the many chemical and neurological processes associated with it.

The physical body and its component parts are made up from billions and billions of cells, and even though there are many types, shapes and sizes, the one thing they all have in common is a requirement for energy. According to the holistic concept, for instance as found in TCM theory, if this internal energy is obstructed, deficient or in excess in any way the cells function less effectively. In reflexology, during a treatment session the therapist will utilize those pathways of energy that already exist in the human body and they return the imbalanced or deficient energy flow safely back into harmony. Reflexology treatment is given to look after and nurture the body, and is often likened to the constant maintenance and preservation that a machine needs to keep it in good running order. We know for any effective control of any manmade apparatus it needs power or energy and maintenance. The first often can only be achieved by giving it a motor or engine that drives it, and this in turn must be maintained. The engine may be driven or powered by electricity or another substance.

Two opposing systems are also usually needed to make it work, for instance in a car engine the brake and the accelerator. This again is paralleled in many of the systems within the body. Locomotion is the result of the co-ordinated action of muscles on the limbs. The muscles of the body work in antagonizing pairs. The same is true of hormones which interact in a biofeedback system that enables them to regulate the body towards an almost constant state. For example, glucagon raises the level of blood glucose, while insulin has an opposing effect and lowers the glucose levels. High levels of oestrogen are secreted by the ovaries to stimulate ovulation but (in the absence of egg fertilization) are counterbalanced during the monthly menstrual cycle by progesterone, which in turn is only secreted under the control of other hormones from the pituitary. These gonadotrophin hormones thus work in unison. From this we see how the body must be in balance. Hormones are responsible for certain changes in the body, and work together with the nervous system to monitor and control blood pressure levels. Hormone responses are not so quick as those of the nervous system, and they function more on a long-term basis. By these physiological processes all the internal systems of the body (for example blood pressure, body temperature, the acid–base balance) are maintained at equilibrium despite variations in the external conditions. If there is a homeostatic imbalance in the various systems then disease will eventually occur.

Since all the systems of the body interrelate, only one area needs to be slightly out of balance to lead to disorders in other areas. These problems can often be observed to travel up and down a zone and even affect other parts of the body. Ill-health often falls into what is known as the 'vague symptom' category: a general malaise is often felt, every part of the body aches with general stress in neck and shoulders, the person may be irritable, not sleeping properly, picking at or eating too much food, making them feel ill or tense. Such a person may be unsure whether to go to their doctor or not, in case they are labelled neurotic, and the symptoms often continue for a long period of time. It is only when a problem becomes chronic do they begin to be more concerned.

Many complementary therapies, among them reflexology, are natural, non-invasive, and drugless paths to self-help, helping to restore a person to a more tranquil temperament, improve their mental condition and enable the person to cope better with life's demands. Reflexology treatment encourages a generally healthier body by facilitating the proper functioning of the circulatory system, so enabling the supply of nutrients and oxygen to reach all cells of the body.

Imbalance of our internal environment is often caused by stress (*see* chapter 10 for a detailed discussion of this). The excitatory process of a stress stimulus often changes this internal environment, causing high blood pressure, pain in many parts of the body because the muscles become tense, depression, brooding or morbid thoughts, a change in our circadian (or daily) rhythms and other regular biological body rhythms (eg daily body temperature variations, sleeping and waking patterns, the female menstrual cycle). The hypothalamus and the medulla oblongata (*see* figure 2.23, page 70) contain the main brain centres controlling such homeostatic functions. While in a healthy body slight changes can be coped with, major changes such as going on holiday abroad (time change) can cause a very real problem. Also shift workers, for instance nurses or people who work nights, often find this interference with regular rhythms of the body leads to the so-called psychosomatic disorders (ie mental and physical disorders such as asthma, eczema, peptic ulcer, irritable bowel syndrome, headaches, back stresses). All these are caused by the body's automatic responses to stress, mediated by the autonomic nervous system.

Theories and philosophies

What is energy?

The general definition of energy is 'power', 'vigour', 'vitality' or 'force'; in physics the definition of energy is the work that a physical system is capable of doing. Energy cannot be destroyed but it can change form. The body's processes utilize electrical and chemical forms of energy. Kirlian photography is a special form of high-voltage photographic process which apparently records the energy field around the body on light-sensitive paper. This process has demonstrated changes in the energy field before and after a reflexology treatment. The exact nature of this energy field is a matter of debate. Eastern and Western systems have tended to have different views on this.

Reflexology is a method of contacting the electrical centres in the body. It aims to create a smooth flow of 'vibratory energy' throughout the body. By contacting various points on the feet this energy is thought to travel to the spine and then out to the organs, glands or cells, following set paths, although these are thought not to correspond to the Chinese meridians. However, the nature of the energy is thought to be the same.

Polarity therapy is another therapy based on the Yin and Yang principles (*see* chapter 1). Its theory is that life energy flows between the two poles, one positive flowing to a negative pole and vice versa. This concept was applied by Doctor Randolph Stone to the general condition of the human body and mind. He likened the movement of energy in the human body as energetic currents; he referred to this as the 'wireless anatomy of man'. The ancient Chinese looked at the living body as being one of the expressions of tension between two poles, heaven and earth. Heaven is found above the head, the Creative, awakening our higher nature, our source of ideas. Earth lies beneath the feet, the Receptive. The head and feet, and the hands, can be viewed as mediators channelling Qi energy to various organs or glands that need revitalizing.

The body field can be demonstrated by the following exercise. With your palms facing, rub your hands together quite gently, then move your hands very slowly a few inches apart, you should feel a sensation of warmth, or flow, or a magnetic type of pulling sensation in the fingers between the two hands.

Reflexology aims to stabilize elements lacking or unbalanced in a person's basic energy; the touch of the practitioner's hand on a person's feet can also be thought to create a flow of energy between them. This particular technique of touch has a great ability to calm down and completely relax a person.

In reflexology the distribution of energy in the whole body is considered to correspond to the distribution of energy in the hands and feet. So by holding a person's hand or foot you become very aware of their internal structure: the limbs, bones, joints, muscles, arteries, nerves, skin and nails. You also begin to feel you can 'read' the energy structure within.

Life energy can mean many different things to people working in different traditions. Perhaps we should not try to explain it, but be satisfied with being aware of its existence. We should also keep in mind that we not only touch tissue, muscle and bone but we also 'touch' the very life force of the body.

How the nervous system works

Receptors

We know that any part of the skin is sensitive to touch. Touch has been used therapeutically over thousands of years. The skin is also very responsive to heat, pain and pressure, whether by touch or by other means. Even pressure from air or water brings about a responsive action in the physical body. Each and every area of the body is connected to the incredible nerve network within the brain that acts like an overseer, guiding and supervising as well as modifying the output when necessary.

Study of the body's anatomy and physiology tells us how these nerve signals are transmitted from the specialized sensory receptors and how they respond to different stimuli. Sense organs are groups of cells that are connected to the brain or spinal cord by nerve fibres (or neurones) running along particular pathways. Those sensory nerve messages originating from the hands and the feet are received in a relatively large area in the brain's sensory cortex compared with those from other locations, showing the innumerable nerve endings that we have in these areas. An anatomical figure (figure 2.1) depicting the size of the sensory areas in one of the paired, halves of the cerebrum that contains the sensory cortex and associated areas shows how tactile the hands and feet are. The fingertips and toes are particularly susceptible to touch because the tactile receptors called Meissner's corpuscles are in abundance in the uppermost part of the dermis in this area of non-hairy skin. The free nerve endings found in most parts of the body enable sensations of pain, touch, pressure and tempera-

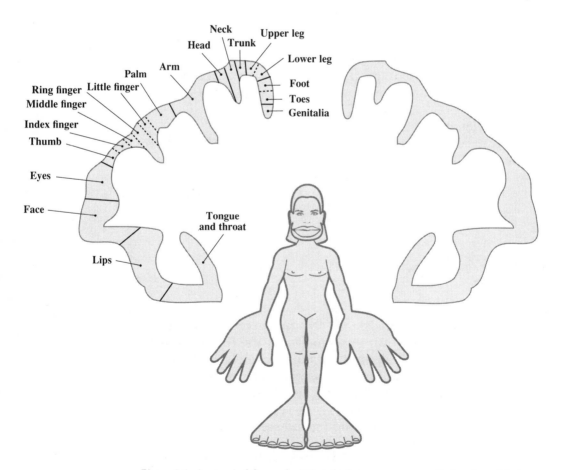

Figure 2.1 Anatomical figure depicting the large sensory area the hands and feet occupy in the brain

ture also to be relayed to the brain. Even hair plexuses respond to pain and touch, while Pacinian corpuscles in the dermis immediately respond to pressure and send their messages to the sensory cortex of the brain.

If there is a stimulus to any of the simple receptors, including all the touch, pain or pressure receptors, this sets off an electrical impulse; a strong stimulus will produce a stronger sensation – for instance, we know how a headache can develop very quickly when we stub our toe. Pain receptors in the skin are known as nociceptors: these include many of the free nerve endings found in the tissues.

The sensory nerve endings lie in the corium, the true skin; they are found within the tiny projections of this deeper layer. Each nerve fibre enters a small rounded bulb. These Pacinian corpuscles, responding to deep pressure, are abundant in the palmar surface of the hands and the plantar surface of the feet, and in all the digits, also around the tendons and ligaments. The smaller corpuscles, the tactile corpuscles of Meissner, are richly abundant in the pads of the fingertips and toes and also in the palms of the hands and soles of the feet; these are in the papillae of the skin.

Every time we stretch the tissue or muscles we contact the group of cells called the mechanoreceptors, found in the basal epidermis, in the form of Merkel's discs. They adapt very slowly to stimulation and they trigger impulses in the sensory nervous system. The reflex action helps to adjust the tone of muscles and the activity of the internal organs. (The isometric exercises carried out during a reflexology treatment session involve active voluntary contraction of muscles without producing movement of a joint. There is also a passive exercise known as neuromuscular facilitation, used to enhance contraction or relaxation of muscles.)

Nerve transmission

In the very simplest of reflexes a sensory neurone on the skin's surface, when palpated or pressed, will react by sending a signal along the nerve fibre belonging to it; this signal will pass to the central nervous system (*see* pages 36–7); once at its terminal end it will connect with another nerve cell, which in turn is also stimulated. The action within this second cell is enough to cause a muscle to contract or to even increase the secretory function of a gland (figure 2.2).

A nerve signal is an electrical impulse produced by chemical reactions on the surface of the cell body of a neurone (a nerve cell). Nerve signals traverse the whole nervous system, both electrically

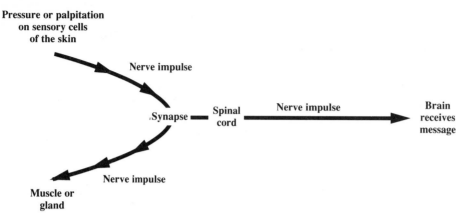

Figure 2.2 Transmission of nerve impulses

and chemically. Electric signals or impulses are carried from one end of a nerve cell to the other end. However, to cross the gap (the synapse) between nerve cells, chemicals called neurotransmitters are released from the end of the cell in response to the electrical impulse. These chemicals move across the synapse and bind on to the receptor sites of the adjacent cells. This sets off another electrical impulse in the next neurone, and so on.

Afferent (sensory) fibres transmit impulses to the centre from the skin, muscles, bones and joints. (However, not all afferent action is consciously perceived.) Efferent (motor) neurones innervate muscle fibres, conveying messages from the brain or spinal cord to muscles, glands or other effector organs (figure 2.3).

When pain or another stimulus is detected the electrical signals are sent to the spinal cord and often ascend to the higher centres within the brain (figure 2.3). The areas in the brain then correlate the information, sending the information by way of the midbrain (a small portion of the brainstem) to the hindbrain, or medulla oblongata (*see* figure 2.23, page 70). These brain areas are involved in the co-ordination of sensory and motor impulses within the body. The returning neural impulse travels back down a motor nerve pathway to where the pain communication came from, when it may stimulate release of endorphins – natural opiates that are often referred to as 'mood enhancers'. This may be why people often report a wonderful sense of well-being after a reflexology treatment. Stimulation of these touch or tactile corpuscles triggers a motor reaction. Consideration of an automatic reaction (such as the reaction when you receive a burn) shows how quickly the nervous system can react to stimuli.

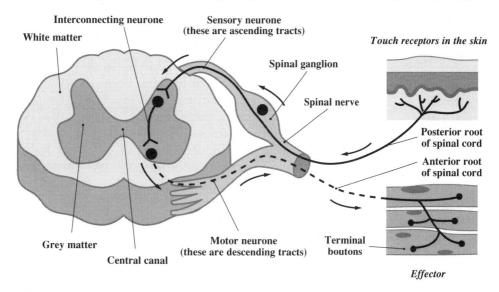

Figure 2.3 A section through the spinal cord, to show sensory and motor pathways

Normally when resting there is a relatively low level of electrical activity in the brain because it acts as a switchboard, receiving impulses from the many sensory organs of the body and correlating these various stimuli and interpreting them accordingly, sending off motor signals to supply a muscle or a gland into stimulation or relaxation, and so on (*see* figure 2.2). Reflexology may act as a stimulant, by increasing the rate of activity in an organ or system, or it may act as an energizer giving the person more vitality and zest. It is also evident after treatment that it has a calming influence, acting as a relaxant to such a degree that it enables the person to unwind and be totally rested and with muscles that are less stiff or tight.

Pain is a sensation we get when our sensory nerves are irritated or inflamed and injured. We all relieve our pain in a similar way when we rub the affected part or area that is hurting. This stimulates the firing of nerve fibres that inhibit the pain signal. This phenomenon was observed by Dr William Fitzgerald prior to his developing the 'zone concept'. However, in reflexology the pressure treatment helps to relieve disorders themselves as well as just relieving pain. Because during treatment the patient is able to relax, the pain of a stiff neck or low back pain, or even abdominal discomfort, is able to just ebb away during the treatment. The medical profession often say any benefit is due to the placebo (or 'expectation') effect because the client has faith in the powers of the therapist or therapy; if that is so then that is in itself a marvellous phenomenon. However, I feel that its mechanism is far more profound than that. I have treated many sceptics who on the first visit state something like, 'I am sure you will not be able to help me, but I have tried everything else, so I thought it would not hurt me if I came', or 'I only came because my wife suggested it, but I cannot see how fiddling with my hands, feet or ears is going to help my stiff knee'. These are just two examples of typical comments one may get from a sceptical person in the first instance. But even so if a good response is obtained such clients will virtually sing it from the rooftops. My most ardent supporter has recommended more patients to me than any other person to date, but at his first session he was almost disdainfully sceptical, and told me he had only attended at the request of his wife. Reflexology is now part of the lives of many such patients because they see it as a preventative against recurrence of ill-health.

Divisions of the nervous system

The nervous system is divided into a number of parts. First, there is the division into the central nervous system (the brain and spinal cord) and the peripheral nervous system. The peripheral nervous system distributes to the skin or peripheral parts of the body. The spinal nerves emerge from the spinal cord; the cranial nerves emerge directly from the brain. (*See* figure 2.5 and page 40.)

There is a functional division between the somatic nervous system, supplying the skeletal muscles, and the autonomic nervous system, supplying the glands, cardiac muscle, and smooth muscle of the internal organs. Reflexology contacts the autonomic nervous system, more than any other therapy, balancing the parasympathetic nervous system and the sympathetic nervous system. These are the two subdivisions of the autonomic nervous system. They exert opposite effects on the end organs, so that homeostasis is maintained. Sympathetic impulses tend to stimulate, and parasympathetic impulses inhibit; for instance, the first increase the heart rate, while the second slow it down. (*See* figures 2.4 and 2.5)

The spinal cord gives off 31 pairs of nerves in its course from the base of the skull to the lumbar region, each of these nerves arises by two roots, an anterior and a posterior root, one being sensory, the other being motor; these unite prior to leaving the spinal canal, forming a mixed nerve that then separates, supplying the front and back of the body respectively. The nerves that form plexuses are from the top and the bottom of the spinal cord; out of these plexuses a number of branches arise to supply the arms and

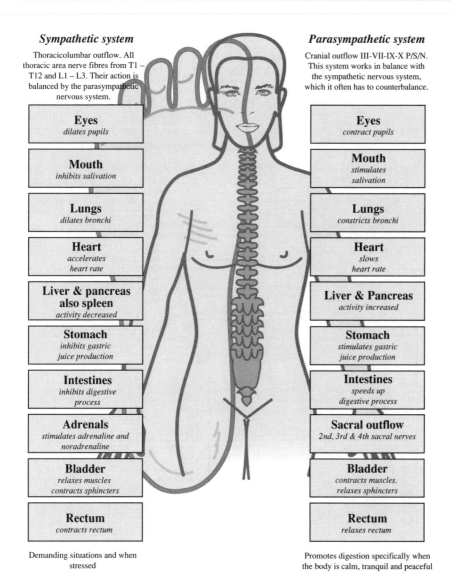

Sympathetic system

Thoracicolumbar outflow. All thoracic area nerve fibres from T1 – T12 and L1 – L3. Their action is balanced by the parasympathetic nervous system.

Eyes	*dilates pupils*
Mouth	*inhibits salivation*
Lungs	*dilates bronchi*
Heart	*accelerates heart rate*
Liver & pancreas also spleen	*activity decreased*
Stomach	*inhibits gastric juice production*
Intestines	*inhibits digestive process*
Adrenals	*stimulates adrenaline and noradrenaline*
Bladder	*relaxes muscles contracts sphincters*
Rectum	*contracts rectum*

Demanding situations and when stressed

Parasympathetic system

Cranial outflow III-VII-IX-X P/S/N. This system works in balance with the sympathetic nervous system, which it often has to counterbalance.

Eyes	*contract pupils*
Mouth	*stimulates salivation*
Lungs	*constricts bronchi*
Heart	*slows heart rate*
Liver & Pancreas	*activity increased*
Stomach	*stimulates gastric juice production*
Intestines	*speeds up digestive process*
Sacral outflow	*2nd, 3rd & 4th sacral nerves*
Bladder	*contracts muscles. relaxes sphincters*
Rectum	*relaxes rectum*

Promotes digestion specifically when the body is calm, tranquil and peaceful

Figure 2.4 Functions of the autonomic nervous system

legs with a network of sensory and motor nerve fibres. These are the cervical, brachial, lumbar and sacral plexuses; the thoracic nerves from T2 do not form plexuses, but supply the skin and muscles in the corresponding area. The eight cervical nerves are divided into two. First there is the cervical plexus, formed from the upper four nerves (1–4); these also communicate with cranial nerves X, XI and XII. They have cutaneous sensory branches and penetrating muscular branches. The lower four (5–8) unite with the first dorsal nerves to form the brachial plexus.

The cranial nerves include the vagus nerve, which contains

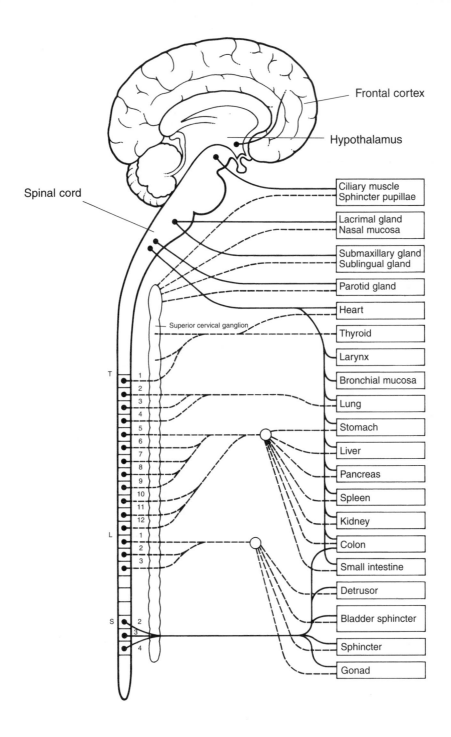

Figure 2.5 Sympathetic and parasympathetic innervation of the spinal cord

parasympathetic fibres that help the function of the viscera of the thorax and abdomen, motor nerve fibres to the muscles of larynx, sensory or somatic stimuli to the auditory canal, and also sensory (visceral afferent) stimuli of the thorax and abdomen. These cranial nerves comprise some motor nerves and some mixed nerves. There is also the trigeminal nerve, which has three branches; the ophthalmic nerve, passing through the superior orbital fissure (affecting the areas around the orbits and certain parts of the nasal cavities), the maxillary branch (affecting sensation below the orbits down to the upper jaw and teeth) and the mandibular nerve (again sensory to lower part of face, lower jaw and teeth, and the motor nucleus of this nerve serving the muscles of mastication). These nerves are attached to the brain stem at different levels. The major nerves all originate from nuclei inside the brain.

Note. It is important that the practitioner is aware of the cranial nerves at all times. There is a simple way of remembering these. I think of a very dear friend of mine from the early days – this lady's name was **OOOTTA FAGVSH**. The letters of this name correspond to all the cranial nerves. The cranial nerves are given roman numerals, I–XII. We only have three sensory nerves (S), five motor (M), and four mixed (MX) both sensory and motor. Of these cranial nerves, four are parasympathetic nerves (P/S/N) – these are nerves III, VII, IX and X. The nerves are as follows:

I   **O**lfaction – the sense of smell (S)
II   **O**ptic – the sense of vision (S)
III   **O**culomotor – the muscles of the eye (M. P/S/N)
IV   **T**rochlear – the muscles of the eye (M)
V   **T**rigeminal – the forehead, cheek sensations, and lower jaw (MX)
VI   **A**bducent – the muscles of the eye (M)
VII   **F**acial – impulses of taste and facial expression (MX. P/S/N)
VIII **A**uditory – the sense of hearing (S)
IX   **G**lossopharyngeal – sensations from the tongue and to the pharynx (MX. P/S/N)
X   **V**agus – the larynx, trachea, oesophagus, heart, respiratory, all digestive organs, the small intestine, spleen, ascending colon, kidneys and the blood vessels (MX. P/S/N)
XI   **S**pinal accessory – the muscles of the neck, the sterno-cleidomastoid and trapezius muscles (M)
XII   **H**ypoglossal – the hyoid region and the muscles of the tongue (M).

By remembering the above name you will always ensure you never miss out on a brain region as it is so important.

The functioning of the autonomic nervous system is closely linked to the pituitary, the adrenal gland and many other specialized nerve cells that secrete their hormones at the nerve endings. Our sensory system makes us aware of changes; these elaborate sense organs receive stimuli from outside of our body. These are then transmitted to our brain. An enormous amount of information is fed into our nervous system; all this sensory information allows the organism to change and correct the internal environment. Interpretation by the brain depends on the connections through the many nerve pathways. If these connections are not co-ordinated the parts of our body fail to respond.

The autonomic nervous system (*see* figure 2.4) depends on the co-ordinated and opposing regulatory functions of the sympathetic and parasympathetic divisions of the nervous system. Each of the organs of the body is supplied with a dual set of nerves from each of these branches; the overall commander of the autonomic nervous system is the hypothalamus, which ensures the interdependence and co-ordination of functions within this system. We do not need to think consciously of which branch of the autonomic nervous system we need to stimulate during treatment, because the brain centre decides which section of it will be dominant when the system is stimulated. If the person is tired, lethargic or sluggish the sympathetic stimulation results in an improvement to all activities, with the person having more energy and sparkle. The body has remarkable powers to protect and heal itself. If the need is for the body to be calmed down, then the parasympathetic branch comes to the fore, slowing the heartbeat, inducing deep physical relaxation, promoting the digestion and increasing the tone and motility of the whole gastrointestinal tract and its eliminating process. If there is also a depletion or loss of energy, the parasympathetic division will help to conserve and restore the energy we need while we sleep. It is only when we are physically or emotionally stressed that the sympathetic nervous system may override the parasympathetic nervous system. This action may inhibit many functions, and the whole gastrointestinal tract may slow down, often decreasing motility and tone – hence the many digestive disorders that are evident in people who are extremely stressed.

The overseer of this dual innervation is the hypothalamus, which lies at the back of the forebrain in the floor of the third ventricle (*see* figure 2.23, page 70). This small portion of the brain controls the vital processes, acting as a regulatory centre of thirst, hunger and temperature, thus moderating the water and food intake. It also regulates the emotions and our sleep patterns and it governs the pituitary body, the major endocrine gland that releases many regulatory hormones directly into the bloodstream. If there is an imbalance in these hormones there can be a decline in the state of health. Ill-health can take many forms, from the simple headache to a complete breakdown in many of the functions of the body.

When the body is totally relaxed, its healing mechanism is given a chance to right itself as blood flow and nerve transmission are allowed to occur unimpeded. The benefits of reflexology are therefore manifold; all parts of the body can be reached through precise stimulation of the reflexes through the feet and hands. A return to homeostasis can be achieved after approximately 40 minutes of such stimulation.

The autonomic nervous system is not separate from the central nervous system; there are many interconnections. It was once thought that we have no control over the autonomic nervous system as most of its responses are involuntary. However, the Hindu system of yoga exercises appears to develop some degree of control and influence over it. Also the Chinese exercises of Tai Chi and Qigong (Chi Kung), popularly practised for health and relaxation, demonstrate that relaxation of the mind improves the natural flow of energy, which in turn stimulates all the internal organs. It seems that the health benefits are considerable when the body is relaxed, and many disorders benefit from the reduction of anxiety or stress.

Dermatomes

Every area of skin is supplied by a spinal nerve, and each segment supplies a dermatome (figure 2.6), the deeper layers of the skin and its underlying connective tissue. Each individual dermatome is designated by the number of the spinal nerve root (cervical, dorsal, lumbar or sacral). If an area of skin is stimulated and there is no response, it is assumed that the nerve supplying the dermatome may be damaged.

Sclerotomes

There are also areas of division of the nerve supply of a bone, called sclerotomes. Each muscle fibre is served by at least one nerve fibre, which ends in a neuromuscular junction. (This is where the stimulus to contract is passed to; almost the meeting point of a nerve fibre and the muscle fibre that it supplies.)

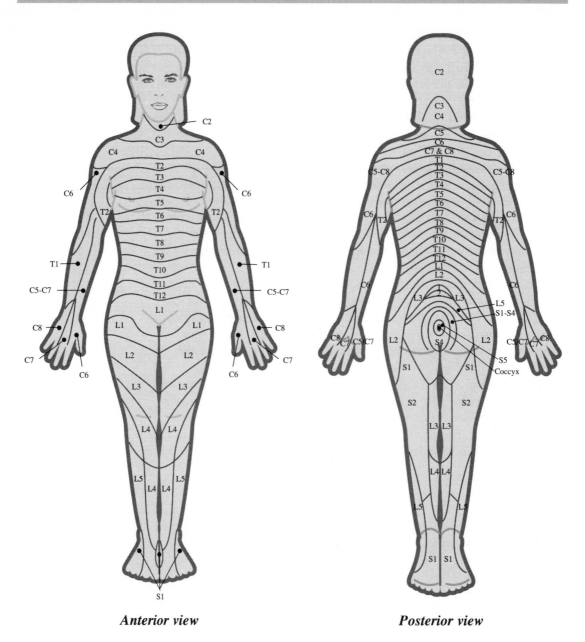

Anterior view   *Posterior view*

Note: The dermatomes are arranged in bands. The areas are enumerated according to the spinal nerve root, indicating the sensory pathways.

Figure 2.6 Dermatomes

Peripheral nerve innervation of a muscle is very closely followed by innervation of the appendicular skeleton. Any injury of these peripheral nerves may lead to fibrosis, a thickening or scarring of the connective tissue, most often as a result of injury or in the healing stage of inflammation. This often accounts for the referred areas of pain felt in the skin.

Neurotransmitters

An essential part of the working of the nervous system is a group of chemicals known as neurotransmitters. There are excitatory and inhibitory neurotransmitters in the parasympathetic and sympathetic nervous systems. Excitatory transmitters stimulate action; inhibitory neurotransmitters inhibit it. When an impulse passes down a parasympathetic nerve, acetylcholine appears at nerve endings and then it transmits the effects of the parasympathetic impulse. This system is involved in maintaining normal levels of activity. The same happens with the sympathetic nervous system, which works in conjunction with the former. At the nerve endings the chemical noradrenaline (a hormone closely related to adrenaline) is released as a neurotransmitter by sympathetic nerve endings. Among its many actions are constriction of swollen blood vessels, often leading to an increase in blood pressure. Increasing the blood flow through the coronary arteries and slowing of the heart rate increases the rate and depth of breathing and complete relaxation to the smooth muscle of the intestinal walls.

Even today there is still a lot to learn about their different types and what each individual chemical does. Most nervous disorders are linked to the homeostatic imbalance of these substances. Many of the 50 or so neurotransmitters of the nervous system are thought to be neuromodulators; the largest group is known as the neuropeptides, which are thought to include both excitatory and inhibitory factors. One particular neuropeptide found within the sensory nerves, the spinal cord pathways and certain portions of the brain is known as substance P; it is thought to stimulate the perception of pain. It is also thought to be involved in the spinal cord pathways and certain portions of the brain that are associated in pain transmission. Conversely, it is known that substances called encephalins have their powerful analgesic effects on the body by inhibiting pain impulses; the endorphins also possess strong analgesic and behavioural effects. The analgesic compounds are concentrated in the thalamus, the hypothalamus and the pituitary gland. This correlates with what

Fitzgerald said in those early years, that stimulation to the pituitary gland reflex point is thought to block or suppress pain. He also elaborated: 'these functions were carried out by the pituitary body and multiple nerve pathways from it'. It may be that stimulation of the pituitary reflex causes the pituitary body to release adrenocorticotrophic hormone (ACTH), which is released in response to stress, and which controls the release of corticosteroid hormone from the adrenal cortex, a powerful anti-inflammatory substance that helps many of the disorders of the body.

Reflexes

Another function of the autonomic nervous system is that of reflex nervous action. A reflex is an automatic involuntary activity brought about by a relatively simple nervous circuit without conscious control being involved. Thus a painful stimuli will bring about a reflex of withdrawing even before the brain has had time to send a message to the muscle involved. This is a reflex action that has been conditioned by other considerations, it is a protective reflex.

Reflex actions are extremely important. They adjust the tone of muscles, particularly those used in posture. It is for this reason I think reflexology has such a dynamical effect on all the spinal nerves of the vertebrae, improving all back and neck related problems.

The medical profession use reflexes for diagnosing many disorders of the nervous system. The most used one, often referred to in reflexology, is the Babinski reflex sign or plantar reflex; this is brought about by drawing a blunt instrument or stroking the lateral side of the plantar area of the foot from the heel to the little toe. In any person over the age of 18 months old, the normal flexor response would be a downward bunching of all the toes. When there is a reverse upward action of the great toe this is indicative that there may be some evidence of a disorder in the brain or spinal cord.

The hypothesis of reflexology is that the medical fraternity expect a reflex on the foot to indicate some clinical significance enabling them to assess a condition in the body (ie they are 'reading' the message coming out); a reflexologist uses the same sensory pathway of stimulation to send a message into the peripheral nervous system, which is a two-way circuit, and on into the central nervous system, a vast nerve network, and through the many interconnections here to reach the autonomic visceral reflexes of the sympathetic and the parasympathetic nervous systems that adjust the activity of the organs of the body cavities in the torso.

As reflexologists we work on the feet, dealing mostly with the minute reflexes. The nerve pathways are thought to traverse through the feet and body. Because of this, often when working on patients they feel a shock or stimuli on the opposite side of the body. This is considered to be crossed reflexes. The term 'crossed reflex' is often used in zone therapy and reflexology. The original neurological term refers to a response that is brought forth on the opposite side of the body to that on which the stimulus was administered, from ascending nerve tracts entering the opposite side of the brain. The term 'crossed reflex' in reflexology indicates an area of referral. This connection affects not only the corresponding organ that has an anatomical connection but also the represented area of the body; for instance, in the case of the head area, we know that if we stub our toe a headache may often develop. Cross reflexes can be used when it is unsuitable to work on a corresponding area, especially if there is any injury or damaged skin; for instance, if the patient has a broken toe, you could get an equal relief of pain by working on the thumb, so the injured part can be avoided. These reflexes can also be used as an area of assistance if the corresponding area is too tender. An area of assistance or helper area is another part of the body that may support or relieve the organ that is injured or has an imbalance through its anatomical connections.

Fitzgerald spoke of the following anatomical correspondences (figure 2.7)

- arms and legs correspond
- palms and soles correspond
- dorsal hands and dorsal feet correspond
- fingers and toes correspond
- wrists and ankles correspond
- hips and shoulders correspond.

This anatomical connection has always been part of TCM.

We know these reflexes are highly complicated and are still not fully understood. As therapists we need to have a knowledge of all these systems of the body thus enabling us to have a greater understanding of how reflexology works. For instance, why is the relaxation on the solar plexus area done on both feet? It was traditionally explained that it was concluded together so as not to cause an imbalance, even though we have only one solar plexus. When we rotate the pressure on the solar plexus point it can be

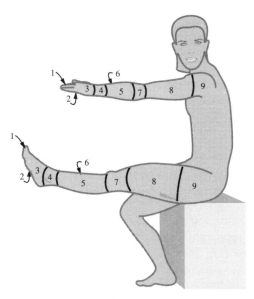

*Figure 2.7
Corresponding cross
reflexes*

1 Fingers – Toes; 2 Palm – Sole; 3 Dorsal hands – Dorsal feet; 4 Wrist – Ankle;
5 Forearm – Foreleg; 6 Under (lower) arm – Calf; 7 Elbow – Knee; 8 Upper arm –
Thigh; 9 Shoulder joint – Hip joint

explained in two ways: stimuli to the foot between zones 2 and 3
has a direct connection to the coeliac plexus because we are also
rotating on the same area on the right foot. This area on the feet
and hands is important when treating depression. The reason for
solar plexus relaxation must be that both feet benefit from this
dual stimulation. We know that the solar plexus is a strong
network of sympathetic nerves and ganglia located high at the
back of the abdomen. On the feet and hands the corresponding
area lies between zones 2 and 3, just below the diaphragm line.
This same area on the feet is the first point of the Kidney meridian
(KI-1) according to TCM; it is an essential point for all acute
problems, and it is a very effective point for all cases of any
urgency. The corresponding point on the hands is PE-8; this is also
a very potent effective point and is very dynamic in clearing
excess heat from the heart and it has a wonderful calming effect
on the mind. The Pericardium meridian originates from the chest
area and descends through the diaphragm to the abdomen,
another branch shoots off to the nipple and then to the axillary
area to descend down the arm to terminate in the large finger (*see*
figure 2.10, page 53); this channel is often considered to be
connected to the emotions of elation and contentment.

Also when working on a person why does the heart rate slow

down? We know that normally cardiac muscle contracts rhythmically without nervous stimulation. The pace is controlled by the autonomic nerves supplying a microscopic group of cells in the upper wall of the right atrium near the entry of the superior vena cava called the sinoatrial node. This area is supplied with parasympathetic fibres from the vagus nerves (tenth cranial nerve) and sympathetic fibres from the cardiac plexus and both end at this point, again receiving this dual stimulation. When stimulated each releases a different neurotransmitter; parasympathetic stimulation releases acetylcholine, slowing the heart rate, and sympathetic stimulation releases adrenaline and noradrenaline, speeding up the heart rate so the rate and depth of breathing are also increased. When working on the reflex points that correspond with these organs the body's systems know whether the heart needs a boost or needs to be calmed down.

Pressure is known to relieve pain. Fitzgerald spoke of how he induced a state of inhibition throughout a zone when he used pressure, and then many of the pathological processes would disappear. He said, 'We know lymphatic relaxation follows pressure'. He was repeatedly being called upon to expand on the theory of zone therapy and he stood by the idea that certain control centres in the medulla oblongata are stimulated, or more shocked, when pressure is applied to corresponding areas; alterations in function are then carried out by the pituitary body secretions affecting the many nerve pathways. He believed man to be of chemical formation but controlled by electrical energy and vibration. When Fitzgerald was in Europe he must have come into contact with many articles and papers that were published in those days, by the many neurologists who were studying the disorders of the nervous system.

Fitzgerald stated in his book *Zone Therapy* that manipulation of the fingers or hand over any injured place prevents a condition known as venous stasis, a state in which the injured surface becomes discoloured. Pressure helps inhibition of the nerve pathways to the brain; also when applied over any bony prominence that corresponds to the location of injury it will tend to relieve pain. If the pressure is correct and long enough it will produce a condition of anaesthesia. This is what led to the discovery of zone analgesia. Fitzgerald also emphasised that it made a difference whether the upper, lower or side surfaces of the joint were pressed. He stated that this pressure therapy had a great advantage over any other method of pain relief because this zone pressure not only relieved the pain, it also removed the cause of pain, no matter where it originated from.

Meridians and nerves

The philosophy of acupuncture and acupressure relies on the connection between a specific area on the skin and a specific organ (*see* chapter 1). Traditionally these are through the meridian pathways that link the organs. According to some TCM authors, these meridians are not the same as the neural pathways; however, that is a theory expounded by some Western acupuncturists. For example, according to Dr Felix Mann in *Acupuncture, How it is Used Today*: 'Nowadays acupuncture can be explained by a wave of electrical depolarisation that travels along a nerve'. This author also refers to the similarity between the TCM idea of Qi transmission along the meridians being like water flowing along a river bed, and the propagation of a nerve impulse along a nerve. Further on in the same book he states:

> The mechanism of acupuncture is elusive. Nevertheless, I have developed the following theory which I think will soon be generally recognised as the scientific basis of acupuncture – albeit with modifications and considerable clarification in detail.
>
> If a patient has a pain in the head or neck, it may under certain circumstances be alleviated in one second, by putting an acupuncture needle into the correct acupuncture point in the foot. This speed of conduction, from one end of the body to the other, is only possible in the nervous system. It would take about half a minute for the blood to flow such a distance, and the lymphatic system is even slower.
>
> Acupuncture is based on the fact that stimulating the skin has an effect on the internal organs and other parts of the body.

Many of the meridians follow the line of a nerve, so the neural pathways must be involved; the above theory is open to conjecture, but the evidence is almost conclusive. The same hypothesis is appropriate for reflexology. By stimulating the precise point a response is felt in the body. In an example that Dr Mann gave, if a person had a headache one would work on the brain reflex and head-related areas; the trigeminal nerve reflex has a definite effect on head-related problems, and these points are on the big toe. Also the liver reflex would be worked as the toxin levels would be quite high; this point is on the plantar area of the foot, but there is no meridian depicted here, showing that the response obtained is from the nerve pathways.

Looking at each meridian in detail reveals that many of them follow nerve pathways; these connect with all the structures along their course: the bones and the deeper muscular branches of their respective muscles, organs, arteries and veins. Thus the pathway could be seen as a direct line to the area of the problem and everything connecting with this pathway is potentially helped. Also, a particular nerve pathway goes in one direction, but a two-way transmission is set up through returning nerve pathways. The following looks at each meridian in detail, typical associated disorders and the nervous connections.

The Lung meridian

The Lung meridian (figure 2.8) is a Yin channel with 11 points. This meridian originates in the stomach and then communicates with the paired organ, the large intestine. As it ascends it connects with the relevant organ, the lungs, the first surface point on this meridian is above the nipple in the first intercostal space. The meridian then passes to the throat from the chest and clavicle along the radial border of the arm, to the middle of the elbow, back to the radial border descending to the thenar eminence and ends at the thumb on the lateral edge of the nail bed. This channel not only communicates with its paired organ the large intestine, but also associates with the kidneys and stomach. So points on this meridian (eg LU-10) will help fluid problems as well; it is ideal for oedema and retention of urine.

The nerve line arises from the lateral cutaneous branches of the

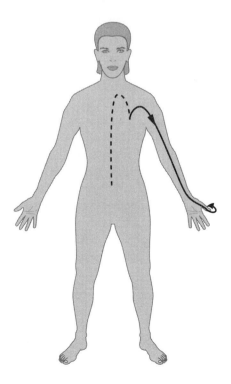

Figure 2.8 The Lung meridian (the dotted line shows how it connects with its paired organ, the large intestine)

first intercostal nerve, the medial and lateral pectoral nerves, median, radial, interosseus and cutaneous nerves of the arm, which then connect with the dorsal digital branches of the palmar digital nerve.

Disorders of this meridian, with signs and symptoms, include: chills, fevers, hidrosis, anhidrosis; pain above the clavicle, or in the chest, upper back, shoulder, forearm, elbow, wrist and hand; headaches; any nasal obstruction, asthma, cough, dyspnoea; fever; sore throat; trigeminal neuralgia, or any twitches in the face. The thumb point is helpful for any cerebral congestion, insomnia, headache, or nervous anxiety.

The Large Intestine meridian

The Large Intestine meridian (figure 2.9) is a Yang channel with 20 points. It commences on the tip of the radial side of the index finger. It ascends the arm on the lateral surface up to the shoulder connecting to the cervical spine and the Governing Vessel on the back. From here it descends to the clavicle and communicates directly with the paired organ, the lungs, and passing through the diaphragm it connects with the relevant organ, the large intestine, to terminate on the face near the nose.

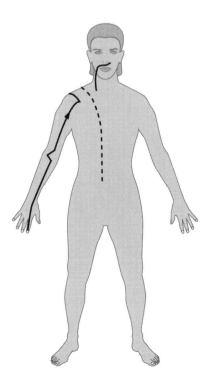

Figure 2.9 The Large Intestine meridian (the dotted line shows how it communicates with its paired organ the lungs and connects with the large intestine)

The nerve line is along the palmar digital nerves, the median nerve, the radial nerve, the ulnar nerve, and the lateral and posterior cutaneous nerves of the forearm; then the branches of the supraclavicular and suprascapular nerves; then the sterno-cleidomastoid nerve; finally the facial and orbital nerves.

Disorders of this meridian, with signs and symptoms, include: all problems related to the head, face, ear (but note that a more powerful point is TB-1 and TB-2) and mouth, including tooth-ache in upper and lower jaw; fevers, sore throats, laryngitis, pharyngitis, influenza; neuralgia of the shoulder and arm, especially the humerus and deltoid, pains to and from the fingers to the upper arm and shoulder; intestinal disorders, constipation and diarrhoea, abdominal pain (because of the calming and antispasmodic action it helps any pain and discomfort arising from any of these disorders); salpingitis; inflammation of the uterus, insufficient menstruation, amenorrhoea (*see* Note below).

Note. There is a vital point, LI-4, that is known as an empirical point to promote delivery during labour; hence it must not be used if the person is pregnant. There are many cautionary warnings on this point.

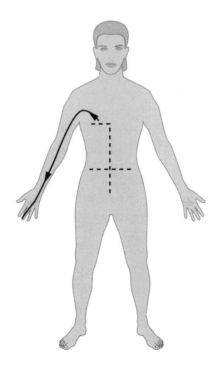

Figure 2.10 The Pericardium meridian (this communicates with all three areas of the body through its paired organ the Triple Burner)

The Pericardium meridian

The Pericardium meridian (figure 2.10) is a Yin channel with nine points. It originates in the thoracic area lateral to the nipple, where it connects with the relevant organ, the pericardium. It then passes through the costal region to the axillary area and runs along the medial aspect of the arm to the cubital fossa. It enters the palm to pass through the muscles, palmaris longus and the flexor carpi radialis to the tip of the middle finger and terminates at the medial side of the nail bed. This channel communicates with all three areas of the body through the paired organ, the Triple Burner.

The nerve line is along the fourth intercostal nerve, the medial and lateral pectoral nerves; then the median, interosseus and cutaneous nerves; it then connects with the palmar digital nerves of the median nerve.

Disorders of this meridian, with signs and symptoms, include: mouth disorders, tongue rigidity; spasms in the hand, wrist or elbow; angina, cardiac arrhythmia, tachycardia; chest disorders, costal neuralgia, pleuritis, mastitis; problems of the mind such as epilepsy, hysteria; heat stroke, fevers. Working it has a wonderful, calming action on the mind.

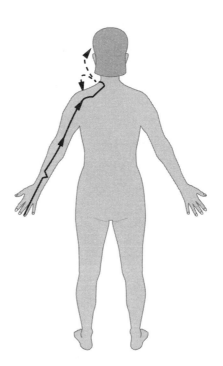

Figure 2.11 The Triple Burner meridian

The Triple Burner (also called the Triple Energizer or Triple Heater) meridian

The Triple Burner meridian (figure 2.11) is a Yang channel with 23 points. It commences on the ulnar side of the ring finger just below the nail bed. It ascends between the fourth and fifth metacarpals in the dorsal side of the arm, between the radius and ulna bone, to the shoulder region where it contacts the Gall Bladder channel, covering the chest. It communicates with the paired organ, the pericardium; then it descends through the diaphragm to connect with all the areas of the body. The point from the shoulder, which enters just above the clavicle, then goes to the neck and the auricle to terminate at the lateral side of the eyebrow. This channel connects directly to the Pericardium meridian.

The nerve line is along the palmar and dorsal digital nerves; then the ulnar and cutaneous nerves of the forearm, connecting with the radial nerve as the meridian ascends. It follows the supraclavicular, suprascapular and axillary nerves, also the first thoracic nerve. There are tributaries of the great auricular and the lesser occipital nerve; also many of the facial nerves, the zygomatic and trigeminal nerves.

Disorders of this meridian, with signs and symptoms, include: headaches and related problems; eye problems, conjunctivitis; ear pain and tinnitus; sore throats; facial problems and toothache; stiff neck and shoulders. The Triple Burner helps all levels of the body, including problems in the chest, upper and lower abdomen, all digestive problems, and intestinal disorders. As it connects with the 'Lower Burner' it also benefits liver, stomach and bladder problems.

As a speculative comment, Fitzgerald would raise the nail of the ring finger on the lateral side to stop unilateral tinnitus; that is the first point on this meridian for any ear problems.

The Heart meridian

The Heart meridian (figure 2.12) is a Yin channel with nine points. It originates at the heart to the medial side of the upper limbs near the axillary area and then descends to the paired organ, the small intestine. There is an offshoot from the heart to the oesophagus, which then ascends to just below the eye. The principal channel ascends from the heart to the lungs, to the axillary area, and follows a line down the ulnar side of the arm to the wrist between the carpals (capitate bone) between the fourth and fifth

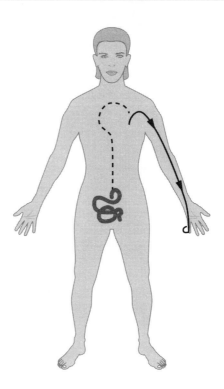

Figure 2.12 The Heart meridian (the dotted line shows how it communicates with its paired organ the small intestine)

metacarpals on the palmar side to the little finger; here it terminates at the medial side of the nail bed of the little finger. This channel connects directly with the lung and the kidneys.

The nerve line is along the intercostobrachial nerve, the radial, ulnar, and the median nerve and its branches, also the palmar digital nerve.

Disorders of this meridian, with signs and symptoms, include: headaches, hysteria, insomnia, mild psychiatric problems, disturbing dreams, depressions or anxiety; problems of the tongue such as glossitis, toothache; all arm and wrist pain; chest, respiratory and breast disorders, angina, mild heart problems, irregular heart beat, palpitations; uterine disorders, dysmenorrhoea.

Note. If you suspect any heart disorder, never treat yourself. Seek help first from your medical practitioner. If they are happy that you receive reflexology, this will have a wonderful calming action on the heart.

The Small Intestine meridian

The Small Intestine meridian (figure 2.13) is a Yang channel. It commences on the ulnar side of the little finger, on the lateral side

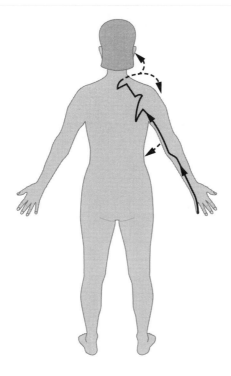

Figure 2.13 The Small Intestine meridian

of the arm to the shoulder, passes around the scapula and goes deep to the supraclavicular fossa connecting to the heart, the paired organ, then descends to join the small intestine. An off-shoot passes up from supraclavicular fossa to the neck and then on to the cheek; from there it connects with the Gall Bladder and Triple Burner channels and then terminates at the front of the ear.

The nerve line is along the dorsal digital and palmar nerves, the ulnar nerve, the cutaneous nerves, the radial nerve, the second intercostal nerve, the suprascapular nerve, the eighth cervical nerve, the first and second thoracic nerves, the great auricular nerve, the auriculotemporal nerve, the superior cervical ganglion, also five of the cranial nerves: the vagus (X), spinal accessory (XI), hypoglossal (XII), trigeminal (V) and facial (VII) nerves.

Disorders of this meridian, with signs and symptoms, include: headaches, febrile symptoms (work on this channel helps to clear the mind); stiff neck and torticollis; wrist, arm and shoulder problems; acute lumbar strain; colic and constipation.

As a speculative comment, Fitzgerald stated that the fourth and fifth zone merged in the head. Note that the three meridians on the third and fourth fingers all deal with head-related disorders: Triple Burner, Heart and Small Intestine. Also the three meridians on the feet, Gall Bladder, Bladder and Kidney, are all points for head-related problems. The first Kidney acupoint arises on the little toe to emerge on the plantar aspect of the foot. In reflexology we would use this point for stiff necks or shoulder problems; just pulling on this toe will help to relieve a stiff shoulder or neck. The spinal accessory nerve supplies the sternocleidomastoid muscle and the trapezius muscle, both of which are involved in neck and shoulder movements. (*See* figure 7.2.)

The Spleen meridian

The Spleen meridian (figure 2.14) is a Yin channel with 21 points. It commences on the medial edge of the base of the nail bed of the great toe and ascends the leg on the medial side to enter the abdomen; there it communicates with the Conception Vessel (see figure 7.6, page 227) where it connects with its relevant organ, the spleen. From here it connects with some of the internal organs, the stomach – its paired organ, liver and gall bladder. The meridian continues up through to the diaphragm, one offshoot going directly to the heart and the other ascending into the throat and root of the tongue.

The nerve line is along the cutaneous medial dorsal nerves of

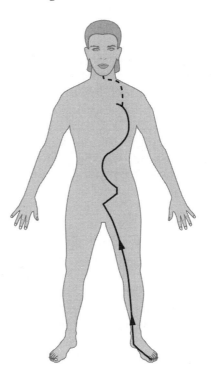

Figure 2.14 The Spleen/Pancreas meridian

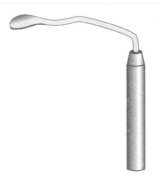

Figure 2.15 This tongue pressor was used on the posterior wall of the pharynx to give relief during menstruation. (Fitzgerald made a statement to the effect that while he had not heard of any miscarriages he cautioned its use in pregnancy.)

the foot and plantar nerves, then along the saphenous, tibial and femoral nerves, which arise from L2–L4 of the spinal trunk; there it connects with the thoracic nerves, then it continues on up to the intercostal nerves and pectoral nerves.

Disorders of this meridian, with signs and symptoms, include: anything concerned with the brain and central nervous system; spinal problems; all genitourinary problems; abdominal and intestinal disorders, such as flatulence, any abdominal pain, gastric pain, painful haemorrhoids, diarrhoea, constipation, irregular menstruation.

As a speculative comment, SP-3 is used for all lung problems. This point is on the lung area in reflexology. SP-4 is a point that is widely used for all excess problems of the stomach and the spleen; this area corresponds to the upper abdominal area in reflexology. Also the Spleen meridian ends in the root of the tongue; Fitzgerald use to apply a tongue pressor (figure 2.15) to reach as far back as possible on the root of the tongue for amenorrhoea, also for painful menstruation. This point is a good point to regulate menstruation, and the former helps in strengthening the spine.

The Liver meridian

The Liver meridian (figure 2.16) is a Yin channel with 14 points. It commences on the lateral edge at the base of the nail bed of the great toe and ascends the dorsal aspect of the foot to the medial malleolus; then it ascends the leg on the medial side following the line of the Spleen channel. It traverses around the pubis area and the genitals, where it meets the Conception Vessel, then moving onwards and up to its relevant organ, the liver, where it links with the gall bladder. It has branches that serve the lungs, the trachea, the larynx and the upper palate of the mouth, and an

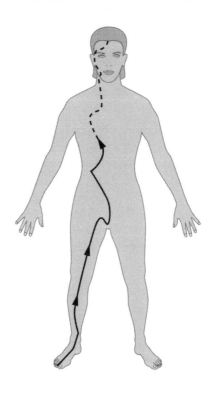

Figure 2.16 The Liver meridian

offshoot serves the lips. The meridian also distributes to the tissue around the eye, and also the forehead; it meets the Governing Vessel at the vertex of the head.

The nerve line is along the cutaneous medial dorsal nerves of the foot and the deep peroneal nerve, then the saphenous, and femoral nerves, which arise from L2–L4 of the spinal trunk; there it connects with the thoracic nerves, then continues on up to the intercostal nerves.

Disorders of this meridian, with signs and symptoms, include: headaches, vertigo and tinnitus; throat disorders, toothache; any colic or abdominal distension due to gastrointestinal disorders; lumbago; and problems in all four limbs; all problems relating to the genitourinary tract.

The Stomach meridian

The Stomach meridian (figure 2.17) is a Yang channel with 45 points. It originates on the cheek at the side of the nose, and passes through the roots of the teeth on to the lips, descending through the thorax to the abdomen, where it communicates with

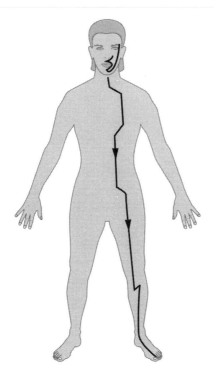

Figure 2.17 The Stomach meridian

the spleen and connects directly with the heart. It passes down the thigh to just below the knee on the anterior part of the leg to terminate on the lateral edge of the second toe at the base of the nail bed.

The nerve line is along the branches of the facial nerve, then the oculomotor, the trigeminal, and hypoglossal cranial nerves, and the auricular nerve, continuing along the cervical nerves that supply the clavicle, and the first thoracic nerves that supply the pectorals through to the first lumbar nerve, which supplies all the abdomen, and the femoral nerve, which splits into many cutaneous branches supplying the area from the inguinal ligament down to the toes.

Disorders of this meridian, with signs and symptoms, include: all mouth and facial problems; problems of the lower extremities. There is a distal empirical point that can be used for shoulder problems. (*See* ST-38, figure 5.41, page 180.)

As a speculative comment, in reflexology we use the ST-45 and ST-44 for all mouth or facial problems, and these reflex areas are wonderful for toothache. ST-43 is used for all digestive disorders; this lies on the hypochondrium area according to the reflexology map of the body.

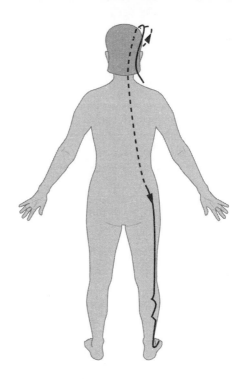

Figure 2.18 The Gall Bladder meridian

The Gall Bladder meridian

The Gall Bladder meridian (figure 2.18) is a Yang channel with 44 points. It originates on the lateral side of the eye at the point known as pupil crevice. The meridian contours the head and neck, with an offshoot passing to the inner ear; it then passes through the diaphragm with branches going to the breast, then it connects with the liver and gall bladder, and emerges in the groin area and runs along the lateral aspect of the thigh down to the lateral edge of the fourth toe at the base of the nail bed. There is also a connecting channel, which links the instep to the first toe, connecting the gall bladder and the liver, its paired organ.

The nerve line is along the branches of the fifth cranial nerve, the largest cranial nerve, whose offshoot the zygomaticotemporal nerve serves the facial area, then along the occipital, and auricular nerves, continuing along the supraclavicular nerve, connecting with many of the intercostal and many of the thoracic nerves, right down to the first lumbar nerve, where the femoral nerve lies, and branches of the peroneal nerve, connecting with many of the muscles of the calf, the dorsal surface of the ankle, the tarsus, the fourth metatarsal and the third, fourth and fifth toes.

Disorders of this meridian, with signs and symptoms, include:

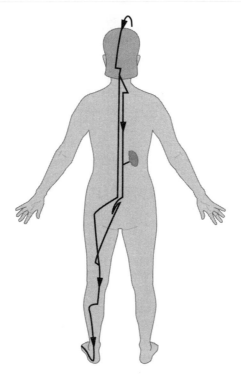

Figure 2.19 The Bladder meridian

all head-related disorders, facial pain, eye, ear and mouth problems, mastitis or oedema of the axillary areas; any pain of the costal region, or neck, arm and shoulder problems.

The Bladder meridian

The Bladder meridian (figure 2.19) is a Yang channel with 67 points. It originates on the face on the medial edge of the eye, contours the head and the neck then descends the lateral side of the vertebrae to connect with the bladder and the kidney. An offshoot from the lumbar area passes around the gluteal muscles of the buttocks to terminate at the popliteal fossa, the depression at the back of the knee. There is a secondary channel running from the neck area down the vertebrae to this point, but this secondary branch carries on down splitting the gastrocnemius muscle of the calf to emerge on the lateral side of the malleolus to run alongside the lateral side of the fifth metatarsal and terminate in the little toe.

The nerve line is along the ophthalmic branch of the trigeminal nerve, the fourth cranial nerve, the trochlear, and the third cervical nerve. It then descends the thoracic nerves that serve many muscles of the back, carrying on to connect with all the lumbar nerves 1–5 and the sacral nerves; it continues down through the

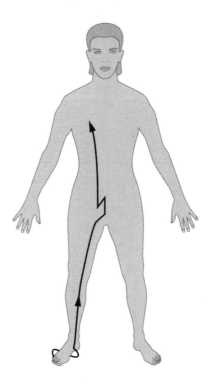

Figure 2.20 The Kidney meridian

buttocks, serving all the hamstring muscles, and along the peroneal nerve, connecting to the digital plantar nerves of the foot.

Disorders of this meridian, with signs and symptoms, include: all head and neck problems; some urogenital disorders; lumbago; foot and leg problems.

The Kidney meridian

The Kidney meridian (figure 2.20) is a Yin channel with 27 points. It originates on the fifth toe and emerges on the plantar surface of the foot, passing to the medial edge of the internal malleolus where it ascends the leg, entering the body at a point at the coccyx. There it runs deeper to connect with the kidneys and bladder through the lungs, to be lost in the roots of the tongue. An offshoot leaves the lungs and connects with the heart to terminate in the clavicle.

The nerve line is along the plantar nerves, connecting with the saphenous and tibial nerve, a branch of the sciatic nerve. It then enters the lumbar–sacral plexus and continues on into the upper thoracic, and intercostal and pectoral nerves.

Disorders of this meridian, with signs and symptoms, include: all head-related disorders of an acute nature; distension or pain of the abdomen or gastritis; most urogenital disorders and irregularities; all lower back and knee problems; most of its problems end in 'itis' or are of sudden onset.

Conclusion

By looking at the nerve pathways involved it is possible to answer why working on a meridian or zone has such a powerful outcome. Nerve transmission works on the 'all or none' principle, so that the channel will open to stimuli that are strong or long enough; providing there is no congestion of toxic matter the impulse will travel right along the pathway. If there is a blockage then several treatments are usually needed to clear the nerve pathway.

It has been found empirically that the distal points used for acupuncture and acupressure are particularly efficacious. These are in many ways the same points that we may cross at some time throughout the reflexology treatment session. Comparing the two systems, the point SP-1, for example, the first point on the Spleen meridian, is for the nose. This is also the point for the nose in reflexology. Qi is considered to be ascending in this channel. Equally, the last point of the Stomach meridian, ST-45, is known as the 'sick mouth', because it is an ideal point to treat those problems at the opposite end of the body. Qi is considered to be descending in this channel. So by treating distal points, and regardless of which way Qi or nerve energy is moving, we get a response. This is exemplified by the aphorism that stubbing your toe gives you a headache, and by the Babinski reflex, the foot indicating what is happening in the brain.

A recent hypothesis to explain the effect of acupressure and acupuncture is that when a needle or pressure is applied at a certain skin depth it seems to stimulate the nervous system in a series of reflex arcs, thus releasing endorphins into the system and producing pain-relieving and opiate effects. We know that the Chinese use acupuncture for anaesthesia and pain relief, and this practice often relieves some other physical symptoms in the process. Acupuncture can be explained by a wave of electrical depolarisation that travels along the nerve pathways activating the deep sensory nerves which cause the pituitary and mid-brain to release endorphins, the brain's natural painkillers. The problem the person is suffering from is often alleviated after a few treatments.

Since the early 1960s, electroanalgesia has been used as a safe and effective method of pain control, regardless of whether it is acute or chronic. There are many manufacturers of electroanalgesic instruments. The theory regarding this therapy is that stimulation by a small electric current, like the stimulation caused by insertion of an acupuncture needle, activates descending inhibitory neurones that block the transmission of pain signals. It is said to 'close the pain gate', so this theory is known as the 'gate control theory'.

The Chinese state in many books that the meridians follow the pathways of the major nerves, and needling or acupressure will activate a point. The nerves lie very close to the bones, and we know that peripheral nerve innervation of the skeleton closely follows muscle innervation. This shows that the same nerve innervates muscles that are attached to that bone. Did Dr William Fitzgerald simplify this whole concept? He stated that pressure over any bony eminence or on the corresponding zone to the location of injury or problem would relieve pain. One of the theories he put forward was that certain control centres in the medulla are stimulated, or that the function is carried out by the pituitary body and its multiple nerve paths from it. He went on to explain that we induce a state of inhibition throughout the body when pressure is brought to bear. When inhibition or irritation is continuous, many pathological processes disappear. He also stated that it was certain that lymphatic relaxation followed lymphatic pressure.

Today there is no concise explanation of the rationale of how or why reflexology works. We as practitioners just accept and know that it does. A recent hypothesis for the effect of acupuncture is that when pressure or needles are applied at a certain depth it stimulates the nervous system in a series of arcs or reflex actions; this may send a motor impulse down a nerve to supply a muscle or gland into stimulation, either contraction or relaxation. One other theory is that this technique stimulates production of pain-relieving endorphins within the brain. These recent theories confirm Fitzgerald's early thoughts and writings.

The zones and the divisions of the feet and hands

The zones and divisions of the hands and feet according to contemporary reflexology are shown in figure 2.21 and plates 1 to 4. (Note that in the anatomical texts the person is depicted standing upright with the feet on the ground and the palmar surface of the hands are facing the front. In the zonal or reflexology position the body is depicted with the palmar surface of the hands facing towards the posterior part of the body. However, this is not adhered to in all representations of the

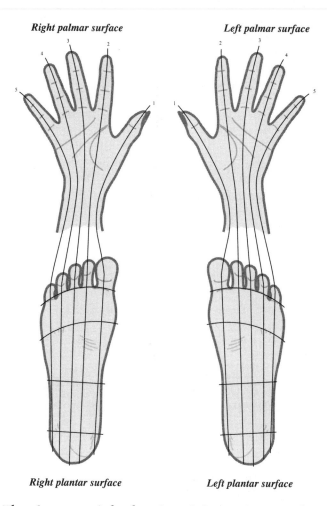

Right palmar surface Left palmar surface

Right plantar surface Left plantar surface

Figure 2.21 The ten longitudinal zones on the hands and feet

zones.) The dorsum of the hand and foot represent the anterior surface of the body. The palmar surface of the hand and the plantar region of the foot depict the posterior portion of the body. Each numbered line represents the centre of its respective zone (*see* figure 2.21). There is considered to be an imaginary line showing the division between the anterior and posterior parts of the body. (Fitzgerald said this was so that when treating any of the viscera, it was usually preferable to treat both anterior and posterior zones simultaneously.)

The theory behind reflexology is that the feet and hands are not just the extremities at the end of our body; these appendicular organs are a somatic reproduction of the entire condition of the body. However, many books show the picture of the human body superimposed on just the foot or hand. This is to outline the need to know the location of the appropriate point for all the principal

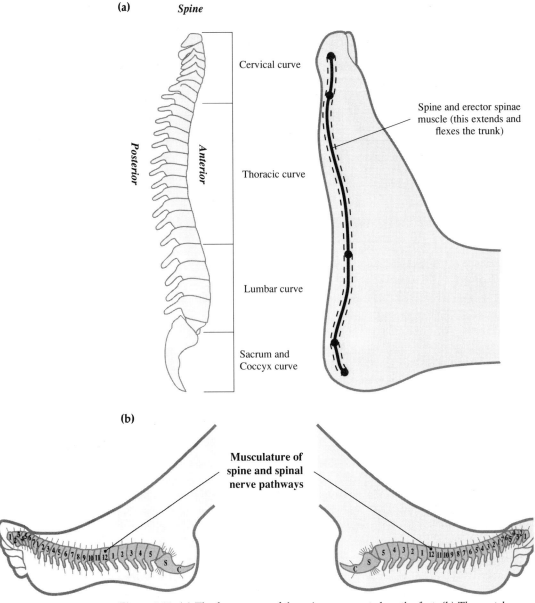

(a)

Spine

Cervical curve

Thoracic curve

Lumbar curve

Sacrum and
Coccyx curve

Posterior

Anterior

Spine and erector spinae
muscle (this extends and
flexes the trunk)

(b)

**Musculature of
spine and spinal
nerve pathways**

*Figure 2.22 (a) The four curves of the spine represented on the foot. (b) The vertebrae
and spinal nerves represented on the foot.*

organs and glands so that they can have pressure applied on the
correct area. The distal limbs are not usually shown other than
where there is an area that is supposed to connect to the area to
work on.

The feet and the spine

The feet are extremely important to the general health of our body, and because of certain similarities reflexology theory considers there to be a relationship between the body and the foot. For instance, there are 26 bones in each foot and there are 26 bones in the adult spine. Further, the vertebral column has four natural curves when it is viewed from the side: the cervical curve is rounded forwards, the thoracic curve is gently curved convex towards the posterior, the lumbar spine is also curved convex forwards creating a hollow, while the sacrum curve is like that of the thoracic curve, convex towards the posterior. The foot appears to have four natural curves also, almost imitating the line of the spine. So the curves and the bones of the foot are designated in reflexology as representing the curves and the bones of the spine (figure 2.22a). From this, particular areas of the foot are considered to represent areas of spinal innervation that correspond to those bones (figure 2.22b).

The following four curves or divisions of the feet represent the four body divisions as follows (the two feet symbolize the whole human body including the limbs, not just the torso).

1 The phalanges of the feet represent the head, the uppermost division of the body, containing the brain and chief sense organs.
2 The metatarsus represents the thoracic cavity from the neck to the abdomen, containing our breathing apparatus, the lungs, also the heart and other structures within.
3 The tarsus represents the abdominal cavity, which is between the thorax and the pelvis area, and all organs and structures within it. The tuberosity of the cuboid bone represents the waistline.
4 The calcaneus and talus represent the pelvic cavity, the almost bowl-shaped area that is formed by the pelvic girdle and the adjoining bones of the spine; this creates the central support for the body, and is composed of the two hip bones, the sacrum, and the coccyx and organs and structures within.

Reflexology and the body systems

The theory of reflexology is that a congestive state creates blockages of energy pathways; it has been conjectured that this blockage causes crystals to become deposited around the nerve endings, causing congestion right through the zone. The deposition around the nerve endings also causes a painful area when pressed or palpated. Over a period of treatment these areas become less sensitive as changes are induced within the circulatory and the nervous system by means of pressure stimuli. Such stimuli trigger the body's inherent ability to move back to a state of correct balance and positive health and well-being. Working all areas of the hands, feet or ears and using a combination of reflexes will therefore eliminate most of these blocked energy pathways, energizing and revitalizing the recipient.

The natural homeostasis of living things can be disturbed by stress, which upsets the internal environment. Every part of the body is involved in maintaining this environment within the normal limits. It is only in cases of extreme or severe stress that the body is unable to cope. Homeostatic functions are maintained by nervous and chemical connections, with the pituitary body and other endocrine glands all working in unison. Feedback systems detect even the slightest change, setting off an immediate response in the form of neural impulses which are sent to neutralize any stress this may cause and to counterbalance the organ in question. If the body systems are not functioning at peak efficiency then disorders may manifest.

In the brain, three areas, the medulla oblongata, the hypothalamus and the pons Varolii (figure 2.23), are very important for this

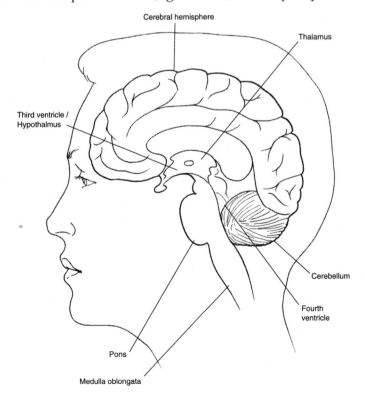

Figure 2.23 A section through the brain

process. The first contains vital centres that control the rate and depth of breathing 'respiration', the rate of the heart beat and blood vessels, and not so vital centres that control reflexes such as swallowing, sneezing, coughing and vomiting. It also forms the major pathway for nerve impulses entering and leaving the skull. The hypothalamus also contains vital centres controlling body temperature, thirst, hunger, eating, water balance and the libido, and is also closely connected to emotional activity and sleep. The pons Varolii contains many nerve tracts running between the cerebral cortex and the spinal cord; it is where the trigeminal nerve emerges and also the sensory fibres relaying information about pain, touch and temperature.

We can therefore see that reflexology might assist the homeostatic function by removing obstruction at the level of the autonomic nervous system. Fitzgerald said all zones must be free from irritation and obstructions for best results. He spoke of all existing pathological conditions being relieved and some even cured by zone therapy. He stated, however, that his work was not a panacea to all ills, but he was glad to offer his knowledge of zone therapy to physicians, surgeons and patients/clients to aid medicine and surgery and for them to make use of it in the practice of their profession.

Conclusion

This section has examined how the ideas of acupuncture, acupressure and reflexology relate to our present knowledge of the nervous system. The main practical difference between the three therapies is that reflexology and acupressure are less invasive and they use the fingers or thumbs for manipulation on given points; but they are equally powerful, often bringing quicker relief from the presenting symptoms. Acupuncturists use needles to stimulate very precise points located according to TCM theory, and can reach a greater depth. Acupuncture treatment is often thought to have longer-lasting effects than massage treatment, but can take longer to work.

There are also many contraindications to acupuncture: certain nerves must never have needles applied to them, and many conditions cannot be treated if the person is already depleted by a great emotional experience, or if they are too fatigued. However, reflexology and acupressure are completely safe with only a few cautionary warnings of the timing of treatment sessions; they cannot make a problem worse if applied in the correct way.

Western medicine and complementary medicine working together

Western medical science has overcome so many things. The prevention, diagnosis and treatment of disease have benefited greatly by the development of injections and vaccinations, and of sophisticated surgery incorporating pain management, anaesthetics, antibiotics, and vital organ transplants. However, it is still powerless to treat a lot of the common everyday ailments, and is still largely unable to relieve the emotional and stress-related problems that we suffer from today without resorting to the use of drugs.

The definition of medicine does not include only substances used for treating disease; it also involves the wider art and science of treating and understanding disorders, which includes their prevention, and the maintenance and restoration of health. We need to realize there are alternatives to drugs. Drugs suppress rather than cure the problem; also, they form only part of the total care of the patient. It is not my purpose here to emphasize the differences between reflexology and Western medicine, but to show that the two should work hand in hand and share their knowledge. However, disquiet about the safety of some of the day to day medicines has led to a growing refusal by people to accept the attitude of some doctors that 'you will have to learn to live with it'. They also may find it frustrating when visiting their general practitioners (GPs) to find that only a few minutes can be spent with them. Not all GPs are so rushed, though, and, more than ever, many are now adopting a more holistic approach to their patients. Many treatments formerly considered 'alternative' are now being included in some general practices. For example, GPs may often incorporate counselling, hypnosis, psychotherapy, but also include some of the complementary therapies; the latter include reflexology, which can be administered by non-medical but qualified practitioners.

Even so, often powerful drugs are given, which take away symptoms fast, yet may do nothing to correct the underlying cause. The real cause could be that you are angry with your partner, or that you are having problems at work, or you could be in a non-fulfilling job. All of these types of problems create stress, and in turn many disorders such as troubles with the digestion, headaches or back problems. The drugs that are prescribed may provoke new problems or cause more side-effects than the original illness. For instance, tranquillizers are often given in times of extreme stress, but can easily become addictive. As reflexologists know, side-effects of such drugs can cause sore spots in the reflexes of the hand, feet and ears.

The medical profession themselves are still uncertain as to the safety of the chemicals referred to as medicine or 'prescription drugs'. No drug is 'safe' in the sense that it can never harm anybody; the dose may be critical, and one person may not be able to take the same amount as another. Furthermore, regardless of how clear instructions are, human error can create difficulties with proper usage. Patients are more aware now of the possibility of side-effects and contraindications to some drugs than ever before. However, many people buy vitamins, patent medicines and other remedies over the counter and these also are not entirely free from side-effects. For instance, vitamins are important for good health, but if taken in excess can cause toxic effects and sometimes an allergic response. It is common knowledge that we have become a nation of pill takers, and often the temptation to take medication is at its greatest when we are unable to seek medical advice. There is always a temptation to indulge in self-medication, but a sensible selection of basic medications for everyday needs is all that is required. No drug should be taken casually or carelessly.

Drug dependence is a term that is now used daily; it indicates that the person suffers in some way if the medication is stopped. This effect is typical of the benzodiazepine group of drugs, which act as a depressant on the central nervous system. These common tranquillizing and antianxiety drugs cause the body to become tolerant to a given dosage, so the dosage has to be increased, causing the person gradually to become dependent. As holistic practitioners, we have a responsibility never to encourage patients to come off any drugs, as this issue is between the medical practitioner and the patient and usually drug treatment must be decreased gradually. However, it is possible to encourage patients into making sure the GP is aware of their feelings if they wish to pursue a more holistic approach, as there are alternatives. Natural healing therapies may be time-consuming in the long term, but are generally less invasive and in many cases far more effective. Complementary treatments such as reflexology are a sensible idea for the busy GPs in these situations, and may even save the medical profession a lot of extra expense and time.

Patients are also guilty of pressuring doctors, and some people expect to be given a prescription, feeling that they must not leave empty-handed. These type of people are often not receptive to the concept of holistic medicine. However, drugs and surgery should be used as a last resort, not as a routine measure. The members of the medical profession themselves are now becoming more hesitant in the use of operations, for instance the removal of tonsils, which used to be a standard childhood procedure, or appendectomy, which was formerly often performed routinely when doing other routine procedures for abdominal surgery. Even the extent of vital radical surgery such as a mastectomy or a Caesarean is being re-examined for necessity.

When the British Medical Association set up a committee to look into alternative medicines, they were interested in looking at the effects of alternative therapies as measured by science-based research, which demands measurable proof that a patient's condition has been improved. To date, however, there have been very few clinical trials. Therefore a scientific inquiry is needed into the efficacy of reflexology, to test the fact and to elucidate on our theories, different levels of pressure must be adopted for true verification of relief of symptoms and pain. As practitioners, we know reflexology is a therapy that gives measurable benefits and in some cases relieves the problem completely. However, for the scientific community just feeling better is not enough proof.

Many doctors now use acupuncture for pain relief. That said, many do not use the TCM ideas of affecting the energy flow to give a complete comprehensive treatment of the whole person. They adhere to scientific research showing that acupuncture works by stimulating nerve fibres to send out pain-blocking messages stimulating production and release of endorphins and encephalins. Reflexology cannot be so wholeheartedly and equally accepted by them unless it can also be explained in this way. This may be at odds with the ideas of complementary therapists who claim that their sensitive hands or fingers feel 'blockages'. Nevertheless, as practising complementary practitioners, healing the whole person is of paramount importance.

Within the therapy session, sympathetic listening and talking become a way of communicating and healing, in which anxieties are reduced and a more positive attitude of mind is encouraged to bring about swift healing, in which individuals also adopt more self-help measures. Relaxation is a must and it is an essential part of acquiring physical and mental well-being to relieve day-to-day tensions and stresses. There are so many techniques that can be encouraged for relaxation: for example, simple breathing exercises calm the mind and body, and many ancient traditions used breathing to alter mental states. Many methods use this, including meditation and yoga and, over the last decade, Tai Chi and Qigong; the latter ancient arts also include focused awareness and relaxed exercises. Daily use of these methods is reputed to increase a resistance to ill-health and in many cases cure the disease, improve the digestive and circulatory systems, enhance many of the internal secretions and increase vigour. Some research seems to substantiate these claims.

A reflexologist working on the solar plexus and diaphragm reflexes points also often induces a state of calm. It is recognized that different breathing patterns are connected to general health problems and anxious people often breath more rapidly, causing shallow breathing, which robs the tissues of oxygen and nutrients. Reflexology is not a cure-all, but it has been used to treat many common ailments and apparently can significantly reduce anxiety and stress.

3 Basics of consultation and diagnosis

The Fundamentals of Good Practice

This chapter analyses the process of consultation and diagnosis, which are the essential prerequisites to deciding on the correct treatment.

The first steps in consultation are to observe, question and listen to the patient/client in order to understand the problem. All the information gained should be recorded in a case history, using a consultation card or index card.

There needs to be a thorough diagnostic analysis prior to commencement of treatment, through a methodical appraisal of the feet, hands and ears (*see also* chapters 5–7 for specific areas). The therapists should be aware of behaviour patterns and how they may affect the patient/client's health. Other factors that may be important need to be considered also. For instance, environmental factors may be affecting the patient/client. These processes lead to a differential diagnosis to understand the cause of the patient/client's problem.

Finally, the therapist needs to decide on and recommend a treatment. However, there may be patients/clients for whom treatment is contraindicated, and the reflexologist needs to be aware of these.

The general order of the consultation process is therefore as follows:

- observation
- questioning and listening
- diagnosis
- recommending treatment.

Clinical observation

Observation should include both observations of the body generally, and detailed observation of the feet.

General observations

General appearance should always be noted; this can only be achieved by a methodical scrutiny of the person as described below to give some idea of their problem.

Being aware of and paying attention to the movement and the physical mannerisms of the person entering the room is of the utmost importance, as many things are noticeable in the first few minutes. These are important as people do not consciously adjust their movements or their mannerisms whilst unaware that they are being observed.

When walking, for example, do they walk on their heels? This could indicate hypersensitivity in the plantar region of the foot, which may indicate peripheral neuropathy. If there is a spring in the step it indicates that the supportive ligaments and muscles are well developed and there is less probability of a spine problem. Is the person flexible in movement when walking? This is a good sign and it shows there is little tension in the body. If the reverse is evident it often indicates the patient is stiff and rigid, and shows that the muscles are tight. This could be due to a muscle injury, a neurological disorder and even arthritis affecting the joints.

The position of the head is important to note. When the body is in the correct position the head is straight and lifted up, the shoulders are relaxed, and this indicates a lack of tension in the person. When the body leans forward it may create pressure on the cervical region, and pressure on the frontal area of the brain; this is thought to be a contributing factor to depression. It also causes pressure on the lower lumbar spine because the weight is not central. The word 'depression' means 'pressure' or 'weighing down'; a posture with a dropped head and hunched shoulders may signify that the person is in a low state of mind. Such a posture can in turn cause pressure on the thoracic cavity and abdominal organs. If the shoulders are drawn in the breathing capacity is also diminished; this lowers and impairs the ability of the circulating blood to reach all areas of the body. Many of the problems associated with rounded shoulders are those linked with respiration, such as asthma, bronchitis and upper respiratory infections.

When clients are seated, the therapist should note the following. Are they relaxed? Are the hands held still and at ease, showing a state of calmness and peace, or are they fidgeting, squeezed or twisted in a wringing action, showing unease and discomfort? Other visible signs of unease include plucking of hair and other movements. For instance, do they cross and uncross their legs, cross their feet, or move around? Attention should also be paid to clients' speech. For instance, do they speak fast without drawing a breath? What is the tone of the voice; is there modulation, or is it high pitched?

All of these behaviour patterns could indicate unease, but there are other explanations. For instance, continual leg movements could be due to discomfort in the lower back or hip area. We should not make a hasty diagnosis, or jump to conclusions. However, the initial observation should enable the therapist to begin to form an assumption of what the problems may be.

A number of specific features can also be observed and are particularly significant.

Facial skin colour and tone

Difference in skin colour is due to the amount of melanin pigment in the skin. However, a good pink facial colour in fair-skinned people is a sign of a healthy circulation and general good health, as the colour of the skin also depends on the quality and quantity of blood moving through the capillaries. Erythema or redness of the skin can be due to many factors; for instance, the client could have rushed to make their appointment, they may be a little embarrassed, or there could be some allergic reaction (as in hives where the skin is often red and irritating). Any undue redness of the skin should be therefore investigated further. Pale skin may indicate a reduced blood flow, or excess time spent indoors, or just that person is enervated by their problems. A grey appearance may indicate illness or total exhaustion; it could even be caused by a lack of oxygen due to respiratory problems. A greying colour can also occur after a sudden shock.

Dry skin or moistureless prematurely aged skin may be indicative of a hormonal imbalance or that the diet is lacking in some nutrients. Any acne, pustules, pimples and spots is nature's way of discarding toxins through the skin. They indicate that the endocrine system may be out of balance, and diet, hygiene and lifestyle may need to be addressed. If the problem is acne, the sebaceous glands may have become blocked, or it could also be due to an allergic reaction to other substances.

Ears

The ears should have the same colour and tone as the facial skin. However, if there is a slight red tinge around the edges this could indicate an uneven blood circulation. If there is a bluish discoloration it may indicate a lack of oxygen and a deficient circulation. Pallor of the skin here in comparison to the face also shows inadequate circulation. (Note, however, that the outside temperature must be noted when doing ear analysis.) Dry skin or exfoliation of the upper layer indicates a possible imbalance in the diet. (*See* chapter 7 for more information on the ear.)

Hair quality

Good health is shown by bright shining hair; poor health is indicated when the hair is dull and lifeless. If the hair is thinning excessively there could be an immunological disorder; this could also occur after an illness, or even excessive dieting. Brittle hair could signify a mineral deficiency or endocrine imbalance, because the endocrine system is responsible for the stimulation of the sebaceous gland – sebum helps hair from drying out, but too much sebum can create oily hair.

Lips (labia)

The lips should be moist and of a pink healthy colour; this indicates good health and good circulation to the peripheral parts of the body. As the lips are extremely sensitive and have numerous sensory receptors they are often prone to allergic reactions from cosmetics, which can make them appear cracked, dry and sore looking. Also it is necessary to see whether the person produces sufficient saliva (*see below*), as this also aids lip moisture. How lips and mouth are held gives a good indication of how the person feels; tight pursed lips often indicate tension or unhappiness.

Mouth (buccal cavity)

A dry mouth can be due to incorrect breathing through the mouth, or lack of saliva. This watery secretion containing enzymes begins the process of digestion, and a lack of this secretion could cause constipation or sluggish bowel action. The secretion is entirely controlled by the nervous system, so can be affected if the person is overstressed. It usually indicates that the sympathetic and parasympathetic nervous systems are not in tune with each other.

Tongue

It is not in the remit of the therapist to take over the diagnostic role of the medical practitioner. However, certain signs do help make an overall assessment of the client's general health. A large flabby tongue often indicates general weakness or possibly the onset of some debility. A furred tongue is often evident if the person constantly breathes through their mouth or is a heavy smoker. In some cases a thick tongue coating could signify a gastric disorder or some other disorder that may be in the process of manifesting. An even, red and shiny tongue could be due to a nutritional disorder. Constipation or an imbalance in the bowels can also cause cracks and crevices together with a heavy coating that appears yellow and brownish.

Eyes

Note should be taken of the general appearance of the eyes. Iridology is an ancient diagnostic tool; the iris patterns, just like fingerprints, are unique to each individual. They help the therapist to see whether the patient is predisposed to ill-health or is generally in good health. As this is quite a complex subject it cannot be covered in any depth here. However, the iris is like the feet and hands a microcosm of the body; each organ has its corresponding position in the iris, and anything abnormal such as a mark or discoloration is an indication of an imbalance. There is in particular a close connection between the central nervous system and the eyes. White 'nerve rings' around the iris may be due to some emotional upset or trauma. Small pupils indicate some nervous irritation.

Bright, clear eyes with a clear sclera or outer coating indicate good oxygenation to the eye and general good health. Lacklustre eyes indicate an indisposition. Dry eyes may be due to a nutritional imbalance. Yellow discoloration is symptomatic of a toxic system.

All the above observations should be taken together and are useful in assessing the overall well-being of the body. For instance, four of the senses are used throughout the analysis of the feet: hearing, sight, smell and touch.

- Hearing – this is used during the initial consultation and assessment process. If the breathing is laboured it could mean a respiratory problem. If the breathing or speech is too fast this could indicate the person is stressed. If a patient sighs this could be indicative of depression.
- Sight – observations are utilized throughout an assessment session, particularly noting behaviour patterns and imperfections.

- Smell – this is a vital factor that is often overlooked and should be used throughout the assessment session.
- Touch – this is an essential factor to help assess the client's vitality and to note whether there are any imbalances.

Observation of the feet

By looking at the body and comparing it with the feet or hands we get a complete picture of the size and shape of the person. The term 'mirror image' when applied to the feet or hands is misleading as this implies that the representation is seen with the right side of the body appearing on the left foot or hand and the left side of the body on the right foot or hand. The term 'microcosm' fits the description much better, as the feet and hands represent *all* the characteristics and attributes of the body. Each organ or part has its corresponding area on the feet, hands or ears.

If the person is short and rotund the feet will show these characteristics also, while if the person is tall and thin this will also be seen in the feet. Even the length of the toes are exactly like the proportions of the neck. If there is an imbalance on one side of the body this is immediately duplicated in the foot.

The longitudinal arch of the foot parallels the shape of the adult spine. The vertebral column also has four natural curves when it is viewed from the side, and the foot has four natural curves almost imitating the line of the spine (*see* chapter 2 for more details). So if the person had a flat foot (pes planus) this would indicate a bad spine, which would interfere with the flow of nerve energy and the circulation.

The foot areas are represented in figures 2.21, 2.22a and 3.1 and plates 1 and 2. The phalanges (toes and fingers) correspond to the cranial cavity, which houses the brain and all its principal parts. Each toe or finger should be in the same plane when you look at the person, if one toe or finger is higher than its opposite partner, that corresponding eye is also set higher on the face. If the little toe or finger curves in towards the fourth toe and third finger respectively is somewhat tucked under, it invariably reflects an imbalance in the shoulder area.

The metatarsals in front of the ball of the foot correspond to the thoracic cavity, the upper trunk between the neck and the diaphragm, housing the lungs, heart, oesophagus and their associated structures.

The abdominopelvic cavity is represented by the foot between the ball and the heel. It is divided into two parts: the first,

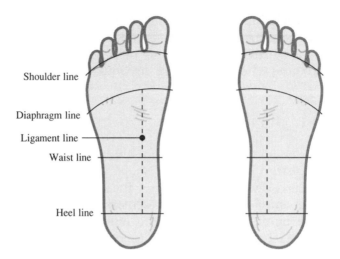

Figure 3.1 The lines of the foot

between the ball and the midfoot, signifies the diaphragm down to the umbilical area, containing the organs of digestion: the stomach, liver, gall bladder, pancreas, spleen and a small portion of the small intestine. The second, from the midfoot to the heel, represents the central and the lower portion of the abdominal cavity to the pelvic cavity containing the small intestine and most of the large intestine. (There is a slight overlap of the three cuneiform bones into the abdominal cavity.)

The tarsals (the seven bones of the ankle) correspond to the pelvic cavity, which contains the genitourinary tract and the last portion of the large intestine.

So there are four natural divisions of the foot and we can also divide the hand into four parts. In addition, specific lines on the foot are believed to represent lines on the body. These are as follows (figure 3.1):

- Shoulder or neck line – this divides off the phalanges, and the head-related and neck muscle areas.
- Diaphragm line – this includes the distal point of the metatarsals and metacarpals, covering the upper part of the body: the chest, lung and breast, also heart and upper back muscles. (*See* plates 1 and 3.)
- Waist line – the waist line is measured on the foot from the fifth metatarsal tuberosity (the protuberance at the proximal base) on the lateral aspect. On the hand it is measured from just below the fifth metacarpal on the ulnar side (*see* plate 4). This is found when the fist is clenched to form a transverse crease. The area between the waist line and the diaphragm line covers the

middle section of the body: the liver, gall bladder, kidney, adrenals, stomach, pancreas, spleen and solar plexus.

- Heel line – the waist line down to the heel line covers the intestinal areas, also the bladder, pelvic and buttock areas. It is found in line with the medial malleolus encircling the heel to the lateral malleolus. On the hand, it is taken from the trapezium bone and the proximal point of the first metacarpal where the muscles bulge at the base of the thumb (thenar eminence), to the middle of the hypothenar eminence on the ulnar side.
- Ligament line (on the foot) – this is a guide line. First work either side of it; at the end of the treatment session you should be able to work on it.

As an example for diagnosis, you can examine the fifth metatarsal notch to assess the waist line. If there is a greater proportion of the foot in front of this imaginary line it denotes that the person is long waisted, but short in the leg; if the reverse is true, this denotes that the person has very long legs. If the medial malleoli at the lower end of the tibia are not level it indicates a low lumbar problem.

Questioning

This aspect of diagnosis, whether using a Western or an Eastern system, can be summed up by an old Chinese quotation called the 'ten askings':

- One, ask chill or fever
- Two, ask perspiration
- Three, ask head or trunk
- Four, ask stool or urine
- Five, ask food intake
- Six, ask respiratory
- Seven, ask deafness or thirst
- Eight, ask past history
- Nine, ask energy
- Ten, ask causes (nowadays we would look at behaviour patterns and lifestyle).

This ancient Chinese system is still used today even in the West. In reflexology we must ask questions, not necessarily to find the nature of the disorder, but to ascertain which organ or part of the body may be in a disturbed state. When palpating on the feet, hands or ears we can also diagnose imbalances by tender spots; however, painful reactions can be caused by all sorts of variables.

During questioning the reflexologist should note carefully what the patient is complaining of. Specific questions may include the following:

- Onset – is the disease or disorder acute or chronic?
- Is there an overactive or deficient organ?
- Are there tender spots on the feet, hands or ears? These can be a signal of a functional problem that is not yet evident.
- Is the person suffering from overtiredness?
- Is there an inherited tendency?
- Are there any foot complaints?
- Have there been any injuries or accidents to consider?
- Where is the site of pain? Does it radiate up or down?
- What is the nature of the pain? Is it sharp or dull? Is it constant or intermittent? Is the pain bearable?
- Is it a slight problem (this means that the patient can still attend to their daily tasks with a little discomfort)? Is it severe (meaning that the patient cannot carry out the normal daily tasks)?

Listening

One of the keys to effective therapy work is the skill of active listening. Active listening could be said to consist of:

- Looking at the person who is talking, and sitting quietly with them
- Responding naturally with gestures and expressions
- Doing nothing else but listening to their particular problem
- Reflecting back the essence of what you just heard so that you can explore any inconsistencies (as a means of helping the client to understand their own problems)
- Asking only a few questions.

For reflective listening skills, the practitioner must develop the ability to concentrate on each individual's problems during consultation, and to give as much space and attention to each and every patient as required. Try and listen and do not be judgemental or too critical of patients' problems. Take note of their tone of voice and watch their body language; it often tells you more than their speech. Awareness and perception play an important role and patients must be allowed to go at their own pace, as the healing process can be slower than you may have allowed for. Never rush a person through their experiences as this will only force the process. Part of the therapeutic encounter is to develop a mutual trust of each other; as well as becoming a teacher and a guide, it is useful to remember that we can learn from our patients. The holistic healing process is aimed at treating the whole person, the mind as well as the body. Make sure in particular that you are ready to deal with their emotions, as during a reflexology treatment emotional release is often likely to happen. This can take many forms: agitation, anger, anxiety, distress, laughter, often slightly uncontrolled, and tears. All of these are the result of an emotional overload. This release is very important and plays a part in the curative process.

Listening is the key to communication; there is a real art in being a good listener. Some people do not listen. Not listening is much more common in our society than listening. Think about your own experiences. When was the last time someone gave you their complete attention while you were talking? The following situations are indications of not listening:

- Interrupting someone while they are talking
- Taking over a conversation that someone has started
- 'Switching off' while someone is talking, or fidgeting and looking at your watch
- Changing the subject, or responding with an inappropriate answer.

These should be avoided during the questioning process.

The case history

The information gained from observation, questioning and specific diagnostic techniques (such as palpation) should be exactly recorded for future reference. This is usually done by keeping a case history. A case history consists of many things that might be related to the patient's disorder. It allows for a methodical evaluation.

It should record the following at the first consultation or treatment session:

- Date of commencement
- Date of birth
- Name and address
- Telephone number
- Sex

- Occupation
- Name of medical practitioner
- Brief medical history
- What medication the person is taking
- What the complaint is and any other health problems
- Dates of all treatments, with a brief evaluation.

The medical history usually consists of information about past severe complaints or medical problems that the person has experienced. Some of these may relate to the present disorder. It is also imperative that the family medical history is explored in case there is some connection. A general social history (eg occupation) to give some background information is also advisable.

It is not necessary to have a ticklist of topics to note, but attention can be given to the following:

- Skin quality (feet, hands and ears)
- Nail quality (feet and hands)
- Hair quality
- Weight – obese or underweight
- Posture
- Exercise, also hobbies and relaxation
- Joints – restricted movement or hereditary defect
- Gait analysis
- Muscle tone
- Sleep patterns
- Behaviour patterns and mannerisms
- Diet – nutritive or convenience foods
- Alcohol – regular or occasional drinker
- Tea/coffee intake – if in excess of six cups per day
- Water intake
- Smoker
- General circulation
- Blood pressure
- Allergies
- Hormone imbalance
- Emotional state and stress level

A record should be kept of any tender reflexes so that symptoms and tender areas can be reviewed throughout the treatment sessions.

Finally, a record must also be kept of the patient's attendance and the amount charged. If you ask your client to refer anything to their doctor, make a note of the date and time you advised them and their response.

The above points are given purely as a guide. They indicate the type of information needed for a case history sheet or index card. It cannot be emphasized enough that the keeping of adequate records is a way of professional life. It also covers practitioners in the event of any claims of any incorrect treatment. One should therefore adopt best and safe practices at all times.

Diagnosis

Reflexologists do not diagnose in the allopathic sense, but use a differential diagnosis, taking many other factors into consideration and many other variables to ascertain where there are imbalances within the body. This is why it is important to assess behaviour patterns at work situations and in the home.

Diagnostic techniques

Diagnostic techniques are usually performed in medicine to determine the nature of the disorder by analysis of the signs and presenting symptoms. They usually include tests of blood or urine and other laboratory tests to make a diagnosis or to eliminate other possibilities. The differential diagnosis used in reflexology is drawn from signs and symptoms and close observation, often comparing and analysing the differences between the two hands, feet or ears. The aim is to find areas of the body that are out of balance. The conclusions drawn from this are not necessarily totally conclusive, as so many factors and variables could be causing an imbalance in the patient's health. Therefore perception and skill are required to determine whether there is a need to refer the patient to a medical authority or other discipline.

Palpation

In palpation a practitioner will explore by examining, touching and probing with the thumb and forefinger to find any sensitive reflexes, or feel a change in texture, such as a deposit and crunchy feeling, or an air bubble and popping sensation beneath your finger, which may indicate an imbalance within that zone. This is where astuteness and dexterity are required, also intuition and perception. Reflexologists use a unique and precise alternating acupressure technique or palpation over all areas of feet or hands to detect any imbalances. The slight changes of texture beneath the thumbs and fingers are often likened to crystalline deposits, although there is no medical evidence that this is correct, but it is enough that these 'congested areas' are noted by therapists. Until alerted that there is a tender area, the patient is usually unaware of overuse of a joint. The reaction may include the following: 'Yes, I do sleep on that side', 'I must have at least two pillows', 'I always carry my bag on that shoulder', 'Yes, I do cross my legs as I am sitting at my desk', 'I always support my elbow on the window while driving', 'I only do the breaststroke as I do not like my hair getting wet' or 'I like tucking my legs up on the settee while watching television'. Such comments indicate how behaviour patterns may cause no end of problems (*see below*).

This process also therapeutically stimulates the nerve endings, and the soft tissue palpation has a curative effect throughout the whole zone, that is from fingertips to the brain and down to the tips of the toes. With reflexology there are many different analytical techniques; it does not matter which method is used so long as the areas are covered in a systematic fashion, and the practitioner adapts the pressure used according to the person's needs.

During palpation the strength of the fingers and hand are felt, also the flexibility of joints are noted, and the resilience and springiness of the tissues are observed. All these are of importance in assessing the patient's energy and vitality. Hand and nail care can often also give an insight into the person's self-esteem. All these points need to be observed in a systematic way. The practitioner must also adopt a holistic attitude, seeing the patient as a whole. Physical, mental and social factors must be embraced and not just the individual parts of the body.

Diagnosing the cause of a problem

Illness is a particular state that is produced by many factors. Any excesses in the regular patterns of daily life can cause an instability. The general state of mind is also most important; both our basic attitude and moods, which may change according to the anxieties suffered. Bad temper and anger create stress, which may leave the person disturbed, uptight and unable to cope, creating the right environment for ill-health to manifest. Stress such as repetitive mental tension and emotional strain can lead to many psychosomatic disorders (emphasizing the relationship between mind and body) and other organic changes in body systems such as headaches, migraines, hormonal imbalances, peptic ulcers, irritable bowel syndrome (IBS), neck and low back problems. This is because internal feelings can change the heart rate, causing sweating and rapid breathing. Even muscular tension can be related to stress. It is most important to understand that no two people respond to stress in the same way.

Mental stress from external influences can also cause chronic problems to manifest. The problem may be related to other people. The old saying 'you are a pain in the neck' is so true, as a difficult person can create a problem for an individual. The 'stress syndrome', leading to many complications, can also be caused by work problems. Fibromyalgia, which is often thought of as a rheumatic disorder, can be stress related. It is an aching and progressive stiffness of the fibrous tissue within the muscle; this affects in turn the neck and shoulder joint and even down to the lower back (so the old adage 'you are a pain in the backside' may also be true). So if a patient comes with an acute or sudden onset of stiff neck or lumbago and no physical exertion can explain it, always check to see whether they had any great emotional upset, particular mental strain or work problem prior to the onset of their predicament.

Behaviour patterns that can cause a problem

The old adage 'We are what we eat' and 'We are what we do' are both true, and are wise proverbs that we should all adhere to. By taking an in-depth case history, eating patterns should be discovered. Many food allergies are caused by the very food the person most enjoys. Gastritis is often caused by incorrect eating or lifestyle, and anxiety and stress also play a role.

As many of the daily activities of the patient as possible should be determined. Behavioural adjustment can help an individual to correct everyday patterns and mannerisms of movement that are second nature to the person but that they are often unaware may be causing the problem and over a period of time leading to imbalances occurring in the area of the body concerned. This imbalance in turn can spread until the whole zone is affected. People often comment, however, on which is their 'bad side', referring to whether most discomfort is felt in the left or right side of the body. When a patient comes complaining of chronic neck or shoulder problems, it is essential to ascertain the behavioural activity that is making the problem worsen. Many people do not realize how much they can help themselves. The following are some of the activities that may cause or aggravate an existing neck or shoulder problem or cause other complications.

Watching television. If a person is not sitting correctly and looking straight at the television this can cause neck problems and low back problems. If the person curls their legs up it throws the hip joint out. When watching television the chair should be placed directly in the viewing line, and the neck and shoulder should not be twisted. Never allow young children to lay on the floor and look up to the television as this places undue strain on the back of the neck and spine.

Holding the telephone. Does the patient use a telephone and have to write at the same time? Often people try to grasp the telephone between the neck and the shoulder and do other jobs at the same time, but over a period of time this will cause no end of problems in the cervical region.

Carrying heavy bags. Carrying a bag always on one shoulder means that the person elevates the shoulder to keep the bag in place. This creates an imbalance that is evident in females with a shoulder bag and golfers carrying their golf bags. Carrying a heavy briefcase always in the same hand, or heavy shopping, can also cause elevation of one shoulder. Weight should always be evenly distributed between two carriers, one for each hand. Schoolchildren as young as 9 years of age may suffer with neck and back problems due to carrying books and other classwork in a satchel on one shoulder. Instead they should carry it in a haversack or rucksack on both shoulders, thus spreading the load. Schoolchildren and students should be made aware of how these postural bad habits repeated over any period can create neck, shoulder and back problems.

Incorrect sleeping patterns. Many people do not have the correct support for their necks when asleep. Each individual body is unique and may require more or less support. It is imperative that the cervical spine is not arched or angled incorrectly and this all depends on the width of the person's shoulders. The line of the spine should be as straight as possible. Even though the whole spinal column can move slightly and is quite flexible it is often subject to distortion, rendering it more susceptible to overstrained muscles and ligaments. The body naturally repairs itself while we sleep, and attempts to return to a normal position. Given the right conditions in a correct sleeping position the muscles therefore relax and recover, but if the wrong position is maintained during sleep the muscles maintain their tension and the person awakes tired, wearisome and stiff, along with a stiff neck or suffering from cervicalgia, which in turn can affect all the muscles down the neck and possibly involve the shoulder and arm.

The two main muscles that turn the head are the thick sterno-cleidomastoid muscle and the splenius capitis muscle. These muscles stiffen very quickly if they remain in one position for any great length of time. When a person is asleep the muscles of the neck relax immediately, and that is why it is imperative to have the right support. If the neck is twisted to the side (as in the case of a person sleeping on their front) then over a period of time this may cause a stiff neck or over a longer span of time spasmodic torticollis. This condition would also travel down and involve the trapezius muscle causing general myalgia (pain in the muscle) or even myositis (inflammation of the muscle) in the whole neck and shoulder region, which in turn can travel down the spine to the hip. (Shoulder and hips are always related in reflexology through the zonal pathways.)

Because muscles draw up when there is any sustained involuntary muscular contraction, it is easy to observe the position of the neck of the patient and note whether the shoulders are level; this will give some indication how severe the problem is. All muscles and the surrounding connective tissue need a good nerve and blood supply to supply nutrients and oxygen to the area. Restriction of muscles may cause muscle spasm. If the patient is not aware that a sleeping habit is creating an imbalance to the muscle structure, the problem can only deteriorate further.

If a patient complains that they often feel worse in the morning it is invariably due to an incorrect sleeping pattern. Before treatment, the reflexologist should therefore explore the right pillow support for the person, using the treatment couch for them to demonstrate how they sleep. The pillow should sit in the crook of the neck and the neck should not be out of alignment with the cervical spine; too high a pillow will cause the neck to be raised off the cervical spine, while too low a pillow will cause the neck to drop away because in sleep there is no muscular support. The person should not sleep on their front as this causes acute restriction on the cervical region and all the muscles that move the head.

Office work. Office workers need to be aware of work patterns, such as holding a telephone in the crook of the neck (*see above*). Continuously reaching to one side to lift an object, such as a file or book, can also create neck, shoulder and back problems.

Typists are often prone to wrist problems owing to incorrect chair height or position whilst typing. Tenosynovitis, which is inflammation of the tendon sheath, is also common in people who do a lot of writing or drawing work. Also the second, third and fourth fingers are drawn up into the palm, and this can lead to trigger finger with a total impairment of extension in any one of the fingers.

Tennis elbow. This is not necessarily caused by tennis, as this term covers any overuse of the forearm muscles, which may cause restriction of movement and painful inflammation of the tendons. It is common in drivers who rest their arm up on the right side window while driving. This elevated position of the arm can cause no end of problems to the arm and shoulder (*see also* chapter 8, A–Z of disorders of the body, Repetitive strain injury).

Sitting for prolonged periods, and lack of exercise or movement.
These habits can create some of the following:

- Cramp – this painful spasm in the muscles can be due to an imperfect posture, or it could relate to a circulatory problem, or an imbalance of salts. This can be caused by working in a very warm environment, in which excessive sweating may occur and the person is further depleted by constant coffee drinking and not enough water intake.
- Rheumatic-type pains – these are often in the lower and upper limbs.
- Back pain – this is often due to incorrect posture or faulty seating whilst working.
- Haemorrhoids – these are often aggravated by prolonged sitting and a restriction to the circulation to the rectum.
- Constipation – apart from dietary causes, this can be caused by ignoring the first impulse or sensation in the rectum; it is easy to remain seated when you have a lot of work to do.
- Urinary tract infections, both male and female – these disorders can be further aggravated by prolonged sitting as the bacteria that cause this are also on the skin surrounding the anus, and increased moisture as a result of wearing or sitting on incorrect fabrics allows the bacteria to enter the genitourinary tract.
- Problems in the reproductive system – these may be due to prolonged sitting on synthetic coverings, or in females wearing tights or synthetic underwear, which are more prone to bacteria proliferating.

When palpating the feet, the muscles in the lower arch of the foot may appear soft and floppy; this area corresponds to the low abdomen, and shows there may be a bulging stomach caused by excessive sitting, both in men and in women. This can cause, as stated above, a deficiency in the upper parts of the body, which in turn can create shoulder, neck and lower back stress.

When at home or at work when sitting or driving, people should always be made aware of their seated position. Do they have support for their lower back, or are they slumping in their chair? The wrong position can cause havoc when repeated over a period of time. Is the patient a manual worker, as lifting heavy goods correctly is paramount? Bending at the knees and keeping the back straight, the person should try not to twist or turn when lifting as this will distort the back muscles. It is quite surprising how the obvious does not occur to some people. Equally, decorators, or anyone who works above their head or with arms outstretched for long periods, are prone to lumbar problems; often this is because the posture is altered and the head and neck are off the centre line of the body, so they are either leaning backwards and over their head, or stretched forwards; there is too much armwork in awkward positions.

People cannot change their occupations, but it is necessary to make them aware that they are usually causing their own problems by unvarying uniform movements, and over a period of time these may lead to repetitive strain injury, or RSI.

Standing for prolonged periods with little movement and relaxation of lower abdominal muscles.
These can cause any of the following:

- Varicose veins – these are a mass of enlarged blood and lymphatic vessels that can become tortuous and swollen because of the internal pressures from higher in the body. The great saphenous vein or its tributaries are the ones usually affected; these are on the medial side of the leg and foot. Any occupation that involves long periods of standing with very little movement will not supply the necessary pumping action that is required to discharge the blood from the veins. There is also often an inherited tendency to varicose veins or faulty valves; this contributes to a loss of elasticity in the walls of veins and valves (structures in blood vessels that regulate the direction of flow of blood) making them flaccid, which may cause an obstruction to blood flow. These inherited conditions are often made worse from prolonged standing and the vessels become distended even more because of the pressures from within the walls and the blood accumulates. Constipation can aggravate this further, as well as inadequate exercise.
- Phlebitis – a poor circulatory system can cause phlebitis, an inflammation to the vein, and one should be very careful when palpating or treating the ankle or lower leg area because of this impaired circulation. Problems may often appear about 4 inches (10cm) above the ankle down to the heel area. If there are signs of broken blood vessels, extreme caution should be used when working on the foot or leg; it may be advisable to work on the hands only.
- Problems in the reproductive system – these can be exacerbated by excess weight of the trunk on the lumbar spine and pelvic areas.

- Oedema of the legs – this is a fluid accumulation in the lower parts of the body, often due to varicose veins.
- Disorders of the legs or lower back – these occur if under-garments are too tight or from prolonged sitting with the legs crossed or standing in one spot for too long. Many such everyday activities may cause a restriction to the blood flow and this may cause tingling and even discoloration in extreme cases.

Many times behaviour patterns and sedentary lifestyle or physical inactivity can create a disorder or exacerbate a problem. Too much standing, or too much sitting, or any activity in excess, are contributory factors that the reflexologist should always bear in mind. Being overweight can also cause too much pressure in vessels; that is why it can often be a common problem of pregnancy.

It is imperative that if there is any prolonged inactivity, simple stretching exercises are suggested. Even flexing and rotating the feet and wriggling the toes will promote a healthy return of the circulation. Or you can get up and walk around on tiptoes to relax the shoulders, then walk on the heels for the lower back.

Recommending treatment

Reflexology is beneficial for many of the behavioural problems discussed above, especially vein problems and haemorrhoids, because stimulation encourages the venous return to the heart. It also stimulates the connective tissue and improves circulation generally, and helps disperse oedema, especially if there is swelling in a joint, and alleviates pain in spinal areas, possibly because of increased blood supply so nutritive compounds are transferred to muscles without any overload of toxic lactic acid (which is produced through voluntary muscle contraction). It helps in tissue renewal as it triggers growth hormone release from the pituitary, which stimulates new bone growth, aiding in healing of fractures.

Before commencing treatment, one has to consider many different factors. For instance, is the illness of sudden onset, or chronic? If it is chronic the system would be very depleted. The age of the person is not really important because young and old alike will benefit. Contraindications must always be considered, also the person's threshold of pain, and their reaction to reflexology during, between and after treatment. A patient should always react positively; if there is any uneasiness during treatment one should always stop and use one of the many relaxation techniques. These can be used to calm, tranquillize, balance or revitalize. The body seems to know when it needs invigorating and when it needs to be restful. When treating patients we have to take into consideration all these many factors.

Contraindications to treatment

Specific factors in a patient's condition may make it unwise to pursue a reflexology treatment. These can include medication and some illnesses. Reflexology can often be given on the hands when a person is very sick or depleted as this ensures that there are less toxins released into the body. Every practitioner must learn to be able to adapt their pressure and area to work on, according to each of their patient's individual needs.

If the body is depleted by any disorder and there is a homeostatic imbalance within that particular problematic system, there is often exhaustion and less energy within the body. This condition creates its own toxins as the internal environment has not got the power to fulfil all the feedback mechanisms to ensure normal functioning of all processes.

There should be no need for a contraindication list as reflexology cannot harm anyone. Any kind of massage to the feet will increase a sense of bodily harmony and well-being, however; the unique techniques of reflexology have the ability to enable all organs and systems to function at peak performance. However, with the increase in medical litigations nowadays, it is sensible as a professional to protect oneself. Even a skilled, qualified practitioner cannot foresee some of the outcomes of treatment when the body is in an unstable state. Therefore, there are certain occasions on which a practitioner must be aware that care must be taken as there may be factors in a patient's current condition when treatment may be detrimental to the well-being. In these cases, certain reflex points must be omitted, or the patient should be referred elsewhere.

Pregnancy

In general, the pituitary point should not be worked throughout pregnancy as the pituitary gonadotrophins are blocked, and the corpus luteum maintains increasing levels of progesterone and the oestrogens until about the fourth month, when the placenta takes over. Many other cautionary areas during pregnancy lie on an acupoint, for instance the chronic uterus area, which lies in the pathway of SP-6, a well-known acupoint on the Spleen meridian that is used for irregular menstruation. One can see in the case of an unstable pregnancy why it would be ill-advised to work this area. Another acupoint on the Bladder meridian, B-60, is used for lumbago; it is marvellous for this, but is also a good point for treating placental retention. The placenta is attached to the wall of the uterus and part of its function is to secrete the chorionic gonadotrophin hormones to maintain the secretion of progesterone and the oestrogens that regulate and maintain the pregnancy. That is why it is another contraindicated reflex point to work on throughout pregnancy. The last contraindicated point is LI-4, known as Hegu in Chinese; this is an acupoint on the Large Intestine meridian of the hand, used for amenorrhoea, so again one can see why caution is needed not to work this point during pregnancy as it stimulates menstrual bleeding. (*See also* Pregnancy in chapter 8).

History of unstable pregnancies (or spontaneous abortion)

In the first 12 weeks it is imperative that the fetus develops normally. Because of the great change in hormonal production at this time, progesterone levels should remain normal and not drop. Problems that may occur are: the fetus may have abnormalities, there could be low placental implantation or the person may not be aware that they have fibroids, cervical erosion, or a defect in the uterus such as a bicornate (subdivided) uterus. There could even be an autoimmune disorder or genetic defect. Even certain infections may damage the fetus. The body goes through so many changes, with the increased levels of the hormones oestrogen and progesterone. It is very important that nothing is done to interfere with the normal production of these hormones as it may affect the formation of the baby.

If the client has never received reflexology before and is in her first trimester, it is best to avoid treatment as we are not sure how the pregnancy is being maintained, and most of the hormones are working to maintain the lining of the womb. After the first trimester it is necessary to start treatment quite gently if the person is unused to this type of stimulation. If the person was used to reflexology before conception then as long as the treatment is modified to the person's needs there should be no problem.

(*See also* Pregnancy in chapter 8, page 320, for a more detailed discussion.)

Those persons taking heavy medication

Powerful drugs often have powerful side-effects. Any medical book or formulary will detail the predictable or expected side-effects and unexpected reactions that may be caused by patients' allergic reaction to some drugs. At one time all drugs were naturally occurring; these were taken from plants, some animals, and certain minerals were also used. Nowadays, most drugs are laboratory produced, the theory being that this is safer and more efficient. However, many such drugs inhibit or alter normal chemical reactions within the body. The organs that may be involved are the liver, intestines and kidneys. The majority of drugs also do not act specifically on the target organ, but also involve other tissues or organs. Other drugs to be aware of are those drugs given together with in-vitro fertilization, as strong fertility drugs are used to stimulate the ripening of the eggs; ovulation is also induced with drugs, and because of the amount of drugs involved the person is susceptible to miscarriage.

Heart disorders

Many people with heart disease have more than one problem. Often the drugs given can change the heart rhythm; even the medication for heart problems may cause an imbalance in the heart beat, or eventually may cause damage to the heart muscle. Beta-blockers slow down the heart rate and reduce the force of contractions; these drugs are also used to regulate abnormal rhythms and to reduce the workload of the heart. As reflexology may increase elimination of the drug from the system it is always advisable to refer such patients to their medical practitioner prior to treatment.

In heart problems the systems of the body are having to work overtime to compensate for the inadequate pumping action of the ventricles. The liver and the lungs may become congested, and the body may become totally overloaded with excess fluids in the tissues, causing oedema, and extra stress on the kidneys. In such a depleted system it would be unwise to give a full reflexology treatment in case the person's body could not deal with more toxins being released into the already overburdened organs and tissues. Treatments should commence on the hands only, once a week to start with, gradually building up to one daily, and then work can commence on the feet, with a weekly treatment together with the necessary changes in diet and lifestyle.

In milder heart problems again the hands are a powerful aid in normalizing palpitations and irregular heart beat, and even angina. (*See also* Heart disorders in chapter 8).

Contagious and infectious disorders of the feet and body

Infections are often due to harmful organisms such as bacteria, fungi or viruses. Common sense should prevail here. It is of paramount importance that the therapist does not contract the disorder or transmit it to a third party. In all infections, any increased circulation may move the infection through the body quicker so that the body cannot build the necessary antibodies required swiftly enough. Reflexology will not actually spread an existing infection as it only works to harmonize and heal; however, if the system is so weakened by existing toxins, only the lightest of treatments should be given. Reflexology applied gently can help most problems once the acute stage and the infection has passed. Then it will strengthen the body's immune system. There are a number of points.

1 There should be no physical contact with any open wound, not only for the practitioner's sake but also because the recipient does not want their problem to be exacerbated. In the case of eczema or dermatitis work on the cross reflex (or *see* hydrotherapy of the hands and feet in chapter 9).

2 In the case of damaged tissue there is often a referral area that you can work on, as again direct contact could cause micro-organisms to enter and cause further problems to the patient.

3 In the case of verrucas on the plantar aspect of the foot, or occasionally on the hands, these are very contagious so it would be inadvisable to work directly on them. Either cover them or work on the cross reflex: hands–feet or feet–hands. Sometimes these are very difficult to see, but often they are felt on palpation, so it is important when scrutinizing the feet during foot analysis that care is taken to note them.

4 Inflammation of the venous system such as phlebitis or thrombosis is a homeostatic imbalance of the cardiovascular system. If the tissue is damaged in any way then work on the hands. The already weakened venous system is under a lot of strain so treatment is aimed at reducing the inflammation by working on the adrenal reflex on the hands and the referral point for the affected part; also work the ear points for the powerful anti-inflammatory properties. Some books state that we should not work if there is a blood clot as stimulation would cause it to move towards the heart; this would be contrary to

everything we know about reflexology as the whole process is to normalize and balance, which encourages the body to heal itself.

5 If a patient has a myelogram it is best to treat only after 72 hours have elapsed, as the medium used to inspect the spinal cord in this X-ray is introduced into the body system. As this is a dye and a foreign substance to the body it may cause a headache; this is the reason a patient is kept quietly resting for a few hours afterwards and told not to take any vigorous activity for a few days. It is better not to stimulate this substance to move around the body, but to let the eliminating processes get rid of it in the normal way.

6 Vaccinations or immunizations are often cultured viruses or bacteria and they are given to stimulate the body into producing the appropriate antibodies to confer immunity. These are usually introduced in several stages, thus allowing the body to deal with this antigenic material. If a reflexology treatment is given at this time, because it improves the circulation it will move the medium through the body before the necessary antibodies have been formed and this may cause some unpleasant side-effects. It is advisable to leave 1 week after any vaccinations either for holidays or for influenza.

Schizophrenia or phobias and epilepsy

Schizophrenia is often linked to a degenerative personality disorder and there are many disturbances in the psychological processes, so it is best dealt with by the medical profession. However, there is still some doubt as to the cause, as with many of the other psychoses. Provided that the therapist works with the medical practitioner's advice, then anxiety and confused states can be helped enormously. Also epilepsy in its milder form benefits, as reflexology treatment seems to act as an anticonvulsive. There is a particular acupoint crossed when working the neck reflex, which is a point used for convulsions (*see* Nervous disorders in chapter 8).

Cancers, tumours and AIDS

There are many differing views on reflexology treatment with these disorders. With reflexology it is the person and not the disorder that is treated, so unlike some complementary treatments that would be frowned upon by the medical profession, with the holistic process of reflexology it would be neither unethical or illegal to treat. However, one should always work closely and with the permission of the medical practitioner. Reflexology applied by a very caring and sensitive practitioner and working extremely gently will aid the patient's immunological system and improve their general energy levels, giving them deep relaxation and improving their whole emotional outlook. It may as well considerably reduce pain levels. This treatment also improves all the eliminating processes, thus getting rid of toxins and helping to reduce oedema.

Diabetes, gall stones, kidney stones and thyroid imbalances

These disorders are all dealt with in chapter 8. The reason why they are listed in some books as a contraindication is unknown. Many such imbalances are further aggravated by the clients' own mismanagement of their diet. If these areas are worked properly we can only improve the functioning. Using precise techniques to work the areas of assistance also (that is, those reflexes that are linked to the organs and have an anatomical link in supporting their function), the treatment then becomes a powerful therapy in improving and normalizing the vital body processes.

Support and care of the client

Some final points to remember about supporting and caring for the client during the consultative process are:

- Consideration of the patient or client should take precedence over all other factors. Interruptions should be dealt with so that they cause minimal disturbances. This should include answerphone facilities, or someone else should be available to answer the telephone and deal with other callers and visitors.
- Clients need to be shown sympathy for their suffering, and awareness and understanding, as this inspires the right relationship to establish mutual confidence.
- The treatment should always appear reasonable and the client should both benefit from it and enjoy the treatment, even though it may be a little uncomfortable at times. The therapist should appear to be involved with the patient's progress at all times.
- A consultation is a two-way process, so ensure you do not monopolize the conversation, and allow the client to speak in their own time.

- Where and how the initial consultation is carried out is vitally important to establishing rapport with the client.
- Each client is an individual and should be treated so; an explanation of treatment should be given and the expected conclusion of treatments should be discussed and agreed.
- Only give practical advice if needed; however, knowledge of different local and national support systems is very useful (*see* Appendix I for statutory support systems).
- Always give encouragement and help if a client is trying to give something up (such as smoking); do not decry any efforts.
- Health and hygiene of self and the client should always be adhered to, as the feet and hands are a common site of many fungal infections, usually in the webs of the third, fourth and fifth toes. On the hands this is often seen as a nail disorder.
- The treatment in its entirety is aimed at the client attaining a holistic balance of their health.

4 Basics of the reflexology treatment session

Reflexology as a science is a very powerful tool. The practitioner's role becomes that of a guide to healing, enlightening the patient to control their own healing process. It is preferable that an indisposed body eliminates toxins that may have arisen as quickly as possible, otherwise these will only add to the body's burden causing further ill-health. Stress is a major cause of many of the problems of today, often impeding a person's mental health and physical well-being. Reflexology shows the patient a natural, non-invasive, holistic pathway to better health. As a treatment it is a totally holistic therapy, embracing many varied concepts that have been formed over many years of practical experience. As reflexologists our main approach should be to use simple safe techniques to return the equilibrium to the body, counteracting any imbalance, the main emphasis being the removal of any stress-related symptom that may arise. By totally relaxing the patient, reflexology becomes an effective potent therapy and many disorders are alleviated. Treatment brings about greater metabolic harmony, encouraging a better blood circulation, with increased vitality. The holistic practitioner treats the person and looks at symptoms as an expression of imbalance within the body. Reflexology has the effect of stimulating the body's own natural healing energy, harmonizing and balancing the life force in order to achieve an improved state.

Reflexology treatment works on similar principles to those of acupuncture and acupressure. These are based on the fact that, by stimulating the skin at a specific minute area of the hands, feet or ears, there is an effect on a specific internal organ in another part of the body. The correct stimulation will give prolonged or even complete relief of symptoms without burdening the body with drugs. The theory is if the stimulation is continually repeated over a period of time then many pathological conditions disappear. It does not matter what modality is used to achieve alleviation of discomfort, but pressure and palpation from a professional practitioner using the most potent and precise techniques bring about rapid results. Water pressure on specific points will help to ease a tender point, after which palpation can be applied. Warming the reflex point, or the use of herbs or essential oils applied directly on the reflex point, will also help to stimulate the corresponding organ; these are an added benefit, but they should only be applied if you are qualified to do so.

As holistic practitioners the attitude of reflexologists to their patients encompasses the whole person. Health is the result of harmony between the body, mind and spirit. It is necessary always to take into consideration the physical, psychological and any social pressures that the patient may have. Reflexology can also be used as a preventative treatment to forestall ill-health; this is shown when reflex points are often tender prior to disorders manifesting in the body.

A treatment session begins with assessment of the patient; this can embrace foot, hand or ear analysis. Patients should be properly prepared, and the therapist should have a knowledge of support techniques, protective hold procedures, relaxation techniques and cross reflexes as well as the correct treatment according to the area chosen to work on. This treatment session should last 45–50 minutes if the correct procedures are followed, and it is necessary to be aware of reactions that may occur both during and between treatments. This chapter details the general principles of treatment. Specific treatments relating to the foot, hand and head in turn are dealt with in chapters 5 to 7 respectively.

Preparation of the client and yourself

Correct preparation of the client is necessary before commencement of treatment. The therapist should be aware also of the need to set up a suitable environment in which to carry out a treatment to obtain its optimum benefit. A suitable treatment couch or chair is essential, and a suitable area to work in. Some other points include:

- Always use a support cushion behind the client's head
- Have all utensils to hand, such as cotton wool buds to apply direct pressure on points of the ear
- Have some wipes to clean hands
- Have clean towels ready
- Use a piece of tissue roll under the head to avoid changing pillows
- Have talcum powder ready in case it is needed (although use of this should be minimal)
- Make sure your nails are short and well trimmed

- Use a hair band if the client has long hair
- Remove patient's earrings, if worn, when applying auricular pressure
- Finally ensure your posture is correct as you stand or sit behind your patient when working on the head areas.

Positioning the patient correctly is also important to enhance the effects of the treatment. Patients find it easier to relax if they have cushions supporting them. There should also be available a covering for them. Clothing should be loosened.

Relaxation techniques, support techniques and protective hold procedures

Prior to commencing treatment, many clients will need a preliminary relaxation massage. This is necessary when the patient needs to unwind; such techniques make the muscles and ligaments less stiff or tight and improve circulation generally.

Practitioners should also be aware of the variety of support holds available that enable treatment to be carried out to its optimum benefit.

Relaxation techniques

Some of the many relaxation techniques used are outlined below. Many of these may be classed as massage to the foot or hand as they involve rubbing and kneading. These preliminary techniques will improve the circulation of blood to the area and relax the tight, tense muscles of the hand or foot. Also the more calloused areas may need to be softened prior to treatment, and the correct application will enhance any treatment process. These relaxation techniques can also be used at any time and on either or both feet throughout the treatment session as they often treat a larger area by relaxing the reflexes. However, reflexology itself is not a massage; it is an alternating pressure therapy, a very precise technique applied to minute areas, using fingers or thumbs or knuckles; rotation or palpation on certain points is used as well as firm unmoving pressure (the reflexology 'law of nerves' is that pressure relieves pain).

It is imperative that the initial contact with the foot or hand is very gentle. The first approach sets the whole tone of the treatment session. The relaxation techniques described below can be used on either the foot or the hand but for brevity the holds will generally be described only for the foot. (*See* chapter 5 for details of foot anatomy, and chapter 6 for the hand anatomy and sequence.)

1 Holding. First hold each foot or hand with both thumbs on the solar plexus point. (*See* figure 4.13.)

2 Ankle rotation (figure 4.1). Gently rotate the ankle, supporting with one hand under the heel and the other supporting and comforting the great toe joint. Rotate in both directions several times. The thumb of the supporting hand should be pointing slightly towards the little toe.

3 Side or spinal friction (figure 4.2). This is done on both sides to warm the limbs and improve the energy throughout the body, relieving stress or any tension immediately, before starting the gentle stretching exercise. Both palms are used, one on the medial (inside) side of the foot and one on the lateral (outside) side. Slide your hands up and down the surface alternately.

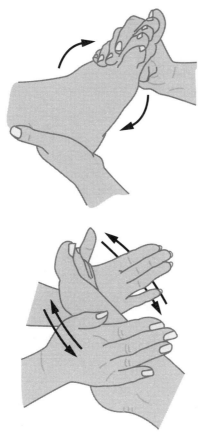

Figure 4.1 Ankle rotation: rotate in an inward direction

Figure 4.2 Spinal friction or side friction

(a)   **(b)**

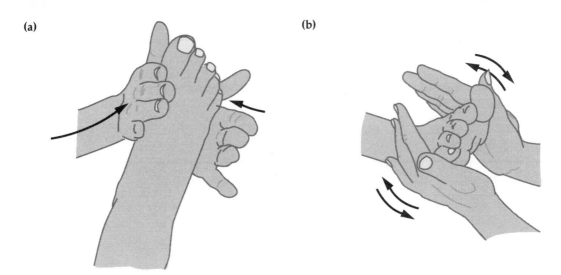

Figure 4.3 (a) Front view of side to side relaxation. (b) Side to side relaxation, showing how light pressure is applied.

4 Side to side relaxation (figure 4.3). This uses the same hand positions as the previous movement, but here the foot is moved alternately backwards and forwards, applying light finger pressure. This loosens the upper part of the body, and relieves stiff tight shoulders and the respiratory tract, thus facilitating the breathing process.

5 Achilles tendon stretch. This is done using the same support hold as ankle rotation (*see* figure 4.1). The whole foot is stretched gently backwards and forwards. This relaxes the calf muscles. Because the Achilles tendon inserts into the heel this movement will have an effect on the wrists, ankles, pelvic areas and the hips. It also helps to relax the arches of the foot. Be careful not to overstretch this at first, as it is often very tight, or even sore or swollen. Do only gentle stretches at first, increasing the force very gradually. Change support hands when working on the other foot.

6 Toe stretching and rotation. Gently stretch and rotate each toe both ways. Then rotate all toes together, while supporting the ball of the foot. This aids the neck and shoulder girdle. Note that stretching the toes or fingers, or rotating them, should be done gently. It is imperative to be aware of arthritic joints, so that you do not hurt the patient or cause further damage to a joint. This technique should only be completed if there are no contraindications (*see* chapter 3, page 95).

7 Diaphragm relaxation. (*See* figure 5.12.) This facilitates the breathing process. Placing the thumb of the working hand on the ball of the foot at the medial edge, apply gentle but firm pressure. At the same time using the correct hold with the other hand to support the upper part of the foot like a crutch, lift it slightly and lightly flex the plantar (under) surface.

8 Metatarsal kneading (figure 4.4). Using a fist with the knuckles in line with the base of the toes on the plantar area and the index finger of the support hand in line with the base of the toes on the dorsal (upper) aspect, push and squeeze alternately. This relaxes the shoulder girdle, as well as aiding the lung and chest area. The working hand should be the hand forming the fist: the right hand to the right foot, the left hand to the left foot. Always work from the lateral edge.

9 Foot moulding (figure 4.5). Both palms working together, place one on the dorsal aspect and one on the plantar aspect. Working from the lateral side only, as this ensures that there is not too much pressure applied to the great toe joint, mould the foot in

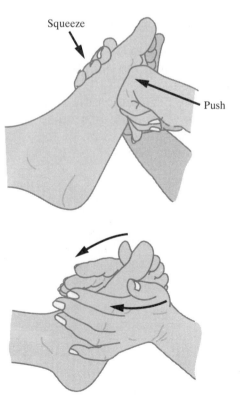

Figure 4.4 Metatarsal kneading (side view)

Figure 4.5 Foot moulding

a rolling action as if you were rolling dough in your hands. This relaxes all the rib cage area, lungs and chest and the shoulders.

10 Rib cage technique (figure 4.6). The thumbs are placed on the plantar surface of the ball of the foot. Now tuck up the first three fingers of each hand and use them in an alternating movement, working horizontally so that they almost meet on the centre line of the top of the foot. Be careful not to pinch the last little bit of skin. This will stimulate the lungs, chest area and shoulder girdle. Repeat this several times starting from the base of the toes and working down to the waist line.

11 Abdominal walking. Using the same hold as for the rib cage technique, finger walk with one, two or three fingers, whichever you find most comfortable, in slight diagonal lines across the dorsal aspect of the foot. This relaxes the abdominal wall, as it stimulates the musculature of the abdomen, the pelvis and the low lumbar area.

12 Working down the dorsum (figure 4.7). This relaxes the whole torso and the chest muscles, so is good for chest complaints. Using three fingers, with the fist supporting the plantar surface, work down to the waist area from the toes.

13 Ankle loosening (figure 4.8). Place the thenar eminence (the padded muscle at the base of the thumb) in the depression of the heel area and move the foot from side to side. This should not be painful, so do not apply pressure on the ankle bone, or shake the foot from side to side. (The ankle is a hinge joint; the sideways movement comes from the interaction of the navicular with the second and third cuneiform bones.)

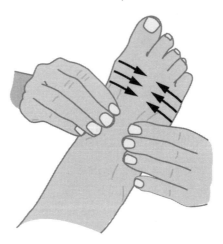

Figure 4.6 Rib cage technique

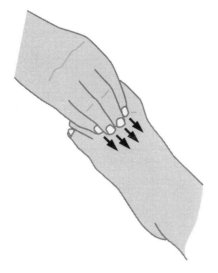

Figure 4.7 Working down the dorsum

14 Uterus or prostate sedation (figure 4.9). Firm unmoving pressure is applied to the heel point (*see* plate 2) with one hand as the other rotates down (always in an inward direction). This helps to sedate the point and alleviate pain; it is very potent for chronic problems.

15 Ovary or testes sedation. This is as 14; these two reflexes can also be worked together, using the thumb on the lateral reflex

(a)   **(b)**

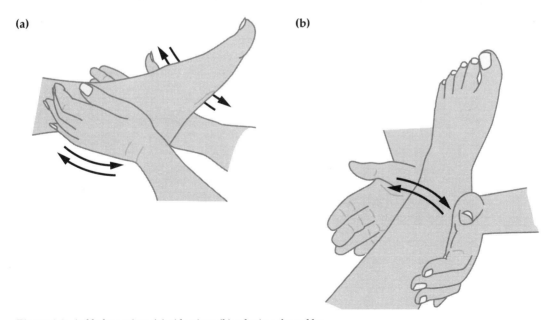

Figure 4.8 Ankle loosening: (a) side view; (b) relaxing the ankles

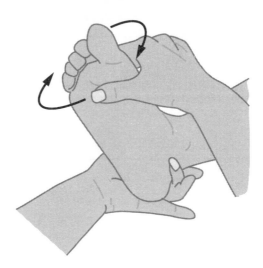

Figure 4.9 Pressure on the uterus/prostate and ovary/testes

point and middle finger on the medial reflex (figure 4.9). Rotate the foot both ways so that pressure is exerted on both reflex points.

16 Overclasp of fallopian and vas deferens areas and lymphatics of groin. Utilizing the web of one hand in a firm unmoving pressure on these points (*see* plate 2), again rotate the foot with the other hand in an inward direction.

17 'Hacking' of the toes and foot. Rhythmically apply a sideways light and brisk stroke up and down the plantar aspect of the foot. It is imperative that you use the fingers (not the heel of your hand) on the ulnar side.

Note. Any rings should be removed prior to striking the foot.

18 Knuckling the foot (figure 4.10). Using a loose two-finger knuckle (index and second finger) sweep down the foot in vertical strips. If the knuckles are used when working a reflex, always use the medial edge of the index finger in a circular movement, and this gives light friction to the area. (This can also be used when massaging at the end of the session.) When knuckling the groin area (figure 4.10b), make rotational movement around both malleoli. This works the lymphatics and pelvic region.

19 Circular friction on the Achilles tendon. Knuckles or thumbs can be used here.

20 Sweeping strokes. These can be applied over the whole foot rhythmically. This helps the blood flow to increase, and to generally disperse any excess fluid, reducing swelling and oedema.

(a)

(b)

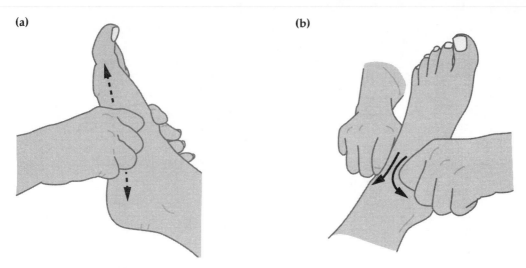

Figure 4.10 (a) Knuckling up and down the spine. (b) Knuckling on the groin area.

21 Pummelling.   Using a closed fist and the heel of your hand, strike the heel area several times. The aim is to soften the solid firm tissue.

22 Metatarsal flexing (figure 4.11).   Both thumbs are placed on the diaphragm area of the ball of the foot (*see* plate 2); the fingers lie on the dorsum. Lift and stretch the toes in a rising and falling movement (like a wave). Both hands apply the pressure. (This can also be used in massage techniques.)

23 Solar plexus rotation (figure 4.12).   Cross the hands, and with the thumbs on the solar plexus reflex rotate the thumbs in an

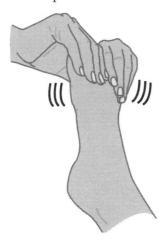

*Figure 4.11
Metatarsal flexing*

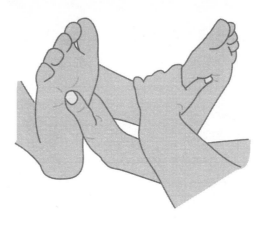

Figure 4.12 Solar plexus rotation

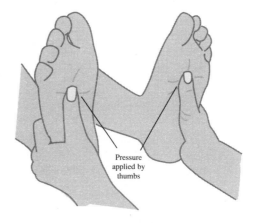

Pressure applied by thumbs

Figure 4.13 Solar plexus relaxation

inward direction three times. (This is easier to do after you have applied a little cream and have massaged the lower leg and foot at the end of the treatment.)

24 Solar plexus relaxation (figure 4.13).   Both thumbs are placed on the solar plexus reflex of the feet. Firm unmoving pressure is applied as the patient takes a breath, and the pressure is relaxed as he or she breathes out. Repeat this three times.

These relaxation techniques can be used in any order and can be repeated whenever necessary.

Self-help tip.   By gently pulling your own fingers, stretching them and rotating them helps all areas of the body, especially a stiff neck or shoulder area.

Supporting and protective hold techniques

It is necessary to provide optimum comfort both for the client and for the practitioner. Different techniques are used depending on the area being worked upon.

If you are working above the waist line area on the plantar surface (on the foot this is the distal area) hold it from above in a comforting firm hold (figure 4.14). Make sure you are applying light pressure with your thumb on the ball of the foot; your fingers encircle the foot. Lightly plantar flex the foot so that the ligament line is not exposed, which would cause discomfort; this allows the skin to relax rather than be taut, allowing deeper penetration without any undue discomfort when applying pressure.

If working on the area below the waist on the plantar surface

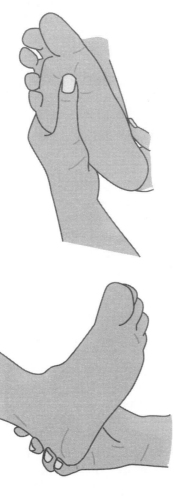

Figure 4.14 Support when working the medial side of the foot and above the waist line

Figure 4.15 Support hold when working below the waist line

(on the foot this is the proximal) support is again important as the correct hold (figure 4.15) allows the heel to rest in the palm of the supporting hand. If the thumb rests on the fifth metatarsal notch it allows you to control the foot so that it does not splay out to the lateral side. As you change support hands, place your thumb on the navicular or the medial cuneiform bone to hold the foot straight. This acts as a guide for the waist line.

When working on the medial or lateral edge of the heel area, keep the foot as straight as possible. This permits the area to be worked without creasing the skin on the heel area, which hinders movement.

When working on the dorsal aspect, it is even more imperative that the correct support procedures are adopted. By making a fist of the support hand you can then rotate this; it also provides an anchor. The thumb of the working hand should be placed loosely in between the thumb and forefinger of the supporting hand, thus allowing a pincer action. This method improves the looks of treatment on this area, whilst at the same time giving maximum comfort to the patient. If dorsiflexing the foot or hand always do it gently.

Finally support can be given simply by the flat of the hand, either the dorsal or the palmar surface. By applying slight pressure with your hand you can move the foot into the required position. Alternatively, encircling the foot in a caressing way take the foot out to the required position.

Support for the hands follows a similar pattern. In all cases the principle should be that it allows both the practitioner and the patient to achieve maximum comfort, and also allows direct access to the reflex for the practitioner.

Some general points about treatment

Some points to bear in mind when treating are as follows:

- Do not touch the nail in case of cross infection.
- Used iced flannels in the summer, if the hands and feet are hot and uncomfortable.
- Use warm towels in the winter to wrap the feet in, or to cover the patient.
- Remember to respect body space, move a leg or arm and do not lean on the patient. Do not allow your hair to touch the client's foot or body.
- The working position of thumbs or fingers should always be towards the direction in which you are moving.

- If working in vertical lines towards the distal point you need to drop your wrist and work upwards, pressing on the metatarsals and between the metatarsals.
- If applying vertical strips on the dorsal aspect, the arm should be elevated accordingly so that you can work in vertical strips downwards, with the correct support behind.
- If making horizontal or diagonal passes on the plantar surface, again sufficient elevation of the arm is needed as this ensures that the correct working position is maintained, safeguarding against repetitive strain injury.
- The arms should also always follow the movement of the thumb or fingers to safeguard against RSI.
- Before treating, practise working on any area, by placing your hands flat with the fingers outstretched, then elevating the palm thumb side. After this loosening up, you are now ready to commence treatment using the alternating press–release thumb movement.

Some books show awkward moves that may encourage injury over a period of time. Work on any area or surface to practise thumb or finger walking. It takes quite a period of time to build up the muscles of the hand and forearm. Always imagine you are working on a pin cushion; making tiny steps makes certain that you have not missed a tiny section out. If the steps are too large then it is possible not to contact the congested reflex area.

Note. If it is uncomfortable to work in any way, then discontinue immediately, and find another angle to work.

Force should always come from the shoulder area and the position of the working hand should allow this to be carried out in the most simplified way. This is why new practitioners are encouraged to use a gas-lift therapist chair, which is ergonomic in design; it is completely adjustable with a five-star double castor base. This enables the practitioner to work more effectively as they are mobile. Unless the reflexologist is free to change position, many of the reflexology moves are not carried out correctly as the hands are put under too much strain.

The treatment couches are also designed so that the practitioner is seated at the correct height with the feet or hands at chest level, and with their feet under the treatment couch (this has no cross struts that catch the legs). The aim is also to position the client so that the head is more or less on the same level as their heart. If the legs are too elevated, as is the case with a 40-minute treatment session in some of the reclining chairs, the action of gravity allows too much blood to flow to the brain, and a U-shaped chair may divert blood flow and create congestion in the pathways of the abdominal organs.

Self-help tip.   Hand exercises can be performed before treating to make your hands more supple, and to strengthen them generally. (*See* chapter 6, page 205 for some of these.)

'Back-up' or cross reflexes, or zone-related reflexes

'Back-up' or cross reflexes are used when it is unwise to pursue a normal treatment on the primary area because of an injured limb. It is important to know which reflex should be worked in order to aid a specific problem. Reflexes are used as an addition to treatment on the primary areas. Such points are related to the primary areas for a particular organ by an anatomical or physiological connection.

The body works as a complete unit at all times. So whenever there is any congestion or tension in any part of a zone this will often travel throughout the zone, and will affect any organ gland or function within it. Such congestion often travels up or down one side of the body. The Chinese empirically observed how one part of the body can affect another, and how each area or limb of the body is related with a corresponding part. Such connections are therefore part of any TCM technique such as acupuncture. With such connected areas if either is out of balance it may affect the other, but it also becomes an area of referral if one of the areas is too painful to work on. The corresponding area in the same zonal pathway would be less painful to use but equally effective. It may also be the distal point on the meridians. According to the TCM theory of treatment, it is often considered more suitable to work the distal point, the furthest point away from the problem. For instance, B-60, which is on the outer ankle, is suitable for back, neck and shoulder problems; it is also ideal for wrists and shoulders as the cross reflex point. This is also evident with ST-41, which is on the front of the ankle, is used extensively for all joints, mainly the ankles, but again is a cross reflex point that can be used for wrists. There are a number of such areas complementing each other, and in each case you can work on one to act on the other.

The specific connections are as follows (*see also* figure 2.7, page 48):

- The shoulders and hips correspond.
- The palms and soles correspond.
- The hands and feet correspond.
- The fingers and toes correspond.
- The wrists and ankles correspond.
- The forearms and forelegs correspond.
- The knees and elbows correspond.
- The upper arms and thighs correspond.

These areas are often referred to as cross reflex or referral areas, and sometimes as areas of assistance or back-up reflexes.

These correspondences relate to the ten equal longitudinal lines running the length of the body, between the tips of the fingers to the head and to the tips of the toes, or vice versa.

Interpretation of painful reflex points

During treatment, it is important to know how to understand and interpret painful points and how they may show that they are areas of dysfunction. These may relate to a number of factors, including incorrect behaviour patterns, medication or food, or stress (*see* chapter 3).

An understanding of each individual client's needs for treatment is also necessary. These include the correct amount of time, the right pressures and how to adapt them accordingly, use of specific relaxation techniques. With regard to pressure, the practitioner should be able to decide how much pressure should be applied to the detoxifying and eliminating reflexes, specifically when the areas for the liver and the kidneys are tender.

Reactions to expect during treatment

These are many different responses that may arise during a treatment. Some of these changes can at times be so subtle that some people are generally unaware of them, so you need to be observant. It is extremely rare, however, for a person to have an adverse reaction to treatment. Reactions may include:

- Sweating of palms of hands or soles of feet (often a release of tension)
- Coughing
- Laughing (release of emotions)
- Crying (release of emotions)

- Sighing deeply (release of emotions)
- Twitching or tingling in the limbs (normal reaction to nerve stimulation)
- Sudden cramp (normal reaction to nerve stimulation)
- Electric-type shock up the zone and sometimes in the opposite area being worked on, and sometimes also on the opposite side of the body (normal reaction to nerve stimulation)
- Warmth in the corresponding area being treated (normal reaction to nerve stimulation)
- Feeling of movement or clawing in the corresponding area being treated (normal reaction to nerve stimulation)
- Great fatigue (natural outcome of treatment)
- Overwhelming desire to sleep, or just close the eyes (natural outcome of treatment)
- Disappearance of all pain and discomfort (this may only last a day but as each treatment session progresses the timespan between the return of the discomfort lengthens).

Reactions that may arise between treatments

The responses that may arise as a result of treatment can again sometimes be so subtle that some people are generally unaware of them. Therefore when evaluating each treatment session it helps if the patient is asked to give a report of any slight fluctuation in the body. Many of these signs are positive signs that the treatment process is working, and are all part of the healing process. This is not the same as a healing crisis, as many books state, but a natural outcome of treatment.

- Symptoms may be slightly exacerbated for 24 hours (this indicates the treatment is working)
- General aches and pains the following day after treatment
- Skin rashes
- Spots or pimples
- Great fatigue for approximately 48 hours
- Flu-like symptoms
- Increased wind or flatulence
- More ease and frequency of bowel movement
- In women, menstrual blood becomes more red, and usually more profuse
- Much better moods
- Improved sleeping patterns
- More energy

- Relief from pain
- Joints appear more mobile
- In the case of respiratory tract infections, mucopurulent (yellow or greenish) sputum becomes clear.

Note. We do not know how any person's body will react or respond to the stimuli of reflexology. The reactions outlined are just a few of the many responses one might expect. A reaction is not a cause for worry; it is a positive sign that the therapy is working. Sometimes these reactions are due to the body not having dealt with the release of toxins from the system; the congested area (a painful or tender reflex) when stimulated reacts by releasing that congestion into the system. Many patients have no adverse reaction, just a steady cessation or withdrawal of symptoms. This is the body's way of dealing with this input of energy. Out of the many thousands of treatments that I have given, I can count on one hand the reflexology treatments that did not agree with people. Most people respond within approximately three to six treatment sessions in some way. In some cases there may not be a complete cessation of symptoms, but certainly a response is felt and there is measurable relief. This is not a miracle cure; however, many long-term and extremely chronic problems respond over a period of a few weeks. Acute problems, especially those of the musculature and skeletal system, are often instant.

Remember, sick people do not become ill overnight, so people who are on heavy medication or those who have been unwell for a long period of time need to be treated gently and with care, as medication and illness can be debilitating to the body, causing physical changes in the efficiency of the detoxifying and eliminating organs. Drugs (medication) may accumulate in the body because the liver cannot process and break down these substances. If the kidneys are not performing at peak efficiency they in turn cannot eliminate these substances quickly enough and they may re-enter the bloodstream. If there is an accumulation of medication in the tissues the patient may get a marked response as their systems are unable to deal with an additional release of toxins due to the outcome of treatment. The strength of any reaction will be in proportion to the force of the treatment. However, as a speculative comment, in China a course of reflexology treatment is over ten consecutive days, with a wonderful response from most treatments.

5 The feet

Anatomy and biomechanics of the foot

Anatomy

The hands and feet have the same basic structure. There are 26 bones in each foot (figure 5.1a). Starting from the distal point (the tip) there are 14 palanges; the big toe has two, a distal and a proximal, while each other toe has three: a distal, medial and proximal phalange. Then there are 5 metatarsal bones forming the foot itself and 7 tarsal bones forming the tarsus (the ankle and heel bones). The latter includes the talus, supporting the tibia and fibula (the two lower leg bones), and the calcaneum (calcaneus), forming the heel. The other bones, from medial to lateral are: the navicular or scaphoid as it is often known (which is boat-shaped, hence its name); the 3 cuneiform bones (named because of their wedged or cuneate shape), referred to as the lateral, intermediate and medial cuneiform bones; the cuboid bone (named because of its cube shape) – this is an important guide in reflexology as it denotes the waist line, and if you do not get this point correct it is easy to miss the reflexes for the two flexures (hepatic and splenic) of the large bowel.

Ligaments are tough fibrous bands of inelastic tissue, but very flexible, between the joint bones; they strengthen and support the joint, but limit movement in certain directions. There are two important ligaments in the foot: the short ligament, which extends from the calcaneum to the cuboid bone, and a longer plantar ligament, which lies nearer to the surface and supports the arch. The latter ligament is the one that practitioners must be aware of, as too much pressure on this point can be excruciating. In fact there are over 50 ligaments in each foot; these are arranged so that the sole is basically hollow.

There are three arches (figure 5.1b and c). These are, first, the two longitudinal arches. The one on the navicular side, together with the three cuneiform bones and the medial three metatarsals, forms the medial longitudinal arch. The one on the lateral side, from the cuboid notch to the distal two metatarsals, forms the lateral longitudinal arch. Secondly, the transverse arch lies across the base of all the metatarsals and is formed by the cuboid and the three cuneiform bones. This arrangement allows the lateral edge only to come into slight contact with the ground when we are walking, the calcaneus and metatarsals and the many ligaments and muscles forming the support structure of the arch.

The ball of the foot lies directly behind the heads of metatarsals. This area is very well protected with an extremely thick pad of fibrous fatty tissue to cushion and support the foot, especially when the heel is raised and locomotion is about to take place. The plantar aponeurosis is a thick mesh of collagen fibres. This not only forms a base but also allows the many muscles and tendons that are attached to it to move the bones. There are tendons to each digit and many around the ankle, all held in place by strong fibrous bands. The foot is richly served with many nerves and blood vessels, making it a vulnerable point for injury. Many people abuse their feet; it is said that each person in their lifetime could have walked over 75,000 miles, which is enough to take you around the world a few times. The pressures on the feet are greatly increased when walking or running; that is why we need this fibrous fatty pad that acts as a shock absorber. Poor posture leads to extra stresses being exerted on the ligaments and the joints, this creates discomfort and in some cases can cause the arches to become flattened or be distorted.

Tendons connect the bones with the muscles. They are made of an inelastic but flexible material. Most tendons are surrounded by a tendon sheath, a double-layered tubular sac lined with a synovial membrane (which contains fluid). The strongest and longest tendon in the body is the Achilles tendon. It commences on the calf on the posterior aspect of the leg and it inserts into the middle of the posterior compartment of the calcaneum. Two of the muscles that play a role in movement of the lower limb are the gastrocnemius and the soleus, and both of these have an insertion into the tendon of Achilles. Even though this tendon is so strong and can withstand a considerable force, it is still one of the most common sites of injury; it is supposed to be very flexible, but often in many people it becomes very tight, sore, or even swollen.

Biomechanics

Biomechanics relates to the forces on the skeleton caused by the muscles and gravity and the resulting movements of the

(a)

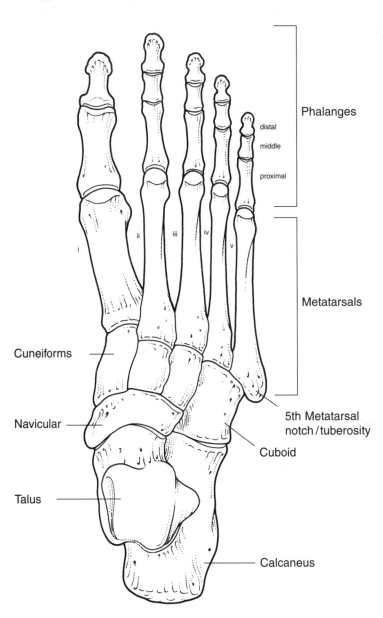

Figure 5.1 (a) The bones of the foot. (b) The longitudinal arches. (c) The transverse arch.

(b)

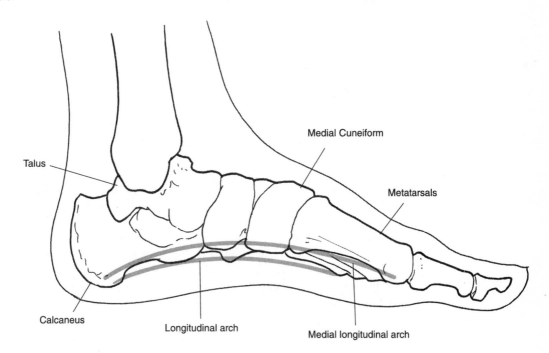

Talus

Medial Cuneiform

Metatarsals

Calcaneus

Longitudinal arch

Medial longitudinal arch

(c)

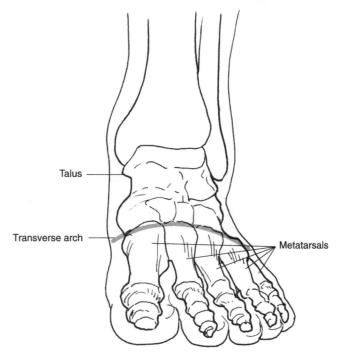

Talus

Transverse arch

Metatarsals

locomotor system. It is generally believed that many foot and leg injuries occur because of faulty alignment, although others may be hereditary.

The following terms are used to describe the anatomy, basic mechanics and movements of the foot, the planes of the feet and body, their motions and positions (*see* Glossary for those not detailed below).

- Anterior • Posterior • Proximal • Distal • Inversion
- Eversion • Superior • Inferior • Abduction
- Adduction • Sagittal

- Coronal (frontal) plane – this divides the body into front (anterior) and back (posterior). It also refers to the divisions of the foot being the hindfoot (proximal) and forefoot (distal); the movement being inversion towards the central body line or eversion away from the midline. A brief evaluation is a part of the assessment procedure.
- Transverse (horizontal) plane – this divides the body into upper-superior and lower-inferior. It refers also to the divisions of the foot being upper-dorsal, lower-plantar; the movement being adduction towards the midline, or abduction away from the midline.
- The sagittal plane – this divides the body down the middle into right and left halves. It refers to the divisions of the foot as the medial-inner aspect and lateral-outer aspect; the movement being dorsiflexion and plantarflexion.

The feet are the basic components of the kinetic chain, producing movement and acting as effective shock absorbers. They also provide the necessary information to the musculoskeletal system, so that impulses from the proprioceptors within the joints, muscles and tendons can relay the correct information to the brain to bring about co-ordinated movement. The feet are the foundations of our body, just like any building or superstructure (figure 5.1). If the underpinning is faulty, serious defects may appear later.

Spinal distortions can be caused by poor biomechanics of the feet or incorrect footwear. The wrong type of footwear, giving little or no support with inadequate cushioning, may eventually cause strain on the spine and overexert the muscles and tendons of the foot and leg. Any tautness or tension on spinal muscles can cause the cervical region to pitch forward relative to the body. If the line of gravity, which should pass through the centre of the body, is out of alignment, this can lead to faulty posture. Backs in action can cause many problems pushing, pulling, lifting, getting

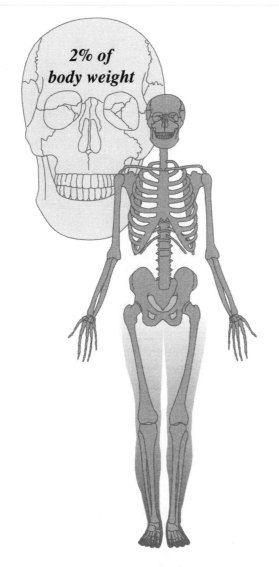

2% of
body weight

*Figure 5.2 How the
feet support the weight
of the whole skeleton*

up and sitting down. The force of all this activity is passed down
your spine to your feet. Even our heads weigh 2% of our body
weight (figure 5.2). It is of the utmost importance to assess these
points at the first consultation.

The ankle joint bears a lot of weight. It also assists in motion
and acts as a shock absorber. Many soft tissue injuries over the
ankle area involve the tendons and ligaments or the tarsal joint
and the arch of the foot. If the foot is inflexible or stiff, it could be
an injury or strain, so move it very carefully when assessing.
Using reflexology directly on the area can often break down
inflammation and swelling, thereby relieving the pain.

Observation and analysis

Three observation and analysis processes required for efficient analysis and diagnosis:

1 Observation as the client enters
2 Assessment through direct observation of the feet
3 Tactile awareness through touch and manipulation.

When analysing the feet we begin to build a hypothesis of the problems that may be causing an imbalance. This is not conclusive evidence, for, as holistic practitioners we need to embrace the whole person not just the feet, but we can combine all these aspects to encompass not only the physical and emotional but also the spiritual side of the individual.

Many indications must be taken into account when we use analysis or 'external reading' of the feet. Common foot faults need to be established first, prior to determining the nature of the disorder or imbalance. A systematic approach should be adopted so that small points will not be missed. Basic analysis of the feet is quite simple if attention is paid to detail.

Common foot disorders we need to be aware of when assessing the feet are as follows:

- Those arising from mechanical or stress defects
- Those arising from footwear faults
- Those arising from hereditary imperfections
- Those caused by infections
- Those evident indications indicative of general or systemic disorders
- Those arising from neurological disorders.

Assessment through initial observation

Mechanical or stress defects

Observational skills are of paramount importance. Evaluation of the many outward superficial signs that are immediately visible may direct you to form a hypothesis regarding the person's ailment. As practitioners, our ability to observe a person in this holistic way will provide many suggestions as to which area or system of the body may be out of balance. This evaluation should not be conclusive, because there are so many other factors. It is just a guide.

Analysis of the feet involves not only assessment of the feet when the patient is seated but also certain clinical observations. As a client walks in you should be studying the gait, noting which foot is used first to step in, as this is often the dominant side of the body. You do not have to be medically qualified to assess whether there is a normal heel strike when the person is walking. The heel should contact the ground first, followed by the forefoot. If the person has had an amputation, or has any paralysis through a stroke or poliomyelitis, this scrutiny is obviously not needed.

Abnormal structure can cause abnormal function, and the opposite is also true. Defects arise from many sources, including hereditary, or anomalies in posture and gait. The latter are being caused by behaviour patterns and other factors due to lifestyles, including obesity and stress (*see* chapter 3).

Footwear faults

Variations in heel heights can cause problems. Note should be taken of the type of shoe worn. If the foot slips forward in the shoe this can cause the toes to be persistently dorsiflexed. This in turn may cause overstrain on the mechanics of the foot, such as the ankle joint, or the Achilles tendon, causing problems in the muscles of the calf. Excessive high heels may cause pressure on toes, and prolonged wearing of high heels does not allow the flexibility that the foot needs. If too high a heel is worn over a period of time, this may cause the body to pitch forward and distort the natural alignment of the body, which in turn can lead to postural abnormalities thus causing strain and tension on the abdominal organs, resulting in possible internal disorders. Faulty posture may also cause pressure to be exerted on the frontal portion of the cerebrum (brain), which may lead to depression or tension headaches.

Assessment through direct observation of the feet

This takes place after a full in-depth case history has been taken (*see* chapter 3, page 81). Make sure the patient/client is seated comfortably. Positioning and presentation are of the utmost importance (*see* chapter 4, page 102). This allows for a detailed examination. The therapist can observe the following suggested procedure for detailed foot observation:

1 Observe the relationship between the feet and the body. The

characteristics of the feet together are comparable to those of the general body shape. For instance, a person with broad shoulders should have broad feet, a tall thin person would have long narrow feet, and so on.

2 Inspect the Achilles tendon for tightness. This tendon is involved in the lower leg muscle complex responsible for plantarflexion. Check the arches of the feet to see whether they are low or completely flat; if so, this is a sign that the spine is rigid.

3 Compare the two medial malleoli at the lower end of the tibia. A difference here indicates that one side of the hip is drawn up (*see* plate 6). You may also notice whether the shoulder is out of line.

4 Compare the arches of the feet, which may be different. If so, this is significant as there could be an imbalance in the musculature of the back, causing a deviation of the spine.

5 Note the suppleness of the arches of the feet. This is a good clue to how flexible the spine is.

Particular attention should be paid to the following:

- Skin elasticity – the state and quality of the skin according to age
- Skin texture – any callosities (corns or dry hard skin), blemishes or scars, lesions and moles
- Skin colour – erythema or rubor, pigmentation, pallor, cyanosis
- Skin temperature – the degree of heat or coldness: hot, warm, cold or cool (always check both feet), using the dorsal surface of the hand
- Skin humidity – sweat or moisture
- Mycotic infections – caused by a fungus (ringworm), athlete's foot, tinea pedis
- Virus infections – plantar warts (verruca)
- Oedema – swelling or puffiness
- Dermatological disorders – eczema, contact dermatitis, allergic rashes and psoriasis.

Note that all these clinical signs may denote an imbalance within the systemic circulation. A detailed chart of clinical signs and the problems causing them is shown in Table 5.1 at the end of this section (page 134).

It is essential that the foot is scrutinized on both the dorsal and the plantar areas for any other abnormalities and clinical signs. This gives an insight into each individual's physical attributes. Observation will provide vital clues to imbalances in certain areas, relating to organs or systems of the body.

Hereditary imperfections

These are imperfections or qualities passed from parent to child, although they may not be visible in all family members. All hereditary factors should be recorded. They include the following (*see* Glossary, page 433, for definitions): pes cavus, pes planus, pes valgus, pes varus, talipes, hammer toe, mallet toe, hallux rigidus, hallux valgus.

Note   that hallux valgus and hallux rigidus can also be caused by faulty footwear, systemic or neurological disorders.

When assessing the feet, disorders of the great toe (hallux, big toe) can often be seen. Hallux valgus, the outward displacement of the great toe, is often associated with a bunion. This lateral deviation may result in discomfort on the second toe, as distortion of the great toe increases the compression on the joint. In the reflexology diagnosis it would be indicative of a problem in the corresponding area of the body, indicating shoulder or neck ailments. It could also cause an energy block throughout the whole zone or part of the zone. Any disturbance in this central zone can reflect on the whole spinal area, interrupting the flow of energy to all body parts. This in turn can affect nerve pathways and the flow of body fluids. Also, the pain and irritation can create abnormal tilting of the body, putting extra pressure on the opposite foot and hip. Even though there may be a hereditary factor here, too narrow shoes with a constricted toe-box can also cause this deformity. Additionally, if the foot is unduly broad, continuous pressure and friction over a period may cause bursitis, the inflammation of a bursa. (Bursae are small sacs of fibrous tissue lined with synovial membrane and synovial fluid, and are usually found around joints and tendons; they allow free movement.)

Vascular assessment

It is essential to give attention to the feet and lower leg to see whether there is any impaired venous drainage, which could indicate a circulatory disorder or failure of one of the valves. If there is any varicose eczema, adopt extreme care, as it is very easy to scratch and break the skin. Watches and rings should be removed for the examination, and nails should be short and well manicured to avoid damaging the patient's skin.

Note. The therapist needs to be aware of contraindications here. For first aid relating to a varicose vein that bursts, *see* Appendix II, page 419.

There is an inherited tendency to varicose veins. Often you will see problems arising about 4 inches (10 cm) above the ankle and at the back and side of the calf. Look at behaviour patterns to help your assessment. Also check the dorsalis pedis point to see whether there is a good pulse. Detect the dorsalis pedis pulse (the average adult pulse rate at rest is 60–80 heart beats per minute). Press gently against the skin over the artery, using one or two fingers only. The vessel wall should feel soft to the touch. If the wall feels very hard when pressure is applied, this may be a sign of arteriosclerosis. If the rate is absent or slow, it could be indicative of some peripheral vascular disorder. If the rate is too fast, it could indicate there is an emotional disturbance caused by stress or anxiety. If unsure whether to pursue any treatment, refer the client to their medical practitioner. (*See* page 180, figure 5.41 ST-42.)

Nail and foot disorders caused by infections

Nails and feet should be pink and healthy, owing to their rich nerve and blood supply. This is a good indication of the client's health. Nail and foot disorders can be caused by several factors such as: injury, infection (bacterial, viral or mycotic), disease, pus formation, inflammation, trauma and, occasionally, nutritional deficiencies. The normal development of a nail depends on the nail's receiving a good and adequate blood and nerve supply. Nails should also be checked to see whether they are ingrowing, involuted, cracked or chipped. Are they soft or peeling? Is the nail thickened, brittle or discoloured? Do they have transverse grooves or longitudinal striations, white spots or marks? All of these points should be noted, as they may indicate an imbalance in the corresponding area of the body (*see* chapter 9).

It is important to be aware of nail disorders to protect yourself and the client from cross infection.

General or systemic disorders

Diabetes mellitus
The most common disorder is diabetes mellitus. This is due to a partial or full deficiency of the hormone insulin being produced, causing a disorder of the carbohydrate metabolism in which sugar is not oxidized to produce energy. There are two types of diabetes: non-insulin dependent and insulin dependent. The former responds to diet changes, and maybe some hypoglycaemic drug medication. Often sufferers are in the older age group.

With the latter, problems are usually more severe. Not only does the diet have to be carefully controlled with adequate carbohydrates, but also the person often needs insulin injections to maintain a normal level of carbohydrate metabolism.

Certain illnesses can cause this disorder, as well as extreme stress and anxiety. Complications the reflexologist may come into contact with are eye-related problems, so always check eye zone on the second or third toe. Kidney problems may also often arise in this disorder, and this reflex area will be very tender when we begin to apply pressure and palpation. This can be due to high blood pressure or other cardiac disorders. Tenderness may be felt all through the same zone as the eyes. The liver and pancreatic areas will also be tender. It is imperative that care is taken so that there is nothing that can scratch a patient's skin, as loss of feeling, and conversely hypersensitivity, are common in the feet. Handle the foot very carefully and apply only the lightest of touch.

Particular problems to be aware of with this disorder include: open sores or other lesions, ulcers on the foot, vascular abnormalities, peripheral neuropathy with unexplained loss of sensations, paraesthesia and pain. These ailments make the person more at risk to infection; hence the need for extreme care because of the person's diminished awareness of sensations.

Peripheral neuropathy may produce trophic changes (nutritional changes in the skin and other tissue), which may follow impairment of nerve supply. These include:

• Coldness
• Loss of hair
• Thinning of skin
• Abnormal sweating
• Hyperaesthesia of hands and feet
• (Tactile) exaggerated sensibility
• Impairment of sensory pathways

The client should be referred to their medical practitioner if in doubt about any signs or symptoms.

Arthritis

Hallux rigidus is stiffness of the joint between the great toe and the metatarsals. This can be caused by several factors, such as inflammatory joint disorders like gout or rheumatoid arthritis, previous surgery or injury to the toe through trauma, which may damage or injure the medial plantar halluces nerve, resulting in muscle weakness or sensory loss.

Hallux valgus is often due to arthritis, which starts as an

inflammation. It is often followed by complications, which can cause abnormality of the joint. Hallux valgus affects the first metatarsal and the metatarsophalangeal joint, often impinging on the second toe, which then may develop into a hammer toe.

Rheumatoid arthritis is inflammation of the joints (*see* plate 7). The smaller joints of the feet and hands are usually involved, often affecting both limbs. The ankle joints can also be affected, with restriction of movement (*see* Biomechanics, page 120).

Gout

This can produce an extremely tender and painful great toe or ankle joint, and occasionally the knee joint. It is commoner in men, but women can suffer also. It is often due to the body's inability to metabolize nitrogen-containing compounds known as purines, leading to accumulation of uric acids in and around the tissues and joints and also in the bloodstream. Over a period of time, deformity of a joint may occur. Reflexology and dietary advice are very helpful here.

Plantar fasciitis

The client with this disorder may experience deep pain in the heel area, which often arises from the central part of the heel at the point of attachment of the ligament structure. The pain is due to inflammation, and the problem should not be neglected, otherwise the client may develop a heel spur. Reflexology treatment to the area will improve lymphatic and venous drainage. Palpation and massage will help reduce the tensile stress at the attachment of the plantar ligament, relieving the pain and reducing the inflammation.

Neurological disorders

Disorders you may come into contact with are those that affect innervation of the limbs, either directly or indirectly controlling the hands or feet. Every muscle is controlled by a motor nerve, so if there is any sensory disturbance it can cause quite a few problems in the intrinsic muscles. One such condition is drop foot; it is due to neuritis in the anterior tibial nerve. This often causes an absence of sensation in the leg, and there is a tendency to drag the foot.

Without a good nerve supply many of the organs of the body would cease to work properly and their function would diminish. Signs of nerve degeneration include: burning sensations over the feet with itching, or pins and needles; aching in the calf area;

shooting pains, or twitching or jumping in the feet or legs. Any damage or degeneration of the peripheral nerves will cause some peripheral neuropathy. Those affecting only one nerve are named mononeuropathy. The symptoms which a reflexologist may encounter are weaknesses in any of the intrinsic muscles of the foot or hand, and absence of reflexes, which may cause an unsteady gait and poor movement. There are many other causes, such as degeneration of the spinal tracts, but these do not come into the reflexologist's remit. Dysaesthesia is a symptom of dysfunction of the sensory pathways, which may be linked to the spinal tract, causing weakness of any of the four limbs. The spinal cord is in part a receiver and an originator of many of the motor nerve impulses to and from the brain.

Reflexology has a powerful effect on the nervous system, stimulating nerve pathways. However, if there is any muscular weakness or sensory loss, the patient should be referred to their medical practitioner for investigation.

Many of the abnormalities of the feet may be caused by both neurological disorder and hereditary factors. Some abnormalities are depicted in plates 8 to 12.

Table 5.1 contains a detailed list of foot abnormalities and the disorders associated with them.

Assessment through tactile awareness

Touch is one of the vital faculties participating in the assessment technique. It not only allows you to assess and confirm a very wide range of manifestations, it also allows analysis of the tissue when palpating to distinguish whether the tissue feels solid, or whether there is evidence of deposits under the skin, or any change of texture, which may indicate an imbalance in that reflex point or zone. This technique also gives us a guide to the client's pain threshold and will give you an insight into how to adapt your pressures when giving a full treatment session. A very marked cutaneous sensitivity could indicate nerve damage (*see* Neurological disorders, page 132). Always check joint movement, or any spasticity or wasting of muscles.

Just like diagnosis and professionalism, tactile skills and awareness can be achieved only with practice over a period of time. Whilst they are training, and also in the early years of practice, the reflexologist should reflect on experiences and learn from them, to develop the awareness to apply precisely the right pressure to the relevant reflex point in a systematic way.

Table 5.1 Common abnormalities of the feet, and associated disorders

Abnormalities of the feet	Potential disorders
Skin colour	
Erythema or rubor (an increase in the size of small blood vessels in that area)	Imbalance in the corresponding area of the body. Toxins in the blood. Systemic disorder. Inflammation in the tissues of the feet, which may be caused by excessive walking or running. Chilblains. Excess circulation, or in some cases a poor venous return
Erythema on the heel area, and pain when standing	Possibly a heel spur
Red or inflamed in one area	Possibly gout if it is around the base of the great toe, or one of the other joints. Otherwise the patient may have a problem in the corresponding area of the body. Often indicative of an overactive organ
Pallor	Poor circulation and reduced blood flow
Blanched tips of toes or fingers	Possibly Raynaud's syndrome; there is an inadequate blood flow to the extremities
Cyanosis (bluish discoloration of nails or toes)	Inadequate amount of oxygen in the blood, poor circulation and often low energy levels. Maybe a respiratory or thyroid disorder
Pigmentation – yellowing	Excess toxins in the system, liver irritation. Excess bile pigments have not reached the intestines, maybe due to an obstruction such as gall stones
Discoloured brown, mottled	Varicose eczema, itchy skin, swelling
Purple hue	The circulation is poor and the system needs to be stimulated
Temperature	
Cold feet	Often indicates a poor circulation
Isolated cold spots on feet	Homeostatic imbalance in the area related to it in the body. Poor circulation in general or low energy levels.
Isolated hot spots on feet	Possibly an emotional overload in the nervous system. Possibly a homeostatic imbalance in the endocrine system
Moisture content	
Very dry feet	Possibly a lack of water, or a disorder of water metabolism, which may be due to a deficiency of essential fatty acids. Could also be a thyroid imbalance
Peeling skin on the plantar aspect of foot	Check foot hygiene; is there any localized infection? Usually shows an irritation/ allergic reaction in the body. Could also relate to a mineral deficiency
Cracked and dry or marked heels	Not enough fat in diet, or footwear is causing slapping action on the heel, depleting the oils in the skin

Table 5.1 continued

Abnormalities of the feet	Potential disorders
Dry skin on the tips of the toes	Often indicates sinus problem or a tendency to headaches
Cracked skin in between the toes; possibly peeling and sore	Any mycotic infection should be treated as they are very contagious. Usually shows that the immune system is low or depleted
Slightly moist, oily feel to the feet	Overstress or proneness to allergies; often indicates excess stimulation of the adrenal gland
Hyperhidrosis (excessive perspiration)	Possible thyroid imbalance

Swelling

Oedema (abnormal swelling of ankles or legs)	Could be a systemic disorder. Disorder in the lymphatics with poor lymphatic drainage. Prior to menstruation or problems in the uterus or rectum (female). Prostate problems or rectum (male). Hormonal imbalance, circulatory problems
Pitting oedema	Light finger pressure leaves a temporary slight indentation. This shows excess fluid in the area.
Puffy area on toes	Possible imbalance in corresponding area of the body
Painful and swollen big toe	Most probably gout

Skin eruptions

Rashes on the feet	Allergy or contact dermatitis
Infection present on any part of the foot	Possibly poor pedicure, or pressure from shoes
Spots that have broken out, almost like eczema, on the soles of the feet and toes, or the palms of the hands and fingers	Possibly due to the ageing process, as sweat production in many parts of the body, usually the feet and hands, becomes less efficient as we age. Excess strain on the sympathetic nervous system leads to overproduction. Owing to the homeostatic imbalance within the gland it becomes blocked, the nitrogenous waste cannot escape and it builds up and breaks out as an eruption on the skin. Often seen in patients who are under extreme stress

Movement

Stiff or rigid feet	Nearly always indicates a stressed or tense person
Stiff ankles when rotating	Indicates stiff hips and lack of mobility in the lumbar spine
Excessively pronated foot	Indicates a bad back, or even rounded shoulders. Poor posture

Odour

Strong odour	Often shows an imbalance within the nervous system

The systems of the body and their respective zones on the feet

This section reviews each of the body organ systems in turn and locates the foot reflex zones. Common disorders for each system are purposely not listed as most disorders are a result of an imbalance within one or more of these systems, and there can be a slight deviation from normality caused by numerous factors. The body systems do not function in isolation, but are interdependent and also rely on the finely tuned balance of each and every organ within each system. Stress is a common denominator in many disorders.

The zones of the respiratory system

This includes all the organs involved in respiration – the nose and sinuses, mouth and throat, pharynx, larynx, trachea, bronchi, bronchioles, lungs and diaphragm, also the rib cage and the intercostal muscles. The heart and thymus are also in this anatomical area (these are covered under the circulatory and lymphatic systems respectively).

Figure 5.3 shows the organs of the respiratory system and the relevant foot zones.

The nose filters impurities in the air going to the lungs, and mucus produced by the sinuses helps to trap these. The pharynx (throat), and larynx (voicebox) belong to the upper respiratory tract. The lower respiratory tract includes the trachea (windpipe), two main bronchi, smaller branching bronchioles, and alveolar sacs, where the gaseous exchange actually takes place. The lungs receive oxygen from air that we breathe in. This fresh oxygen is transferred to the blood in the tissue of the lungs. In exchange, carbon dioxide is transferred to the lung tissues, and then breathed out. Difficulties in breathing happen when this lung tissue is congested, becomes inflamed, or damaged because of pollution, smoking or infection, or if the air passages become narrowed, as in asthma. Reflexology facilitates the whole breathing process by opening up the airways. In cases of asthma, working on the adrenal glands stems any inflammation and aids the breathing process.

The foot positions for the structures of the respiratory system are shown in Table 5.2.

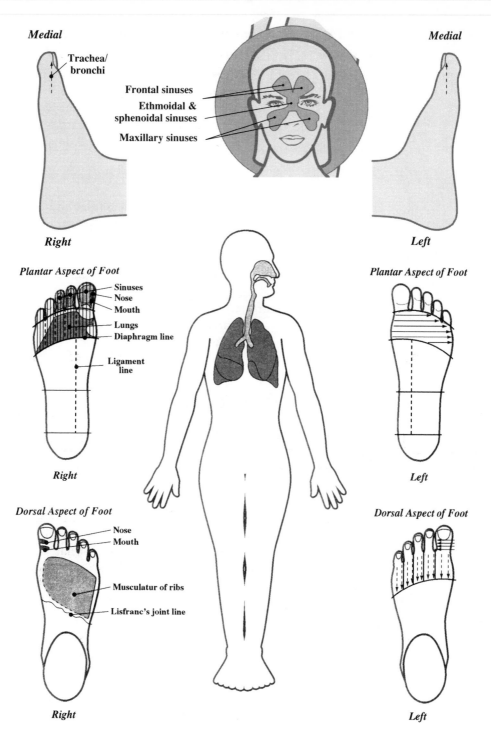

Figure 5.3 The respiratory system and its representation on the feet

Table 5.2 Foot positions for structures of the respiratory system

Referral area	Positions on foot
Mouth/nose	Great toe medial and dorsal aspect, just below the nail bed, zone 1
Sinuses	The first three toes, from the medial edge, plantar and dorsal aspect, zones 1–3
Throat	Great toe medial edge and dorsal aspect, zone 1
Larynx	In the web between the great toe and the second toe
Trachea/bronchi	In line with the spine from nose point to the middle of the proximal phalange of the great toe, zone 1
Lungs	The main part of the proximal phalanges to the heads of the metatarsals, dorsal and plantar, zones 1–4
Rib cage and intercostal muscles	On the dorsal aspect of the foot in the above area and down to the fifth metatarsal notch, zones 1–4
Diaphragm line	Directly on the ball of the foot, zones 1–4

The zones of the head-related areas

The areas of the head include the neurological centres in the brain, which includes the cerebrum (the right foot represents the right cerebral hemisphere, and the left foot the left cerebral hemisphere) and the functional areas of the cerebral cortex, the basal ganglia, the hypothalamus and thalamus, and the epicranium, which covers the muscles of the skull. Facial areas include the eyes, ears, nose (dealt with in the previous system), jaw, teeth, trigeminal nerve, tonsils and upper lymphatics. Neck-related areas and musculature are also covered here. (The brain areas are shown in figure 2.23, page 70.)

The eye

The major structures of the eye are shown in figure 5.4a. The two lids are the protective covering of the eyes. Tears spread over the surface to clean the eye. The sclera is a thick protective outer coating. The under surface of each eyelid is covered with the conjunctiva, a smooth mucous membrane. The retina is a layer of light-sensitive cells at the back of the eye. The front eyeball is filled with a watery substance called the aqueous humour and the back

(a)

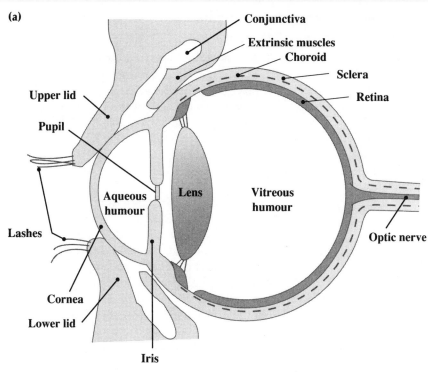

(b)

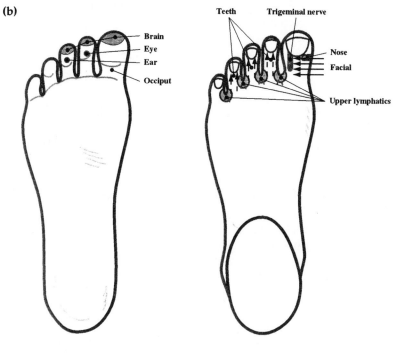

Plantar right foot   *Dorsal left foot*

Figure 5.4 (a) A vertical section through the eye. (b) Representation on the feet.

Table 5.3 Foot positions for head-related areas

Referral area	Position on foot
Brain area	The caps of the three first toes mainly, zones 1–5, as zones 4 and 5 merge in the head and contact the temporal area
Epicranial aponeurosis	The very tips of the first three toes, as near the nails as possible, zones 1–3
Back of the head (occiput)	Pad of great toe, mainly zone 1
Hypothalamus	*See* Table 5.4
Cerebellum and medulla oblongata	Under the ball of the great toe, mainly zone 1
Eyes	On the second/third toes, dorsal and plantar on distal phalanges, zones 2 and 3
Ears	On the third/fourth toes, dorsal and plantar on distal phalanges, zones 3 and 4
Facial area	Dorsal aspect of the first four toes on distal or medial phalanges, zones 1–4
Nose	*See* Table 5.2
Jaw/teeth	On the dorsal aspect of the first four toes, zones 1–4
Trigeminal nerve	On the lateral and dorsal aspect of the great toe, in line with base of the distal phalange to the base of the nail bed, zone 1
Tonsils	*See* Table 5.8
Upper lymphatics	*See* Table 5.8
Neck-related areas	Medial and lateral aspect of all the toes on the dorsum and plantar surfaces, zones 1–5

eyeball with a jelly-like substance called the vitreous humour. The iris is a pigmented layer.

The ear

The structure and function of the ear are covered in details in chapter 7 (page 212).

The foot positions for head-related areas are shown in Table 5.3, and illustrated in figure 5.4b.

The zones of the endocrine system

Many complicated functions of the body, such as body growth and development, sexual function, nutrient distribution and responses to stress, are controlled by a series of glands that produce hormones. These are known as endocrine glands; they have no ducts, and the hormones are released directly into the bloodstream and are carried to different parts of the body, where they control various aspects of the metabolism. These glands are all controlled by the 'master gland' – the pituitary gland at the base of the brain. The glands are scattered around the body with no anatomical link.

Glands in head-related areas include the hypothalamus, a brain area that connects the nervous system to the endocrine system by secreting releasing hormones that stimulate the pituitary gland, the pineal gland, which secretes melatonin, a hormone linked to the light–dark cycle and the body's circadian rhythms, and the pituitary gland, which has two parts, the adenohypophysis and the neurohypophysis. Other glands are the thyroid and parathyroid, regulating calcium metabolism (the latter being four masses of tissue embedded within the thyroid), the two adrenal glands on top of the kidneys, part of the pancreas (*see* digestive system, page 145) and the ovaries and testes (covered in the reproductive system, page 147). The thymus has a vital role in the defence mechanisms of the body and is covered in detail in the lymphatic and immune system (page 150).

The pineal gland is thought to play a role in the light–dark cycle. The pineal gland itself is a small conical body attached by a stalk to the epithalamus on the posterior wall of the third ventricle of the brain. (Pineal is a Middle French word for 'pine cones'.) Many theories are postulated regarding the pineal; it is thought that it may play a part in initiating the development of the gonads and the onset of puberty. The precise hormonal function is still not fully understood, but it is thought also that it may be involved with the metabolism of salt and water within the body. The pineal also contains certain neurotransmitters: noradrenaline, serotonin (thought to be the mood enhancer), histamine and some of the hormonal peptides, somatostatin, and oxytocin, a hormone secreted into the blood only by the pituitary gland that causes contraction of the uterus during labour (*see* Pregnancy, page 320). These hormones are produced in larger quantities elsewhere in the body. Only melatonin from the pineal is released into the bloodstream; it undergoes a nychthemeral cycle (relating to the alternation of a single night followed by day). The Pineal gland is innervated by postganglionic nerve fibres arising in the sympathetic cervical ganglia.

Figure 5.5 shows the endocrine organs and the foot positions for these areas. Table 5.4 details the foot positions for each endocrine organ.

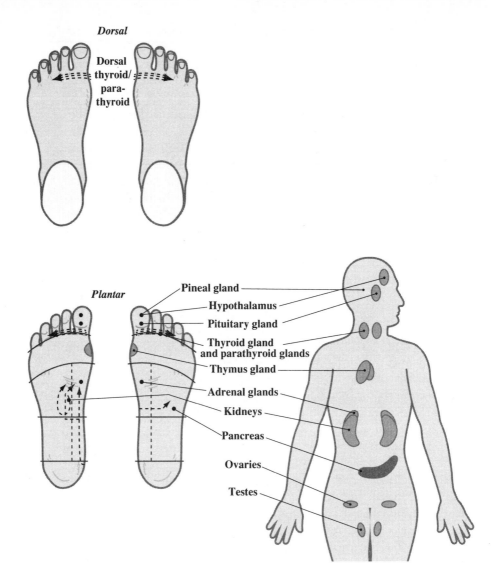

Figure 5.5 The endocrine system and its representation on the feet

There are other endocrine tissues lying in the gastrointestinal tract and producing hormones that are involved in the digestive function. The kidneys release erythropoietin, which stimulates the production of red blood cells. The placenta, an organ within the uterus, provides the embryo with the necessary nourishment and eliminates its waste; its hormonal function is the secretion of certain gonadotrophin hormones that help to maintain pregnancy.

As a speculative comment, since the pituitary lies in the sella turcica (Turkish saddle), the saddle-shaped portion of the

Table 5.4 Foot positions for the endocrine glands

Referral area	Position on foot
Hypothalamus	On the pad of the great toe, zone 1
Pineal	Same area as above
Pituitary	On the whorl of the pad of the great toe, zone 1
Thyroid/parathyroid	Mainly the base of the great toe and the second toe, dorsal and plantar aspect, zones 1–3
Thymus	*See* Table 5.8
Paired adrenals	On top of the kidneys, plantar aspect just above the pancreas, zone 1
Pancreas	*See* Table 5.5
Paired ovaries/testes	*See* Table 5.6
Kidneys	*See* Table 5.6

sphenoid bone, which is found in the centre of the middle cranial fossa, it connects with the occipital bone; this is the reason it is thought to be only contacted by working the great toe. My conjecture is that, as it lays near the sphenoidal sinuses on this central point, it can also be contacted on the facial areas, specifically the LIV-1 point on the middle of the trigeminal pathway. This may be why this acupoint is ideal for all menstrual problems.

The zones of the digestive (gastrointestinal) system

The digestive system includes the mouth, oesophagus, stomach and intestines, both small and large. The small intestine contains the duodenum, jejunum and ileum. The large intestine, surrounding the small intestine, consists of the caecum, vermiform appendix, and ileocaecal valve. The colon has four sections: ascending, transverse, descending and the sigmoid flexure. There are also two other flexures, the hepatic and splenic flexures. The other associated organs involved in digestion are the liver, gall bladder and pancreas.

For food to be of use to the body, it must be broken down (digested) into molecules small enough to be absorbed. Digestion of starch begins in the mouth. Food is further partly digested in the stomach. Final digestion and absorption of nutrients take place in the small intestine. In the large colon, water is removed from the contents to form the faeces, which are excreted from the rectum through the anus. The liver, gall bladder and pancreas are associated glands as their nutrients are absorbed into the body, utilized and metabolized.

The intestinal tract is another term for the gastrointestinal system. The intestines are a long tube, from the stomach to the anus, through which food and faeces pass. Many litres of fluid enter the small intestine daily. Some of this is absorbed in the small intestine, and some of this water and recycled fluids helps to hydrate the body by transferring vital electrolytes back into the system. The large intestine is involved in the formation of the faeces, and further absorption of water and essential electrolytes. Material from the small intestine enters the ileocaecal valve as liquid chyme; the ileocaecal valve is there to prevent any back-flow of contents into the ileum. The ascending colon is most important as the contents have to move against gravity, and because it is a coiled tube all the flexures must be worked, the hepatic, the splenic and sigmoid flexure, so that the contents move towards the rectum. This dehydrated indigestible matter is made up from 30 per cent food waste and 70 per cent dead bacteria such as leucocytes and bile pigments. These are all squeezed along by peristalsis in the colon. The sigmoid colon is a very narrow part of the large intestine; it has no digestive function and faeces can often lie here in the rectum between the sigmoid flexure and the anal canal. The rectum is about 12cm long; if faeces remain here too long the contents can become too hard, making defecation difficult. A good general treatment, with emphasis on the pancreas area, will relieve this problem.

The hydrochloric acid secreted in the stomach has strong antiseptic qualities, necessary because of its storage capacity and its work in the gradual release of food into the duodenum; this kills off any microbes that may be present. Pepsinogen is an inactive enzyme until the hydrochloric acid activates the production of pepsin to further the breakdown of proteins. The stomach also secretes intrinsic factor that is necessary for absorption of B12, often known as the antianaemic factor because of its role in erythrocyte formation. The mucous cells that secrete the mucus are activated to release the correct quantities to act as a barrier or a protective layer. All these substances are so necessary for a balanced functioning of the digestive tract.

The liver plays a vital part in many of the processes of the body; it is our vast chemical factory. This important organ will detoxicate any noxious substances and helps in the general metabolism of fats and carbohydrates.

Figure 5.6 shows the organs of the digestive system and the reflex foot zones. Table 5.5 gives details of the foot positions.

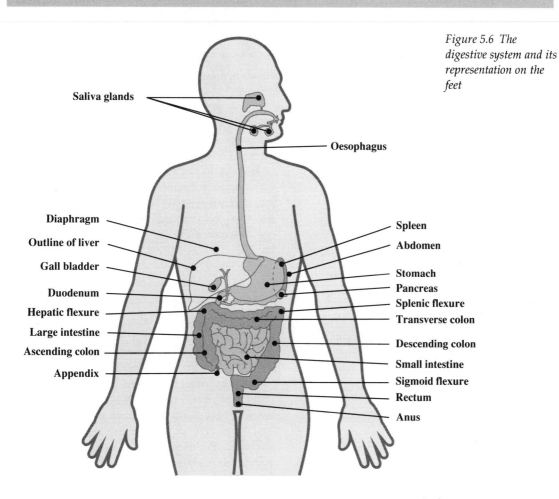

Figure 5.6 The digestive system and its representation on the feet

Table 5.5 Foot positions for the digestive system

Referral area	Position on foot
Mouth/tongue/teeth/salivary glands	The dorsal aspect of the first three toes, zones 1–3
Throat/oesophagus	Connects the pharynx to the stomach, commencing from the base of the great toe just above the seventh cervical on the medial edge and lying behind the trachea, but anterior to the vertebral column, right down to the stomach (*see* note)
Stomach	A continuation of the oesophagus, a J-shaped area lying between this and the small intestine, zones 1–2 (right) and zones 1–3 (left)
Small intestine/duodenum	Starting just above the waist line by the right kidney, above the waist encircling the pancreas, zones 1–2 (right) for duodenum; zones 1–4 (both feet) for the small intestine, plantar surface
Large intestine	
Ascending colon	Working on the plantar surface, right foot only, ascending from the heel line to the waist line in a vertical strip, zones 4–5
Transverse colon	Both feet following the line of the waist line, zones 1–5
Descending colon	Left foot only, descending from the waist to the heel line, zones 4–5
Sigmoid flexure	Just below heel line in a low shallow 'V' on the left foot only, zones 1–5
Rectum/anus	Both feet in line with the bladder, medial aspect, zone 1
Hepatic flexure	Right foot only, on the waist line and just above, zones 4–5
Splenic flexure	Left foot only. As above.
Associated organs	
Liver	Occupying the main part of the area between the diaphragm line and the waist line on the right foot, zones 1–5, on the plantar aspect. The liver is basically prismatic in shape, with the left lobe extending on to the left foot, zone 1
Gall bladder	Right foot on the plantar and dorsal aspect, zone 4
Pancreas	The head lies in the duodenum behind the stomach, tipping up to the spleen on the plantar aspect, zones 1–2 (right), zones 1–3 (left) in line with the first and second lumbar vertebrae, just above the waist

Note. If a person suffers from any oesophagitis, you can sometimes see a few striated lines on the right or the left foot in the area of the liver just under the diaphragm line near the medial edge. If there are any lines on the liver area it could indicate high toxicity levels or an allergy.

The zones of the genitourinary system

The zones of the reproductive system include the paired mammary glands (breasts), paired ovaries/testes, uterus/prostate, Fallopian (uterine) tubes/vas deferens. The zones of the urinary tract include the paired kidneys, the paired ureters, the urinary bladder and the urethra.

In the excretory system, the paired kidneys form and excrete urine through the ureters to the bladder, where it is stored until the bladder fills up. It then passes through a valve to the urethra, and is then expelled from the body. Waste elements in the blood are extracted in the kidneys and transformed into urine; selected substances and some water are reabsorbed. The kidneys also regulate body fluids by controlling the mineral, salt and water content in the blood.

Figure 5.7 shows the organs of the genitourinary system and the foot zones. Table 5.6 shows the details of the foot positions.

The zones of the musculoskeletal system

The vertebral column is a vital part of the skeletal system. As mentioned the joints and musculature allow movement. The body has a complex system of bones, joints and muscles, which allow this great variation of movement. The joints are where two or more bones meet. These are supported and strengthened by ligaments, fibrous connective tissue linking two bones together, strengthening around or inside the joints. Tendons are tough cords that connect the body of the muscle with fixed points on the bony skeleton. Some joints and tendons are lubricated by synovial fluid; this is produced by the synovial membrane surrounding the joints.

The zones of the musculoskeletal system include the spine, the neck, the musculature of the neck, the shoulder/axillary area, the shoulder point, the shoulder muscle, the arm-related area, the elbow/knee area, the hip/leg area, the musculature of the pelvis and the musculature of the buttocks. Treatment covers the

(a)

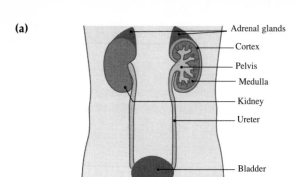

Male reproductive system   *Female reproductive system*

Anterior view (schematic)

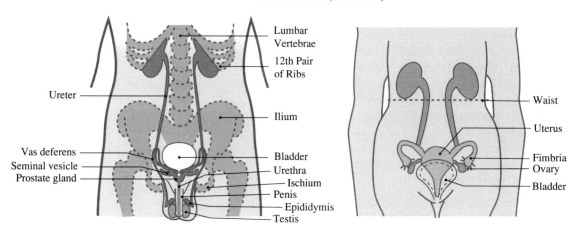

Sagital view (schematic)

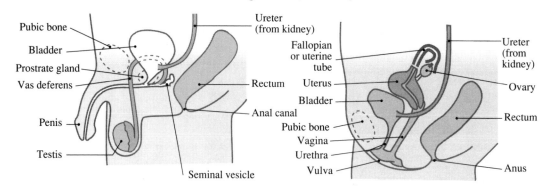

Figure 5.7 (a) The genitourinary system. (b) Representation on the feet.

(b)

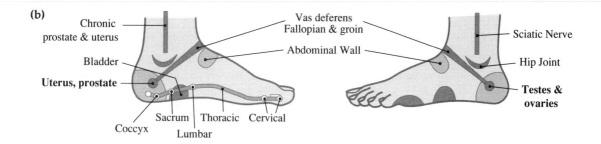

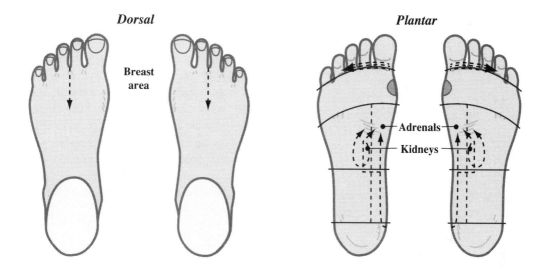

neurological system, brain, spinal nerves and some peripheral nerves and the solar plexus (coeliac plexus).

Figure 5.8 shows the musculature of the trunk and the foot zones of the muscles and skeleton (for the spinal curves *see* figure 2.22). Table 5.7 shows details of the foot positions.

Working the foot positions for the cervical nerves can aid most hand and arm problems, whilst working the positions for the lumbar and sacral nerves can aid most leg problems. Figure 5.9 shows the spinal innervation to the upper and lower limbs.

Note. The solar plexus lies behind the stomach; it is a network of sympathetic nerves and vagal parasympathetic fibres; it lies in zones 2–3. On the right foot, in exactly the same place, the liver receives sympathetic stimuli from an extension of the coeliac plexus and parasympathetic stimuli from the vagus nerve. This basically is one reason why we work the solar plexus reflex on

Table 5.6 Foot positions for the genitourinary system

Referral area	Position on foot
Paired mammary glands (breasts female)	On the dorsal aspect (both feet), zones 1–4, with the nipple in line between zones 2 and 3
Paired ovaries/testes	On the lateral aspect of the heel area (both feet) in the depression midway between the lateral malleolus and the heel area, zone 5 of the pelvic cavity
Uterus/prostate	On the medial aspect of the heel area on both feet in the depression midway between the medial malleolus and the heel area, zone 1 of the pelvic cavity
Fallopian (uterine) tubes/vas deferens	On both feet, dorsal aspect, zones 1–5. A line from the uterus/prostate point to the ovaries/testes point from the depression between each ankle across the dorsal aspect
Kidneys	On the plantar aspect (both feet), zones 1–2 in line with the first and second lumbar vertebrae, just straddling the waist
Ureters	Leading from the kidney point to the bladder, zone 1
Bladder	On the medial aspect (both feet), in line with the rectum and anus point. The slightly raised area in line with the heel line, zone 1
Urethra	As the bladder point

both feet. As a speculative comment, this is the first point on the kidney meridian, and for all acute problems an ideal calming point for palpitations or acute problems. Which point are we working here? Is it the reflexology point? Or the nerves? Or the meridian? Does it really matter, for as previously stated this technique is empirical, and experience has shown us that this point has a wonderful way of achieving equability and restfulness in the recipient?

The zones of the circulatory and lymphatic systems

The zones of these systems include the areas for the heart, lymphatic system, upper lymphatics and tonsils, axillary lymphatics, lymph nodes of the groin, thymus and spleen.

The cardiovascular system comprises the heart and the vast network of blood vessels, the systemic and pulmonary circulations.

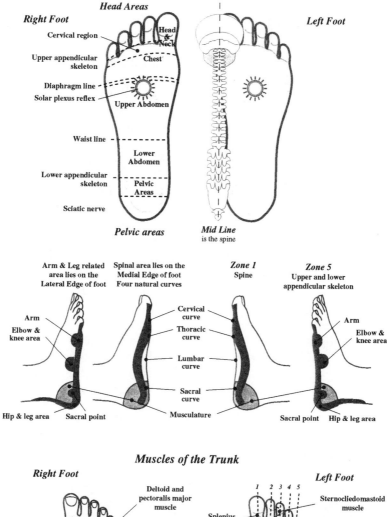

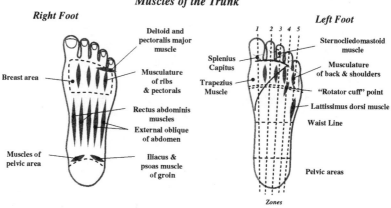

Figure 5.8 Representation of the musculoskeletal system on the feet

Table 5.7 Foot positions for the musculoskeletal system

Referral area	Position on foot
Brain	*See* Table 5.3
Cervical spine	Inner aspect (both feet), from heel to the base
Thoracic spine	of the nail bed of great toe. This area also
Lumbar spine	covers the musculature of the spine as the
Sacrum/coccyx	spinae erector muscle lies above and below the line of the spine. The spinal cord is located within the vertebral column and the 31 pairs of nerves emerge along its length, zone 1 (both feet)
Solar plexus (coeliac plexus)	Zones 2–3 (both feet; *see* note)
Neck	Base of the first three toes, dorsal and plantar aspect, zones 1–3 (both feet)
Musculature of the neck	On the lateral aspect of the great toe. The medial and lateral edges of the second and third toes, zones 1–3 (both feet)
Shoulder/axillary area	From the diaphragm line to the tips of the fourth and fifth toes, zones 4–5 (both feet)
Shoulder point (*see* rotator cuffpoint, figure 5.8)	On the lateral aspect of the proximal phalange of the fifth toe. Plantar and dorsal aspect, zone 5 (both feet)
Shoulder muscle	On the lateral aspect of the proximal phalange of the fifth toe. Dorsal aspect, zone 5 (both feet)
Arm-related area	On the lateral aspect of the fifth metatarsal from the fifth metatarsal notch to the base of the little toe, zone 5 (both feet)
Elbow/knee	Around the fifth metatarsal notch on the lateral aspect (both feet), elbow slightly above, knee slightly below, zone 5
Hip/leg	On the lateral aspect (both feet), from the heel line almost to the fifth metatarsal notch, zone 5
Musculature of pelvis	Following the line of the Achilles tendon from the edge of the heel to the line of the medial malleolus, posterior to the uterus/prostate reflex, zone 1 (both feet)
Musculature of buttocks	Following the line of the Achilles tendon, posterior to the ovary/testes point, zone 5 (both feet)
Musculature of ribs	Dorsal aspect surrounding the lung area, zones 1–5 (both feet)

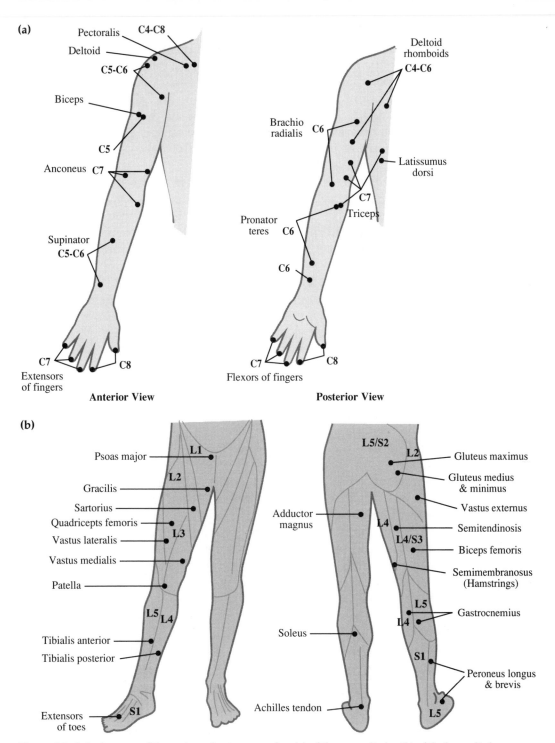

Figure 5.9 Spinal nerves of the major voluntary muscles: (a) of the upper limbs; (b) of the lower limbs

It transports oxygen and nutrients around the body and is also responsible for the removal of waste products. Blood must flow through the circuit in one direction totally without being impeded or hampered in any way. In the vascular system two conditions must be maintained: (1) the competence and rhythmic regularity of the heart, (2) the right condition of all the vessels, especially the small arteries and veins. The nerve supply to these vessels is of the utmost importance as they allow the vessels to dilate and constrict.

At the centre of the circulatory system is the heart. Let's look briefly at what work the heart has to do. It is a four-chambered very hard working double-pumping hollow muscular organ, basically a blood-filled muscular container. It acts as a double pump to drive blood around the body. One pump transports blood to the lungs to be oxygenated; the other pump has to push the newly oxygenated blood out to the rest of the body. The left ventricle receives oxygenated blood from the lungs via the left atrium and then pumps the blood, under pressure, down the aorta to the organs of the body through the arteries. From the main arteries, the blood then passes into a branching network of smaller and smaller blood vessels ending in tiny capillaries, which allow all the nutrients and oxygen in the blood to reach every cell in the body. The right ventricle receives non-oxygenated blood returning to the heart along the vena cava from the peripheral circulation via the veins and right atrium; it then pumps it at relatively low pressure into the lungs. The two sides of the heart have separate functions, but each is dependent on the other. The venous blood is kept apart from the arterial blood by the septum, a thick central muscular wall dividing each cavity. There are also four valves to prevent any backflow of blood. There is no muscle in the body so strong as the heart; each day it pumps blood through approximately 65,000 miles of blood vessels. If you are overweight then there are thousands more blood vessels and the poor hard-working heart has to work twice as hard. The heart is roughly the size of its owner's fist.

The heart muscle contracts about 70 times a minute to pump blood around the body; to do this it needs a good supply of oxygen. It gets this from the bloodstream, not directly because it cannot obtain enough from this flow, hence it needs its own source of blood. This is supplied by its own right and left coronary arteries that arise from the aorta, and these then form branches that encircle the heart muscle. The direction of the blood flow is controlled by valves. If the arteries become too narrow because of a build-up of a fatty deposit called atheroma, the blood supply to the heart becomes restricted, or even blocked in extreme cases; this then becomes coronary heart disease, the two main disorders being angina or a more serious problem such as a heart attack.

The heart has its own intrinsic system whereby the myocardium will contract without the brain being involved, but the pace of contraction is normally controlled by fibres from the autonomic nervous system, which supply a minute area of specialized cardiac muscle located in the upper wall of the right atrium near the opening of the superior vena cava. This is the sinoatrial (SA) node, often referred to as the natural pacemaker of the body; its fibres are self-excitatory and will contract rhythmically at around 70 beats per minute. Parasympathetic fibres from the vagus nerve and sympathetic fibres from the cardiac plexus both end at this node; a fine balance is necessary at all times as it is essential that the heart contracts in a precise sequence. Extrinsic control comes from impulses originating in the cardiac centre of the medulla oblongata in the brain. These impulses from the autonomic nervous system accelerate or decrease the heart rate. Many hormones and excess stimuli of the nervous system can have an effect on the rate, either by speeding it up or slowing it down. The other area in the right atrium is the atrioventricular (AV) node (pertaining both to atrial and to ventricular chambers of the heart); this is situated slightly lower and in the middle of the heart; it receives slower impulses to contract from the SA node, through a mass of modified fibres known as the bundle of His. These originate from the AV node in front of the septum between the ventricles where they divide into two, right and left, one for each ventricle. These fibres convey nerve impulses of contraction and in response this generates tension in the muscle, causing movement in the ventricles, which then pump blood into the arteries. The pulmonary circulation is via the pulmonary artery and systemic circulation via the aorta. The nerve supply to the heart is very easily disturbed; sympathetic stimulation speeds it up, and this can be due to excitement or exercise or stress, all of which may increase cardiac activity. Cardiac activity naturally decreases while we are at rest.

Many reflexology charts show the heart in different positions, but if the feet and hands are supposed to represent the physical body then the heart's apex must be in line with the left nipple or just below it. The heart also lies only 9 cm off the midline resting on the central tendon of the diaphragm muscle, with the left lung slightly overlapping it. The base extends up to the level of the second rib. True, there may be a false impression of referred pain to a particular area, but the reflex point is shown as the anatomy of the body.

If there is an imbalance in the heart we would be more likely to pick it up on the left foot and hand on the heart reflex, as there is more muscular bulk on the left side of the heart as it has to contract much more forcibly than the right side.

Figure 5.10 shows the heart and the relevant foot zones. Table 5.8 gives details of the foot positions.

The lymphatic circulation is part of the vascular system. The clear watery fluid called lymph passes into the blood system through the many lymph nodes and vessels situated at strategic parts of the body; these act as a filtering station, stopping foreign particles from entering the bloodstream. The lymph has to pass

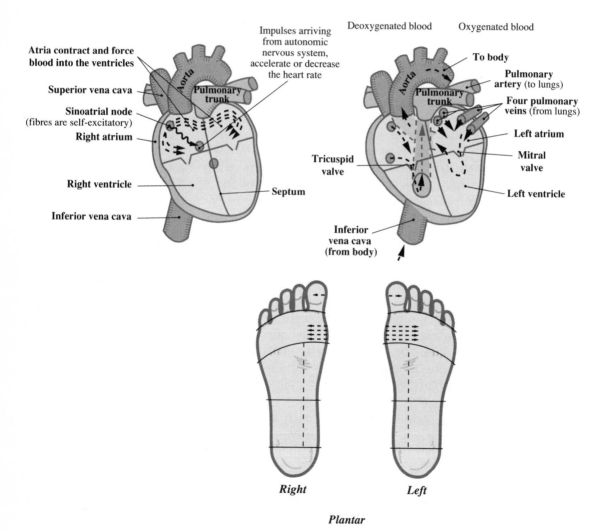

Plantar

Figure 5.10 *The cardiovascular system and its representation on the feet*

through many blind-ended capillaries to drain finally into two large channels: the right lymphatic ducts receive lymph that is drained from the right side of the head, thorax and the right arm; the lymph from the rest of the body drains into the thoracic duct. Lymph carries a rich supply of nutrients to every cell within the body; its other task is to remove toxins and waste. As there is no pump at its centre like the circulatory system, lymph is moved by pressure of the adjacent vessels and by muscular exercise. If it cannot flow from the tissues to the heart because of a sedentary or inactive lifestyle due to illness or injury then excess fluid may accumulate causing oedema. Reflexology is a wonderful way of encouraging the free flow of lymph; treatment helps to disperse any blockages and it also boosts the immunological system.

The thymus, a tiny bilobed organ that plays a vital role in the immune system, produces thymosin, which stimulates the development of lymphocytes and thymopoetin, which inhibit neuromuscular transmission. Inflammation of the thymus gland (thymisitis) is thought to be responsible for myasthenia gravis, an autoimmune disorder. The spleen, another lymphatic organ, produces some types of immune cells. It is a mass of red and white pulp, controlling the quality of the blood supply through its storage of blood and iron.

Figure 5.11 shows the lymphatic system. Table 5.8 gives details of the foot positions.

Note. The general circulation is improved by reflexology, which in turn will stimulate the transportation of the necessary nutrients and hormones to the tissues, and the many leucocytes (white blood cells) to the site of infection. Oxygen supply is improved from the lungs to the tissues, which, together with the nerve and blood supply, helps the general metabolism of the muscles. The waste products of all this activity are eliminated by the excretory organs, mainly the lungs, excreting carbon dioxide and some water, the kidneys, excreting all the nitrogenous waste, principally urea, from the blood, the gastrointestinal tract, eliminating the waste products of digestion, water and bile pigments, and finally the skin, excreting carbon dioxide, some water, and a small amount of urea and salts through the sudoriferous glands.

Treatment procedure

The treatment session should commence only when the foot analysis has been completed. Each area of the foot can be worked

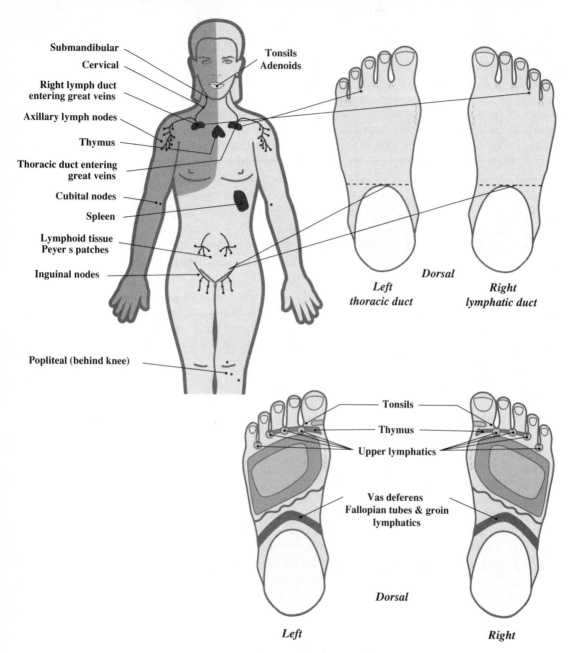

Figure 5.11 The lymphatic system and its representation on the feet

in several ways. If there is a tender spot, go back and work it from a different angle. No one way is completely right, and each time you change direction you may pick up another congested reflex. This is therefore only a suggested order of work.

Table 5.8 Foot positions for the circulatory and lymphatic systems

Referral area	Position on foot
Heart	In the chest area between the neck and resting on the diaphragm line. A larger area on the left foot, reaching the line of the nipple, zones 1–3. On the right foot halfway into zone 1
Upper lymphatics	Webs of the toes, zones 1–5
Axillary lymphatics	*See* Axillary area, work plantar and dorsal, zones 4–5
Lymph nodes of the groin	On both feet, dorsal aspect, zones 1–5. A line from the uterus/prostate point to the ovaries/testes point from the depression between each ankle
Thymus	Just beneath the thyroid gland, in the fourth intercostal space just above the heart, on the very medial edge, zone 1 (both feet)
Spleen	On the left foot only, its base is in contact with the tail of the pancreas, zones 4–5

Start on the right foot

Solar plexus point

Place both thumbs on the solar plexus, as this is a good preliminary start to the treatment session. Not only does it compose you, the practitioner, but it also brings about a feeling of peacefulness to the client and it is a good way to approach the feet for the first time.

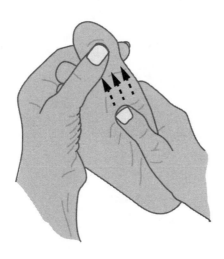

Figure 5.12 Working position for diaphragm relaxation and to commence on the lungs. This also demonstrates the support hold for working above the waist.

(a)

(b)

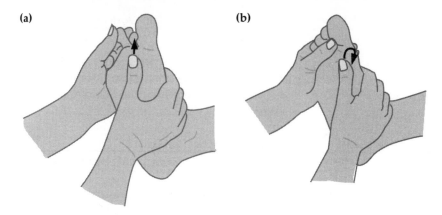

Figure 5.13 (a) Working all chest-related areas; separate toes accordingly, making sure you get into the base of the webs for the upper lymphatics. (b) Working the heart point on right foot. Rotate on point or palpate.

Side to side relaxation – both feet (B/F)
See relaxation 4 (chapter 4, page 106).

Diaphragm relaxation – B/F
See relaxation 7 (chapter 4, page 107) and figure 5.12.

Lungs (figure 5.12)/ plantar/thymus/heart (figure 5.13)
This area can be covered in vertical strips working from the medial to the lateral edge on the metatarsals and in between them; change hands and return the other way. Or this can be covered using circular friction over the whole area, or using horizontal pathways. On the medial edge there is the thymus reflex. It is important to work this area in young children or if the patient is suffering from myasthenia gravis. Change direction and repeat several times. There is a small section of the heart on this area also; again work this reflex by changing your direction. (On the left foot there is a larger area, over to zone three.)

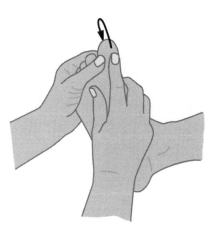

Figure 5.14 Working the toes for all head-related areas

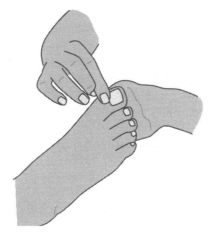

Figure 5.15 Working the nose area. Use firm moving pressure to release a blocked nose.

Note. Remember the area of assistance for all respiratory problems is the intestines as these aid the removal of mucus and they are also paired with the lungs in the meridian system.

Sinuses/head-related areas (figures 5.14, 5.15)

Work all the toes in vertical strips. You can use both thumbs and fingers, making sure every single toe is covered on the medial edge on the plantar and the lateral edge of each toe from the medial edge to the lateral edge, and then repeat returning the other way. When you work make sure you are not in contact with the nails. When working the nose area on the dorsal aspect (*see* figure 5.15), make horizontal strips.

Pituitary

The pituitary is accessible in one of three ways. When you have completed the toes, as you come to the great toe you can push the

(a) **(b)**

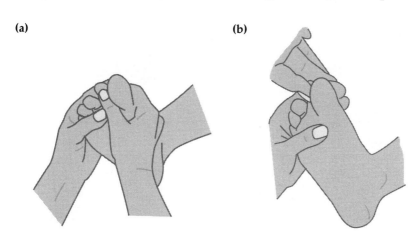

Figure 5.16 (a) Working the eye reflex. Remember the shape of the face; if the eyes are set wide apart this may be on the third toe. Rotate on point. (b) Pressure and rotation on the eye point, showing plucking-up method.

reflex into the middle and rotate, using your left thumb on the right toe and your right thumb on the left toe. The working hand must be on top of the support hand; this ensures that the nails are not contacted. This time, working with the right thumb, pluck up and rotate; alternatively, you can work with the right thumb to right foot, pluck up and rotate – as for the eyes. Or you can apply firm unmoving pressure with your knuckle.

Eyes (figure 5.16) and ears (figure 5.17) – plantar dorsal

This is the same action as on the pituitary. You can pluck up on the reflexes and rotate using firm unmoving pressure on the dorsal aspect. Or, using both hands, press the index finger on the dorsal distal point and the thumb on the plantar distal point; rotate both together.

Note.   Remember the zonal pathway and work the kidneys for eye and ear problems.

Neck/thyroid/parathyroid – plantar

Work in horizontal strips from the great toe medial to the lateral third toe, then lateral to medial. Repeat this procedure several times. If there is a tender reflex apply circular rotation gently on the spot. Working this area also helps the eyes and ears.

Lungs/breast/lymph – dorsal

This is best covered by working in vertical strips on the meta-tarsals and in between. Again this must be covered both ways, from medial to lateral and returning from lateral to medial. Make sure you start from the webs. If there are tender spots, work in horizontal strips, both hands working together, as in the rib cage

(a)   **(b)**

Figure 5.17 (a) Working the ear point; repeat on the fourth toe. Rotate on point. (b) Pressure and rotation on the ear point, showing plucking-up method. Remember, support hand must protect the nails. Working hand is always on top of support hand.

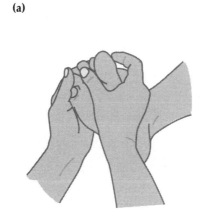
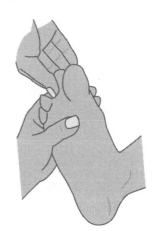

technique (*see* chapter 4, pages 108, 109, figures 4.6 and 4.7), thumbs supporting the ball of the foot. On zones 4–5 you will pick up the shoulder (we will be working that area later).

Facial areas – dorsal (figure 5.18)
Making a fist of the support hand provides an anchor. Now place the thumb of your working hand loosely in between the thumb and forefinger of the supporting hand, thus allowing a pincer action. Work with your index finger in tiny horizontal strips from the nail bed down to the base of the great toe and back. Work the other toes also, as in figure 5.18a.

Trigeminal nerve (figure 5.19)
Supporting with the flat of your right hand on the plantar surface of the foot, bring your other hand round so that you can work up the lateral side of the great toe using your left thumb. Repeat this procedure on all the toes as it is much easier to support without fear of pushing against the tiny joints of the phalanges. Change hands for the other foot, as shown in figure 5.18.

Neck/thyroid/parathyroid – dorsal (figure 5.20)
Making a fist of the support hand provides an anchor. Now place the thumb of your working hand loosely in between the thumb and forefinger of the supporting hand, thus allowing a pincer action. Work with your right index finger in horizontal strips from the great toe medial edge to the lateral edge of the third toe; then lateral to medial. Repeat this procedure several times. If there is a tender reflex apply circular rotation gently on the spot.

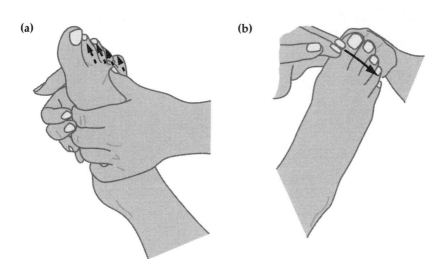

(a)   (b)

Figure 5.18 (a) Position for working the dorsal facial areas, which include the teeth, sinuses, eyes and ears. (b) Working the facial area for the teeth and mouth

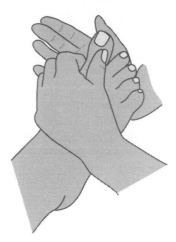

Figure 5.19 Working up the lateral edge of the great toe you will contact the reflex to the trigeminal nerve.

Trachea/bronchi

Using the flat of the left hand, and the thumb in line exactly with the great toe, work with your right index finger up the medial edge of the toe on the trachea/bronchi reflex in line with the side of the nail.

Rib cage technique

See relaxation 10 (chapter 4, page 108). This aids and facilitates the whole breathing process.

Relaxation techniques

Use relaxation 8, 9, or 12 (chapter 4, pages 107, 108). Any one, or all of these, can be utilized.

Liver/gall bladder

The area from the waist to the diaphragm line can be covered in slight diagonal strips working both ways from the medial to

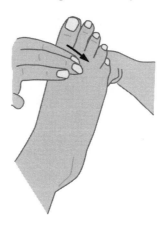

Figure 5.20 Working the reflexes for the neck, thyroid/ parathyroid on the dorsal aspect of the foot.

lateral edge then returning the other way; this is easier than going across in horizontal bands as there is too much loose flesh. If there is a tender spot, change direction or do circular rotations. The gall bladder lies in zones 3–4, dorsal and plantar.

Note. You are working from the waist and above so you should be supporting from above. Watch out for the ligament line at this point as it may be very tender. Plantar flex the toes when working to safeguard against causing any undue discomfort. Remember, the nerve supply to the whole alimentary tract is balanced by the sympathetic and parasympathetic nervous systems; you may need to go back and work the brain areas.

Ileocaecal valve (figure 5.21)
Using your left thumb, hook out on this reflex at least three times. It lies exactly on the heel line, approximately one thumb-breadth in. You can also apply extra pressure by utilising the other thumb as well.

Note. You are now working from the waist and below so you should be supporting from underneath the heel.

Ascending colon
Still using your left thumb, work up the lateral edge of zones 4–5 to the hepatic flexure. (*See* figure 5.6.)

Transverse colon/small intestine/buttocks (figure 5.22)
Working with your right thumb from the medial edge to lateral edge in horizontal strips and making as many bands as you can,

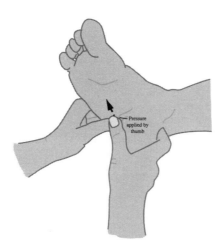

Pressure applied by thumb

Figure 5.21 Applying extra pressure on the ileocaecal valve reflex

carry on right down to the base of the heel. Change hands and repeat the other way. Just to make sure you have contacted the hepatic flexure, go back and apply pressure on the lateral plantar side of zone 5 in line with the fifth metatarsal notch, as in figure 5.21. If there is a tender spot then change direction or do circular rotations.

Abdominal walking – dorsal
See relaxation 11 (chapter 4, page 106).

Bladder/ureters/adrenals/kidneys (figure 5.23)
These reflexes are best worked in unison. Using the thumb of the right hand, make tiny steps on the bladder reflex. This is the slightly raised rounded area on the side of the foot in alignment with the heel line. Repeat at least three times. Then carry on up the medial edge, making sure that you do not press on the ligament line. Go right up to work on the adrenal glands point (this lies approxi-

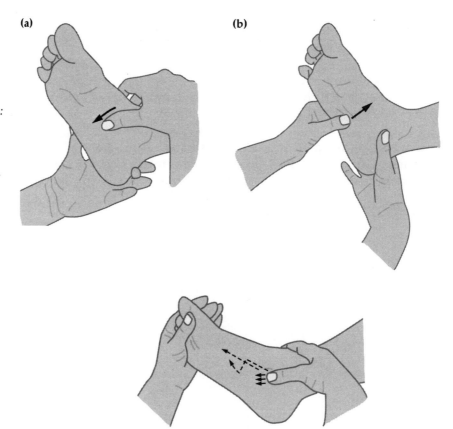

Figure 5.22 (a) Working the intestines: the support hand is on the waist line and acts as a guide for the transverse colon reflex. (b) Working from the lateral to the medial edge: the support allows the skin to be relaxed and not taut.

Figure 5.23 Working the bladder point and kidney point

mately two finger-breadths below the diaphragm line); rotate on this point firmly three times. Come back to the bladder and now complete a continuous circuit from the bladder up to the waist. Lift the wrist so that you can cross the waist to the kidney, making sure that you plantar flex the foot so that you do not apply undue pressure on the ligament. Once you are in zone 2 work the kidney point by rotation three times at least (*see* figure 5.24). This is an area that is often incorrectly worked. Normal kidney function is needed for good health. Look at figure 5.7b to see the recommended pathway for working.

Note. The support hold encircles the foot in a caressing way with the left hand; the right hand is then ready for working. Take the foot out to the required position.

Kidney pressure and rotation (figure 5.24)
Apply firm unmoving pressure to the kidney reflex with the right thumb. This point should lie fractionally above the waist. The left hand rotates the foot down on to the unmoving thumb. You can also use the knuckle in sweeping downward strokes, providing it is not too tender.

Prostate/uterus
This reflex can be worked with two fingers on the medial side of the heel. Work from just before the depression on it and just past it. This ensures the whole area has been covered. (*See* figures 5.7b for area to work and 5.31a for correct support hold.)

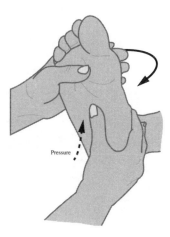

Pressure

Figure 5.24 Pressure on the kidney reflex and rotation to aid in elimination. Right thumb is between zones 2 and 3 on the waist line.

Note. When you are working on the medial or lateral edge of the heel areas, keep the foot as straight as possible; this permits the area to be worked without the creasing of skin on the heel area hindering movement. Remember that in females there is an anatomical and physiological connection between the breasts and uterus, so the breasts will be an area of assistance.

SP-6 on the Spleen meridian shares the same point as the chronic uterus reflex; this can be used providing the person is not menstruating or pregnant, as not only is it an empirical point to promote delivery during labour, but it will also stimulate blood flow.

Chronic areas of the above (for persistent deep-rooted problems)

If there are no contraindications you can carry on from the last point up the leg for about three to six finger-breadths as near to the posterior edge of the tibia as possible; repeat this three times.

Warning! This area can be very tender. There is no need to apply great pressure. If the client is male make sure you do not drag the hairs on the legs.

Testes/ovaries

This is worked exactly the same as the uterus/prostate reflex, but this time you are working on the lateral aspect of the heel. (*See* figure 5.7b for area to work. Change support hand.)

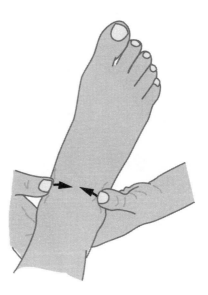

Figure 5.25 Working the vas deferens and Fallopian tubes and groin area

Rectum/haemorrhoids (This also covers chronic areas and the sciatic nerve)
Support above with the right hand, taking the weight slightly off the heel area so that you can work with the thumb and index finger of the left hand. Start in line with the medial malleolus and work at least six finger-breadths up the Achilles tendon. Repeat several times. (*See* figure 5.31b.)

Vas deferens/Fallopian/groin area (figure 5.25) (This also covers the groin lymphatics)
Support is given by cupping the heel with the fingers of both hands, and the thumbs (or index fingers) then work distal to the two malleoli up each ankle to join in the middle. Be careful not to pinch the skin. Carry on over the top with one thumb at least three times. Repeat this procedure, but this time work on the proximal side of the malleolus.

Prostate/uterus/testes/ovaries sedation
The support is from above with the right hand. Put the index finger or second finger on the prostate/uterus reflex and the thumb on the testes/ovaries reflex. Apply firm unmoving pressure as you rotate the foot with the right hand in a medial or lateral direction, as required (*see* relaxation 14/15, chapter 4, pages 109, 110).

Overclasp vas deferens/Fallopian/lymphatics of groin
This is a light hold; a grip is too strong. The web between the thumb and index finger of the left hand is placed on the above reflex, the thumb to the lateral edge. Supporting with the right

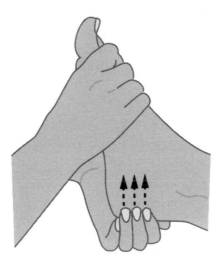

Figure 5.26 How to work the coccyx/sacrum on the medial edge; the support hand and working hand change over to work the lateral edge.

(a)   (b)

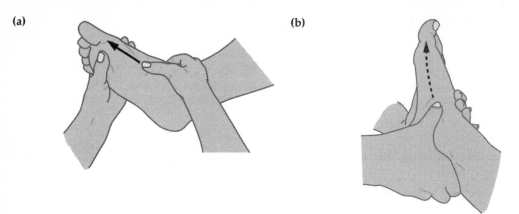

Figure 5.27 (a) Working all spine-related areas, including the erector spinae muscle and nerve pathways. (b) Working the spinal pathway; move the support hand up as you ascend the foot.

hand, rotate in a medial direction, pushing up to make contact with your hand. Do this several times as it relaxes this area (*see* relaxation 16, chapter 4, page 110).

Coccyx/sacrum (figure 5.26), hip/pelvis – medial and lateral

The aim is to cover the calcaneum almost in a 'U' shape. This is achieved by supporting above with the right hand as the left hand encircles the heel. Use the first three fingers starting from the midline of the heel and walk up in alternating steps to the level of

(a)   (b)

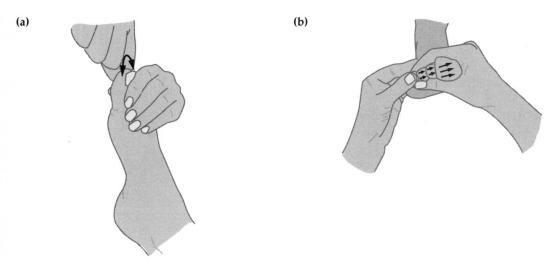

Figure 5.28 (a) Working the brain area. Fingers or thumbs can also be used. Work both ways, rolling the knuckle across. (b) Working the brain area using the thumbs.

the heel line of the medial edge. Change hands and repeat on the lateral aspect for the hip and pelvic area.

Spine (figure 5.27)/brain (figure 5.28)
The support hold encircles the foot in a caressing way with the left hand. The right hand is then ready for working; take the foot out to the required position. The spine reflex can be worked using the thumb following the line of the spine on the inner aspect of both feet, from the heel to the base of the nail bed of the great toe; this includes the cervical, thoracic, lumbar spine and sacrum/coccyx. This area also covers the musculature of the spine as the spinae erector muscle lies above and below the line of the spine. The spinal cord is located within the vertebral column and the 31 pairs of nerves emerge along its length; if we work directly on the arch of the foot and then above and below we contact all the areas of the body. You can also work individual areas crossways, using one or two fingers. The brain area lies on the caps of the first three toes. Work this with the thumb and index finger in alternating steps over the area. Or use the knuckle in a rolling action back and forth to cover all areas. (*See* figure 4.10a.)

Self-help tip. If you are feeling under the weather and do not have time for a full treatment for yourself, partner or colleague, work the spine area for 5 minutes. It is a wonderful first-aid treatment.

Chronic neck area (figure 5.29)
The support is the left thumb on the base of the distal phalange and the third finger on the dorsal aspect in the same area. The second finger can then keep the toes apart. Work the lateral edge

(a) **(b)**

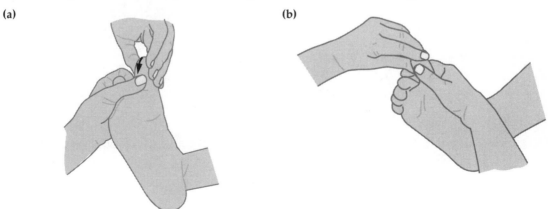

Figure 5.29 (a) Working the chronic neck area down the lateral aspect of the first three toes. (b) You can use your index finger, or the other hand.

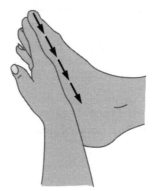

Figure 5.30 Support for working down the spine. Use the thumb or index finger, whichever is more comfortable.

of the first three toes using the index finger or the thumb of the right hand, whichever is more comfortable.

Return down spine (figure 5.30)

The aim is to pick up a congested spot that you may have missed as you ascended the spinal reflex. Support using the dorsum of your right hand to the plantar aspect of the right foot. Your index finger should be in line with the great toe, and your left thumb is going to work all the way down. Be sure to cup the toes as you start; place them on the lateral edge between the great toe and the second toe. If the span of your thumb is insufficient to allow you to come down easily, put the support hand under the heel and elevate the foot towards the working hand.

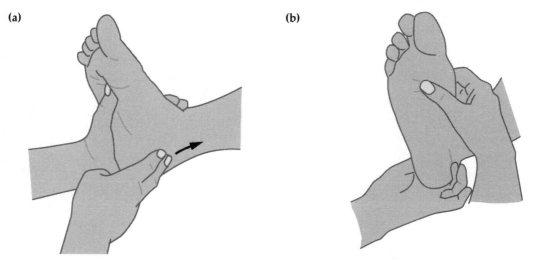

(a)   (b)

Figure 5.31 (a) Working the musculature; make three passes and repeat on the lateral side. (b) Squeezing technique for rectum and haemorrhoids.

Musculature – medial and lateral (figure 5.31)
Work the musculature of the pelvis following the line of the
Achilles tendon from the edge of the heel to the line of the medial
malleolus, posterior to the uterus/prostate reflex of both feet
(zone 1). Then work the musculature of the buttocks following the
line of the Achilles tendon, posterior to the ovary/testes point of
both feet (zone 5). These reflexes lie behind the prostate/
uterus/testes/ovaries respectively in the web of the heel to
the last crease. An alternative is to use a squeezing technique
(figure 5.31b).

Side friction of whole torso
See relaxation 3 (chapter 4, page 105).

The spinal tweak and stretch (figure 5.32)
Both hands are placed on the medial edge of the spinal reflex, in
between the web of the thumb and the index finger. The thumbs
are placed on the plantar area with the fingers lying across the
dorsum. Holding the hand nearest to the ankle stationary, tweak
up with the hand nearest to the toes; repeat this procedure two or
three times. Then applying a stationary firm hold, gently stretch
all spinal areas.

Ankle rotation
See relaxation 2 (chapter 4, page 105).

Pummelling
See relaxation 21 (chapter 4, page 111).

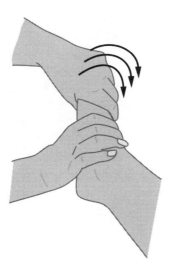

*Figure 5.32 Spinal
tweak and stretch*

Achilles tendon stretch
See relaxation 5 (chapter 4, page 106).

Shoulder/axillary areas (figure 5.33)
By making a fist of the support hand, the left hand knuckles to the lateral edge in a punching action; this can rotate any way and it provides an anchor. Now place the thumb of your right hand, your working hand, loosely in between the thumb and forefinger of the supporting hand, thus allowing a pincer action. If you hold it high enough this should enable you to reach over the top of the foot and work down between the third and fourth toes. As you come in line with the diaphragm line take your thumb out thus allowing you now to continue off to the outside edge in a slightly diagonal direction. Repeat this on toe 4 down the metatarsal, following the same line. Continue in between the fourth and fifth toes and then finally on the fifth toe down to the diaphragm line.

Shoulder muscle (figure 5.34)
Immediately change hands; the support is with the right hand for the right foot this time. The knuckles are in line with the base of the toes, and the working hand is your left index finger. Your left thumb is placed loosely in between the thumb and forefinger of the supporting hand, thus allowing a pincer action. Work the shoulder muscle reflex three times, from the lateral edge to the third toe.

Arm-related area
This reflex lies on the lateral aspect of the foot from the fifth meta-tarsal notch to the little toe. The support is the flat of your right

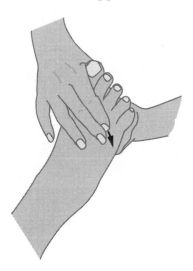

Figure 5.33 Working the shoulder and auxillary areas

hand, the palmar surface to the plantar area of the foot. With your hand apply slight pressure. You can move the foot into the required position encircling the foot in a caressing way; taking the foot towards the midline, work up the arm-related area at least three times.

Note. For all hand problems you are working on the feet, the cross reflex. Work the area that corresponds to the problem; also the nature of the nerve pathways is such that you should also work the cervical spine area for any problems of the upper appendicular limbs. (*See* figure 5.91a.)

Knee/elbow-related area

The support is from above with the right hand; this helps to expose the fifth metatarsal notch. This is a shared reflex, with the upper area serving the elbow and the lower area serving the knee. Using your index and second finger together, work above, on and below this reflex. Repeat and come back up, below, on the notch and above it, covering the area as shown in plate 2, Reflex zones of the feet.

Hip/leg-related area

This reflex is from the base of the heel to the fifth metatarsal notch on the lateral side. The support is the same as the arm-related area; the only difference is that you may need to elevate the foot slightly to make it more comfortable for yourself and your patient. Use the supporting hand to raise it marginally; the fingers of the working hand can add to this and then work the lateral aspect to cover the whole hip- and leg-related area.

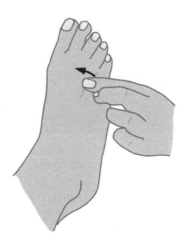

Figure 5.34 Working the shoulder muscle from the lateral aspect

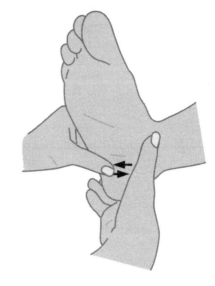

*Figure 5.35 Working
the main sciatic area;
work both ways*

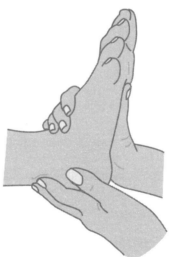

*Figure 5.36 Working
the chronic sciatic area
on the lateral edge*

Note. For all foot problems you work on the hands, the cross reflex. Work the area corresponding to the problem; also the nature of the nerve pathways is such that you should also work the lumbar and sacral spine for any problems of the lower appendicular limbs. (*See* figure 5.9.)

Main sciatic/base of heel

The sciatic nerve arises from the sacral plexus, passing round the buttocks and thigh to divide into two at the posterior portion of the knee. The peroneal nerve descends on the lateral side while the tibial nerve descends on the medial side; hence we can access it on both sides of the foot and leg. (*See* Chronic sciatic.) However, the medial side can be worked only if there are no contraindications (*see* chapter 3, page 96).

The support is the same as for the intestines, with the left hand cupping the heel, and the right thumb working from the medial to the lateral edge three times. Change hands and return from lateral to medial (figure 5.35).

Note.   One of the branches is the sural nerve, which supplies to all the tissue of the heel. This area is very tender if there is a sciatic problem.

Chronic sciatic – medial/lateral aspect (figure 5.36)

If there is any intense sciatic problem it can be worked from two reflexes. It is important to check the contraindication list as there are two acupoints that lie on these pathways: SP-6 and B-60. These can be used only if the person is not pregnant, as they are empirical points to promote delivery during labour.

Ankle loosening

See relaxation 13 (chapter 4, page 109).

Sweeping strokes

See relaxation 20 (chapter 4, page 110).

Now cover the right foot and commence on the left foot.

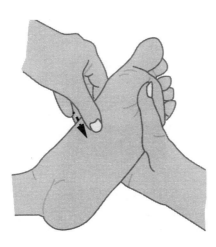

Figure 5.37 The pancreas being worked on the left foot zone 1, just above the waist line.

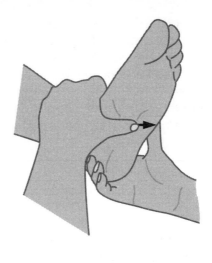

Figure 5.38 Working the splenic flexure: apply extra pressure on the lateral edge when on the descending colon on the lateral edge of foot. Also apply extra pressure on the splenic flexure.

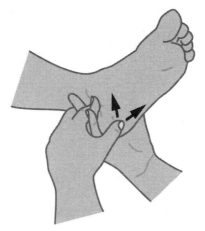

Figure 5.39 Working the sigmoid flexure; change hands to work medial edge.

The left foot

Repeat all the moves, changing support hands as required until heart. This is worked the same way as the right foot, but over a slightly larger area (*see* figure 5.13b); then continue until:

Stomach/spleen/pancreas (figure 5.37)

This is worked exactly the same as the liver area but note that there are three organs here. If you work in diagonals then change direction to pick up the pancreas. This is best worked in a horizontal strip one thumb-breadth above the waist. Work the right foot first zone 1, then zones 1–3 on the left foot, then tipping up slightly into zone 4 repeat three times. The spleen can be contacted as you do the diagonals but if there is any tenderness, work it with the right hand from zone 4 to 3 or rotate on the spot.

There is no reflex for the ileocaecal valve on the left foot, so you commence the intestinal area with the transverse colon.

Transverse/descending colon/small intestine/buttock areas

Working with your left thumb and from the medial edge to the lateral edge in horizontal strips, making as many passes as you can, carry on right down to the base of the heel. Apply slightly greater pressure as you come down the descending colon reflex, or apply pressure using your knuckle. Change hands and repeat the other way. Just to make sure you have contacted the splenic flexure and descending colon (figure 5.38), go back and apply pressure on the lateral plantar side of zone 5 with your left thumb in line with the fifth metatarsal notch, down to the heel line. If there is a tender spot then change direction or do circular rotations.

Sigmoid flexure (figure 5.39)

This is a salient reflex for all colon problems as it aids in defecation (the sigmoid flexure is the 'S'-shaped portion prior to the rectum). It can be worked with the right thumb. Coming down from the descending colon, work down into the midpoint

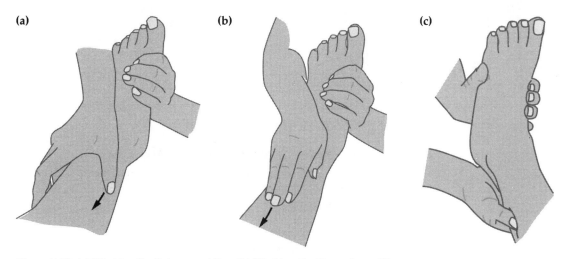

(a) (b) (c)

Figure 5.40 (a) Working the Spleen meridian. (b) Working the Stomach meridian between the tibia and fibula: you can also use your thumbs. (c) Working the Gall Bladder meridian and the nine terminating points of the Bladder meridian to BL-59: this is the same area as the chronic sciatic nerve.

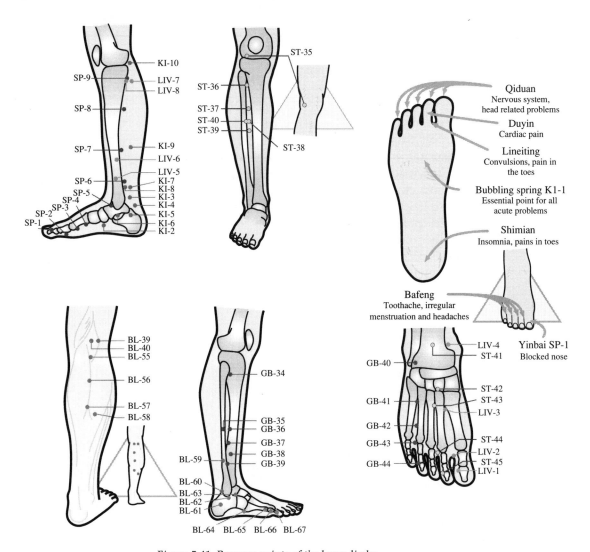

Figure 5.41 Pressure points of the lower limbs

Points of the Spleen channel of foot – Taiyin (SP)

SP-1.   Regulates blood from the nose, stomach, bladder and intestines. It also calms the mind. Relieves spasms in uterus.
On the medial side of the great toe at the base of the nail.

SP-2.   Promotes the digestion and helps general fatigue and agitation in children.
In the middle of the proximal phalange of the great toe.

SP-3.   Strengthens the spine and helps stomach problems, hernias, lung problems. It also helps upper, middle and lower burners and helps lumbar problems.
At the distal end of the first metatarsal joint.

SP-4. This is a very complex point. It helps regulate menstrual problems and is a very useful point in all excess patterns of the stomach or spleen. Cardiac inflammation.
At the proximal end of the first metatarsal joint.

SP-5. Very good for oedema of the abdomen, constipation and any spasms of low abdomen. Constipation, haemorrhoids, spasms in the calf.
In the depression anterior to the medial malleolus.

SP-6. *Vital point. DO NOT USE DURING PREGNANCY.*
The next most important point next to KI-1. It is a meeting point of all three Yin points. KI-8, known as the crossing point and LIV-5. These points will stop any lower abdominal pain, whatever the cause. SP-6 is a major point for all gynaecological complaints, but it also has a strong calming action of the mind.
Four finger-breadths above the medial malleolus posterior edge of tibia.

SP-7. This point helps flatulence and abdominal swelling, also all leg problems.
Eight finger-breadths above the medial malleolus.

SP-8. Lumbar problems. Painful menstruation.
Four finger-breadths below SP-9.

SP-9 All knee problems and urinary problems and oedema of the leg. All adominal pain.
In the depression below the head of the head of the tibia.

Points of Liver channel of foot – Jeuyin (LIV)

LIV-1. All menstrual problems. This point acts on the lower burner and helps bladder problems, constipation and also helps lumbar area.
On the lateral side of the great toe at the base of the nail bed.

LIV-2. Mainly head areas. Secondary genitals, allays insomnia and toothache. Genitourinary tract and palpitations.
In the web between the first and second toes.

LIV-3. Migraines, hypertension, mental calming point, cramp, also helps upper and lower abdominal areas.
Furthest proximal point between the first and second metatarsals.

LIV-4. Genital problems, cystitis, any paralysis.
In the depression, medial side of the crease of ankle.

LIV-5. Genitourinary problems, also colic and spasms of abdomen.
On the medial side of leg. Six finger-breadths above medial malleolus, on the midline of the tibia.

LIV-6. Knee problems and useful point for extreme pain in cystitis.
On the medial side of leg. Nine finger-breadths above medial malleolus, on the midline of the tibia.

LIV-7. Known as the Knee gate, so will help all knee problems.
Almost in line with SP-9. Slightly posterior aspect.

LIV-8. This major point will help all four limbs, all vaginal problems, discharge, pruritis, and abdominal pain.
On the medial side of leg just below SP-9 and in line with LIV-7.

Points of the Urinary Bladder channel of foot – Taiyang (BL)

BL-67. Headaches, vertigo, it is also used as a major point for malposition of the fetus in the eighth month of pregnancy. Paralysis or arthritis of foot.
On the lateral side of the little toe just below nail bed.

BL-66. Bladder problems, major point for stiff neck, headaches and uterine congestion.
On the proximal phalange of the little toe.

BL-65. Headaches, vertigo, good point for releasing necks, torticollis.
On the distal end of the fifth metatarsal joint.

BL-64. All lumbar problems, helps the bladder and calms the mind, cerebral congestion.
Just below the tuberosity of the fifth metatarsal joint.

BL-63. All pelvic problems, bladder and abdominal pain, knee problems.
On the lateral side of the foot just below the external malleolus on the proximal border of the cuboid bone.

BL-62. Major point for movement in lower back. Relaxes all tendons of legs.
In the depression immediately below the tip of the external malleolus.

BL-61. All leg problems.
On the lateral side of the calcaneum, at the point where red and white skin meet in the longitudinal line of BL-60.

BL-60. *Vital point. DO NOT USE DURING PREGNANCY but may be used during labour.* All backache, shoulder, neck and head problems. Sciatica, ankle and leg problems, placental retention.
On the posterior edge of the lip of the external malleolus.

BL-59. Lumbar and thigh problems, muscular and nerve problems of leg.
Four finger-breadths above the external malleolus on the tibia.

BL-58. Helps kidneys and lower leg problems.
Nine finger-breadths above the external malleolus on the tibia.

BL-57. Backache, low lumbar area. Sciatica and leg problems.
On the midline on the gastrocnemius muscle in the pointed depression.

BL-56. Lumbar problems, cramps.
Exactly six finger-breadths below popliteal crease, on the midpoint.

BL-55. As above and knee.
Roughly two finger-breadths below popliteal crease on the midpoint, above BL-56.

BL-40. Lumbago, leg problems, sciatica.
Midpoint of transverse crease of popliteal.

BL-39. Cystitis, and constipation.
Midpoint of transverse crease.

The Kidney channel of foot – Shaoyin (KI)

KI-1. Any acute problems, cardiac, palpitations, vertigo, sterility in females.
To restore consciousness. Prolapse uterus.
On the plantar aspect of the foot between zones 2 and 3. Plantar flex the foot and the point is just below red skin.

KI-2.   Cystitis, all uterus problems, orchitis, sterility, prolapse, dysmenorrhoea, incontinence of urine.
On the medial aspect of foot, just below the tuberosity of the navicular bone.

KI-3.   Helps kidneys, lower back, knees, regulates uterus.
Behind the medial malleolus in the depression.

KI-4.   Uterine spasms, helps and strengthens the back.
On the medial aspect of the foot behind medial malleolus and anterior to the Achilles tendon.

KI-5.   All menstrual problems, helps regulate uterus.
On the medial aspect of the foot immediately below KI-3.

KI-6.   Promotes function of uterus and any fluid problems, dryness in throat or eyes.
In the depression just below the tip of the medial malleolus.

KI-7.   Helps all oedema. Relieves pain and strengthens lower back.
On the medial aspect of the leg, directly above KI-3.

KI-8.   Regulates all menstrual problems and abdominal pain. Dissolves any masses.
Almost in line with SP-6, between the tibia and Achilles tendon.

KI-9.   Extreme calming point, relaxes chest area and relieves palpitations.
Six finger-breadths above and in line with KI-3.

KI-10. Similar action to KI-8, SP-9 and LIV-8.
On the medial aspect of the popliteal crease, press when patient's knee is flexed.

Points of the Stomach channel of foot – Yangming (ST)

ST-45. Known as the sick mouth, all mouth problems, tonsillitis and gingivitis.
On the lateral side of the second toe at the base of nail bed.

ST-44. Lower jaw paralysis, trigeminal neuralgia, facial problems.
Just below web between second and third toes.

ST-43. Hernia, flatulence. Fevers and night sweats.
Lies on the medial side of third metatarsal in the depression between second and third metatarsals.

ST-42. Anorexia, stimulates stomach and spleen. Arthritis of the foot.
On the dorsal aspect of foot on instep where dorsalis pedis pulse is palpable.

ST-41. Constipation, headaches, rheumatism. Helps all joints especially ankles.
It is known as the dispersing stream.
In the depression midpoint of the dorsal crease of the ankle.

ST-40. Known as the abundant bridge it is next to ST-38. It aids the removal of lumps in the thyroid and uterus areas. Also a helpful point for asthma as it eliminates phlegm.

Lies on the lateral side of the tibia ten finger-breadths approx above the external malleolus. A connecting point.

ST-39. Regulates stomach and intestines, relieving any abdominal spasms.
Nine finger-breadths above external malleolus on lateral side.

ST-38. Helps shoulder problems, when moving shoulder and pressing point at same time.
Six finger-breadths below the knee, lateral side of tibia.

ST-37. A good point for large intestine and very good for chronic diarrhoea.
Aids lumbar and leg problems.
Five finger-breadths below the knee, lateral side of tibia.

ST-36. This is a major point to strengthen the whole body and for all abdominal problems. *NOT TO BE USED ON YOUNG CHILDREN.*
Four finger-breadths below the knee, lateral side of tibia.

ST-35. Stomach problems, gastritis, diarrhoea.
On lateral edge of patella.

Points of the Gall Bladder channel of foot – Shaoyang (GB)

GB-44. Alleviates headaches. Aids problems relating to eyes, ears, mouth, breast and lung areas.
On the lateral side of the fourth toe at the base of the nail bed.

GB-43. Helpful in migraine and tinnitus disorders. Aids axillary areas, arms and breast.
In the depression between the fourth and fifth metatarsals middle of proximal phalange.

GB-42. Mastitis and all axillary area. Any pain in dorsum of foot.
Distal end of fourth metatarsal on lateral edge.

GB-41. Important point helpful in relieving pain in the whole body.
In the depression between fourth and fifth metatarsals on medial edge of fifth metatarsal.

GB-40. Sciatica, leg and ankle problems. Pelvic disorders.
In the depression lateral to the tendon of the toes, in front of external malleolus.

GB-39. Weakness of limbs.
Four finger-breadths above the external malleolus.

GB-38. Lumbar problems and knee disorders, or any numbness in lower extremities.
Five finger-breadths above the external malleolus on lateral side of tibia.

GB-37. Leg problems, especially calf muscle and ankle weakness.
Six finger-breadths above the external malleolus on the lateral side of tibia.

GB-36. Leg and ankle problems.
Nine finger-breadths above the external malleolus on lateral side of tibia.

GB-35. Leg problems and sciatica, particularly on fibula.
Nine finger-breadths above the external malleolus on the lateral side of fibula.

GB-34. Knee problems, chronic constipation, sciatica.
In the depression on lateral side of leg, just below the head of the fibula.

of the heel then up to the rectum point. This forms a 'V'. If it is more comfortable you can work from the midpoint to the lateral edge. Change hands and work to the medial edge, again forming a 'V'. (*See* figure 5.39.)

All the other reflexes are covered exactly like the right foot. Just change support hands accordingly. If there are tender areas go back and gently work them again in a different direction.

Remove the towel from the feet. Complete with relaxation techniques 20, 23 and 24 (chapter 4, pages 110–12) as the foot should now be completely flexible. If you do not wish to massage the feet and legs finish off the session.

Optional extra massage of feet and legs

This is an ideal time to work the meridians as you massage. (If it is not convenient to apply cream because the client has tight trousers or does not wish to remove the relevant clothing, you can apply pressure through the clothes.) After applying a small amount of cream, use circular friction up the plantar tendon, and over the whole plantar surface of the feet. Carry on this circular movement in between all the metatarsals and on them, especially in the depression of the crease of the midankle. This is ST-41, a good point for any oedema. Use the knuckles to work gently around the depressions distal to the medial and lateral malleolus. Then, using the knuckles in sweeping strokes, commence up and down the spinal reflex, which is also the Spleen meridian. Also work the lateral aspect of the foot. (*See* chapter 4, pages 104–13.) You should now have contacted all the acupoints on the foot of the six leg meridians. You can now commence up the legs to the knees (figure 5.40).

Note. These are vital and potent acupuncture areas. Check contraindications (chapter 3, page 95) to make sure it is safe to continue working if your client is female. SP-6 and B-60 can be used only if the person is not pregnant, as they are empirical points to promote delivery during labour. If the person is menstruating it is also not advisable to work this point unless the person is aware that it creates a natural free flow of blood; sometimes this can alarm the person if they are not prepared for this.

When massaging, the client does not need to be face down. Massage also helps the lymphatic system by aiding the dispersal of any excess fluid that remains, which could cause oedema. The general blood flow and the whole circulation of the body are enhanced. Think of making three lines up the medial side of the leg on the tibia and posterior to the tibia with firm sweeping strokes. Use friction strokes over the fleshy part; this is best achieved with your hand under the client's leg, thumbs on the medial side. Now, using one or both thumbs, or finger, work from the ankle making a pass up between the tibia (the shin bone) and the fibula (the outer bone) to the point where you cannot pass any further. At the lateral side of the tuberosity of the tibia in the depression lies ST-36; this major point strengthens the whole body. However, it is not thought suitable for use until after the teenage years are over. In the elderly or infirm it helps to normalize functions. On the lateral side of the leg, again using sweeping strokes, work right up to the knee point between the lateral tibia and the fibula, applying pressure with your thumbs as you sweep up the shin bone. The last meridian changes course from just below the calf where it then runs up right between the gastrocnemius to the popliteal fossa; this area on the calf will aid all lower back disorders, so even if you cannot finish on a massage, with the leg bent gently apply pressure through any clothing using your three fingers of either hand. For direct treatment of any acupoint use firm unmoving pressure to suit the patient's tolerance levels for at least 30 seconds. (*See* figure 5.40a, b and c.)

Finish with some metatarsal flexing (*see* relaxation 22, chapter 4, page 109).

Solar plexus rotation
See relaxation 23, (chapter 4, page 111–112).

Solar plexus breathing
See relaxation 24 (chapter 4, pages 111–12).

Metatarsal kneading and foot moulding can be used at any time together with any other relaxation technique and stretching exercises.

Details of the foot and leg meridians and acupoints are shown in figure 5.41.

Foot exercises

1 Shake the feet; rotate the ankles both ways.
2 Wriggle and stretch your toes, fanning and separating them as much as possible (figure 5.42).
3 Extend the great toe as much as possible, pointing the toe then dorsiflexing it (figure 5.43).

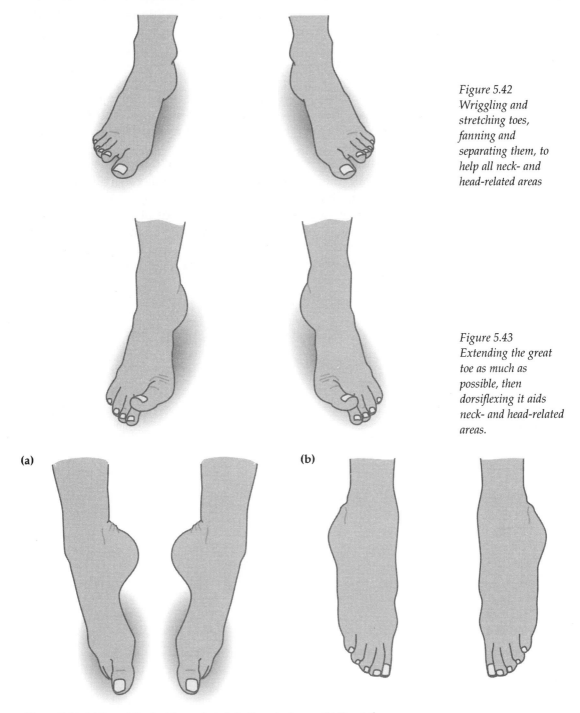

Figure 5.42 Wriggling and stretching toes, fanning and separating them, to help all neck- and head-related areas

Figure 5.43 Extending the great toe as much as possible, then dorsiflexing it aids neck- and head-related areas.

(a) **(b)**

Figure 5.44 (a) Invert the foot inwards to help the spinal area. (b) Evert the foot outwards to help hip, knee and shoulder problems.

4 Invert the feet (figure 5.44a), then evert the feet (figure 5.44b). (Do this exercise while sitting down.)
5 Walk on the balls of the feet; this aids the lungs and is very good for asthmatics.
6 Walk on the heels; this aids the lower back.
7 Apply pressure on the top of your foot by placing one foot on top of the other. Press the top one down and pull the bottom one up; this is very good for the spine and legs and also aids the lung area.
8 Try and pick up a pencil with your toes (figure 5.45).
9 Place a ball or other round object under your feet and roll it the length of the foot (figure 5.46); repeat two or three times.
10 For tired legs and feet, whilst in a comfortable sitting position, place a twisted towel under the arch of the foot. Holding both ends pull gently, straightening the leg and lifting (figure 5.47). This helps to stretch the Achilles tendon gently.

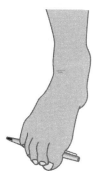

Figure 5.46 Place a round ball or other round object under your foot and roll it the length of your foot several times. This works all the organs at once.

Figure 5.45 Pick up a pencil to aid the lungs and shoulder areas.

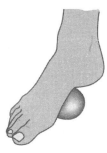

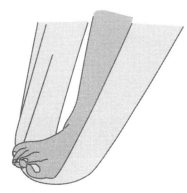

Figure 5.47 For tired aching legs, place a twisted towel under the arch of your foot; pull gently whilst straightening the legs.

6　The hands

Our hands are of the utmost importance in touching and sensing. They are also a most wonderful form of making contact and communicating with each other. Healing touch has been used for centuries. Perhaps that is why the hands are so forceful in the healing process, whether using hand reflexology, acupuncture, acupressure, or another method. Or is the effect explained by the large area the hands occupy in the brain (*see* figure 2.1, page 34)? Whatever the reason, hand reflexology has a powerful effect on the emotions, and because of its simplicity everyone enjoys this treatment and finds it very pleasant and relaxing. It is a convenient and quick method of influencing someone's inner energies and emotions, through the many nerve pathways.

History and theory of hand treatment

Old Chinese writings spoke of a pressure therapy being used and exercises that involved just wringing the hands or rubbing them together to benefit the body in general. Putting the fingertips together would be considered stimulating to the brain; it also contacts some of the meridians on the hands. It is quite instinctive that when we are cold we rub our hands together, and one point that would be crossed when doing this is for invigorating the blood, so this would warm us; this point is also used for whooping cough and digestive disorders. One of the other points contacted is for headaches, or toothache. In fact most areas of the hands when rubbed or palpated would benefit most disorders from sore throats, epilepsy, some mental disorders, all digestive problems, deafness, tinnitus, to arthritis of the hands. Hand acupressure and hand analysis also go back many thousands of years. The Chinese developed hand analysis, but in the latter years it engendered a certain amount of superstitious practice known as palmistry.

The practice of hand reflexology itself goes back 90 years. The modern-day authority on hands was Dr William Fitzgerald. In the early years he worked mainly on the hands, and only later with the feet, but the latter became very popular, and over the years hand reflexology became ignored and used very little. This chapter aims to show that hand reflexology is a powerful tool and should be used far more than it is at present, as it has many powerful points and is particularly invaluable for self-help and first-aid situations.

In his book on zone therapy in 1917, Fitzgerald spoke about working on the palmar surface of the hand for any pains in the back of the body, and working on the dorsum and the top surface of the fingers for any problems on the anterior part of the body. The distal joints were squeezed, then the medial, and then the proximal joints by clasping the hands. Fitzgerald said he could cure lumbago with a comb; his advice was to press its teeth in the base of the palm beneath the second and third fingers. He related the story of Signor Umberto Sorrentino, a noted tenor, who claimed to relieve tightness in his throat by squeezing the lateral aspect of his forefinger and the thumb, as these points helped and governed the vocal cords. Another remarkable hand point that Fitzgerald found was for helping morning sickness in pregnancy, or for stomach upset generally; this was working the first and second zones on the backs of the hands with deep pressure, also the palmar surface of the wrist and forearm (which corresponds with a well-known acupoint). He spoke further of finger squeezing for eye and ear troubles. Thyroid problems were also helped, he said, by pressing upon the joints of the thumb, first and second fingers. In modern-day reflexology these vital zones should not be ignored, as we should embrace both old and new reflexes, as well as the meridians and the acupoints.

Anatomy and physiology

The hands are a highly developed piece of machinery; they have the ability to grasp and manipulate with marvellous dexterity. The bone structure of the hand follows the same basic pattern as that of the foot. It comprises 8 carpal bones forming the wrist, 5 meta-carpals forming the palm and the dorsum and also 14 phalanges (the individual bones that make up the fingers and toes). There are 2 of these in the thumb, a distal and a proximal, and 3 in each other digit, a distal, a medial and proximal phalange. In total the hand contains 27 bones, as well as 38 muscles, 20 tendons, and over 40 ligaments and thousands of nerve endings (including Meissner's corpuscles, Pacini's corpuscles, Ruffini's corpuscles: all pressure receptors).

Tendons and ligaments of the hand

Wrapped around each bone are many muscles and tendons, nerves and blood vessels. The hands have 12 very strong tendons, which stretch from the muscles of the forearms to the front and back of the wrist. Nine of these pass down to the digits, forming around the joints just like a hand-stitched glove. The synovial fluid-filled tendon sheaths particularly enclose the flexor tendons at the wrist, where they help to minimize friction and facilitate movement.

Two very strong ligaments in the wrist form a band of tissue, just like a wristband. They surround all the nerves, blood vessels and tendons, keeping them in place as they pass through the wrist area. They are named the flexor retinaculum on the palmar side and the extensor retinaculum on the dorsum side. Nerve entrapment is common in this area (*see* Carpal tunnel syndrome, page 197).

Muscles of the hand

For the reflexologist the hand is always in the same position as the feet, palmar surface facing to the posterior aspect, just like the plantar surface of the foot, with the dorsum reflexes to the back of the hand and upper surface of the foot. The chief muscles of the hand, fingers and forearm are the extensors and flexors; these allow bending and straightening of the fingers. There is also a supinator and pronator of the forearm and hand. Many of the arm muscles originate in the scapula (shoulder blade) or humerus (upper arm bone) and insert into the radius or ulnar (forearm bones). The muscles on the palmar aspect of the hand and forearm are flexors and muscles on the dorsum surface are extensors; this is the same arrangement as the muscles of the legs. The intrinsic muscles give the finger and thumb joints flexion, extension, abduction, adduction and opposition. The opponens are a group of muscles, the opponens digit minima (fifth digit) and opponens pollices (attached to the thumb joint), that bring these digits opposite to each other in to the palm of the hand, giving flexion, abduction, opposition between the thumb and the little finger, allowing the complex grasping action.

The thenar muscles are the bulging mass of muscles and related tissue at the base of the thumb and lateral aspect of hand, forming the thenar and hypothenar eminence (specifically, the abductors, the flexors, and the opponens), each complementary to the other, allowing the aforementioned action and other functions. The lumbricales are four small muscles in each hand, of which the first and second originate from the lateral sides and the palmar surface of the flexor digitorum tendons to the index and middle finger, and the medial two originate from the adjacent side of these tendons in the other half of the middle finger, ring finger and little fingers. These muscles, together with the palmar and dorsal interossei muscles, give the hand its strength.

Blood supply to the hand

The palmar surface contains the palmar arch; this branches to form the superficial palmar arch and the digital arteries, supplying all fingers with a fine blood capillary network at the tips (figure 6.1). Wherever there is an artery there is a vein. The venous palmar arch drains the used blood from the fingers into the radial, ulnar and median veins together with other smaller veins. These all drain into the axillary vein, which in turn empties into the subclavian vein, then into the innominate vein and at the junction of both innominate veins from each limb is the superior vena cava, returning all the blood from the arms, neck, thorax and head to the right atrium of the heart (*see* chapter 5, figure 5.10, page 156).

As there is so little room in the hand for a large arrangement of blood vessels it is the rich extensive network of capillaries that varies the flow of blood. This is why on cold days the fingers often cool quicker than other parts of the extremities.

Nerve supply to the hand and arm

The nerve supply to the hand and forearm is supplied by the radial, ulnar and median nerves (figure 6.1). The radial nerve is the chief nerve arising from the spinal segment C5–C8 supplying the extensor aspects of the upper limbs. In the arm it supplies the heads of the triceps, the anconeus (behind the elbow), the brachioradialis and the extensor digitorum. It winds itself around the humerus and lateral side of the cubital fossa where it separates into the deep and superficial radial nerve. The median nerve, the major nerve from segment C5–T1, gives flexion to the forearm and hand. It arises as two routes from the brachial plexus (the network of nerves that arises from the spine and supplies the arm, the forearm, hand and parts of the shoulder) and passes deep between the furrow of the cubital fossa; then it descends deeply to

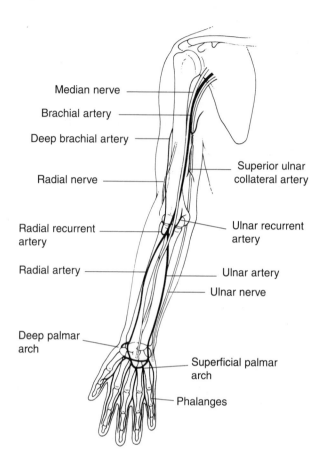

Median nerve

Brachial artery

Deep brachial artery

Radial nerve

Superior ulnar
collateral artery

Radial recurrent
artery

Ulnar recurrent
artery

Radial artery

Ulnar artery

Ulnar nerve

Deep palmar
arch

Superficial palmar
arch

Phalanges

*Figure 6.1 The nerves
and blood vessels of the
arm*

the flexor digitorum and the flexor retinaculum, finally dividing into the palmar digital nerves. The ulnar nerve is a mixed peripheral nerve that also arises from the brachial plexus. It originates from segment C8–T1 and reaches the wrist along the medial surface of the forearm. Its branches are articular, muscular, palmar and cutaneous. It distributes mainly to the skin on the dorsal and palmar surface of the medial portion of the hand, and also supplies some flexor muscles in the forearm. The lateral cutaneous nerve, which arises from segment C5–C6, reaches as far down as the thenar eminence, the muscle beneath the thumb.

We can see from the above that any problems in the upper arm, forearm, wrist, hands and also the fingers are all governed by the cervical nerves and the first dorsal nerve. This shows once again that peripheral nerve innervation of the bones closely follows muscle innervation, the bones being innervated by the same nerves that supply the muscle attached to that bone. This allows us to work the cervical reflexes to benefit the arm, elbow or hand (*see* figure 5.9a, page 153).

The skin on both palmar and dorsal surfaces of the hand is very richly supplied with thousands of sensory receptors that provide information on pain, touch, pressure and heat. In particular, in the fingertips are found a great concentration of sensitive nerve endings, the Meissner corpuscles (see chapter 2, page 35), which lie in groups in the dermal papillae around the hair follicles, each tiny corpuscle being served by several nerves and each nerve serving several corpuscles, thus always spreading any sensations. As we know from the experience of touch, our hands are one of the most highly sensitive areas of the body.

Observation and analysis

Hands

Just as with the foot, we can analyse the hand. By observing the hands closely we get some indication of the patient's imbalances. Hand analysis has been practised by many ancient people far back into history, the most important examples being the Chinese and the Indians. The modern-day finger analysis techniques are known as dermatoglyphics; these are used by doctors, anthropologists and often used in criminology. The ridges and patterns of the thumbs, fingers, palms, toes and soles of the feet are studied for genetic and other abnormalities.

In Chinese hand analysis, the length and size of the fingers are looked at as these often indicate the person's characteristic traits, such as how they express themselves, their creativity, how they communicate with others, whether they can accept responsibility or not; as these were not totally conclusive this practice was discontinued, and in later years, as previously stated, this analysis became more associated with early palmistry.

Each person's hand is individual and unique, and, just like the feet, each shows a similarity to the corresponding part of the body (*see* plates 3 and 4).

The hand should have a healthy colour to it. The skin should not appear dry or lack sheen; if it exhibits a shrivelled impression, if it is scaly and dry, this often indicates that there is a lack of body fluids (*see* plate 13). The moisture and texture of the skin are of the utmost importance. Sweating can be assessed by lightly rubbing the fingers over the skin on the dorsal and on the palmar surface to detect the presence of moisture. It should not be too moist – excess sweating of the palms is symptomatic of a deficiency of the energy in the lungs, or a nervous imbalance. If the tissue around the wrist is reasonably firm this is a good sign that the fluids of the body are in abundant supply and the circulation is good.

If the hands feel cold to the touch it may indicate a stomach imbalance. If there is a bluish colour to the thenar eminence this is even more indicative of cold in the stomach. If this is accompanied by pain in the abdomen, then diet may be one of the main causes, and this must then be analysed from many aspects, such as the type of food, regularity of eating, conditions of eating, all of which give some insight into the cause.

Erythema in the palm of the hand may indicate an imbalance in the liver. It is advisable to check for the following: does the person suffer from constipation, do they have red eyes, do they have a thirst and the desire to drink a lot of cold water? All of these symptoms are indicative of interior heat, due to the lack of movement and undue retention of faeces. The palm of the hand reflects the state of the internal organs, so it is important to look very closely at all points on the palm. Warm pink palms show a good circulation and usually a good metabolism. Cold palms often suggest a sluggish circulation; the person may be a smoker. Always check case history details to gain as much information as you can.

Rings on fingers can often block energies if the rings are too tight. Vertical ridge patterns on the skin of the fingers indicate there may be blocked energies (these are other than the normal creases and folds; *see* plate 14); these ridges or lines are not conclusive but they help in the overall assessment of the person. Heavy vertical lines indicate excess energy being used; this may result in debilitation and fatigue. Transverse lines indicate energy blocks in that zone manifesting as head-related problems, which may be anything from anxiety states to palpitations, neck strain, eye disorders, and nose, throat and breathing problems. The fingertips are also important to observe. A good colour indicates a good circulation. Poor colour could indicate poor nerve and blood supply (*see* plate 13).

Finally, any distortions in the shape or position of the hand or digits should be noted. They can be noticeable in chronic disorders such as arthritis and myasthenia gravis (*see* plates 14 and 15).

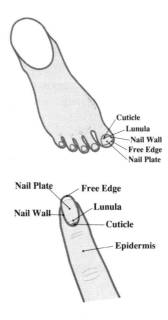

Figure 6.2 The structure of the nail

Nails

The nail (unguis) is the horny keratin structure that covers the dorsal aspect of the distal phalange of each digit. Figure 6.2 shows how nails are constructed.

We examine nails to help in differential diagnosis. A nail free from any disorder should be pink and healthy without striations, or lines, and should be free of any fungal infection. The main points to look at are:

- colour – this gives an indication of the general circulation; blanching may point to anaemia, while blue or purple nails show a lack of oxygen. The moons of the nails often represent the state and health of the heart.
- marks and surface appearance – flecks and ridges are indicative of some trauma, ill health or emotional disorder. Beau's line, a superficial transverse depression appears on the nail plate about a month after any acute illness. If there is an acute illness with a fever this can cause an irregularity in growth often producing a slight transverse groove; this is not so evident as the Beau's line but as the nail grows this groove moves onwards towards the distal end. A fingernail takes between 6 and 9 months to renew itself completely, so measuring the position of the groove can give a good indication of when the problem occurred.
- moisture content – if the nails are moist and healthy-looking, according to TCM this shows that the Liver Blood is in

abundance; if they are dry, indented or cracked this indicates that the Liver Blood is deficient. Brittle nails may point to poor peripheral circulation to the hand in general, if all nails are involved; if one nail is brittle it could be the local circulation to that finger.

- For more specific indications, *see* nail disorders, figure 6.3.

Disorders

Hands

Peripheral nerve lesions of the median or ulnar nerves may lead to eczema or hyperkeratosis of the skin, also the fingernails take on a clubbed appearance, often developing transverse white lines and in some cases becoming thick and brittle.

Trigger finger is an annoying problem in which as a person straightens their finger there is sometimes a snapping sound, or the finger may refuse to straighten. Often the cause is obscure, but stimulation to the cervical reflexes and the channel points will help the problem.

Carpal tunnel syndrome is caused by compression of the median nerve as it enters the palm of the hand. This whole area is a mass of structures, and the carpal tunnel is the space between the carpal bones, which is bound by the transverse ligament above and surrounded by the bony carpus, with the median nerve contained within it. This syndrome can be quite common in women between the ages of 40 and 60 years. Pain can be quite debilitating, often involving the index and middle fingers; intermittent numbness is accompanied by muscle weakness. This may be linked with repetitive strain injury, or prolonged wrist flexion. If the use of the hand deteriorates over a short period it could point to some degeneration taking place in the brain, as in the case of a stroke, in which the hand often suffers more than the leg or face. Digital nerve entrapment is not very common; often if a trauma arises it is linked to occupational factors, such as repetitive strain injury. In other cases it may be due to arthritis of the joints, where osteocytes become embedded in the bone matrix, causing swelling and inflammation. Most arthritic sufferers who receive reflexology state that their joints are less painful and they feel as if the joints have been greased, allowing more flexibility and movement.

Drop wrist occurs when the muscles that raise the wrist become paralysed because of damage to the radian nerve. This is relieved by working the cervical areas for the brachial plexus, which contains the median, ulnar and radial nerves.

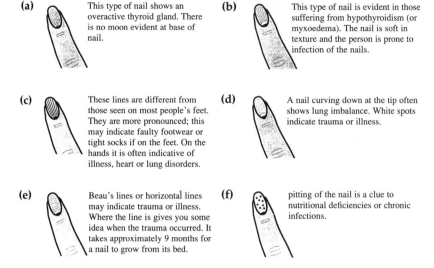

(a) This type of nail shows an overactive thyroid gland. There is no moon evident at base of nail.

(b) This type of nail is evident in those suffering from hypothyroidism (or myxoedema). The nail is soft in texture and the person is prone to infection of the nails.

(c) These lines are different from those seen on most people's feet. They are more pronounced; this may indicate faulty footwear or tight socks if on the feet. On the hands it is often indicative of illness, heart or lung disorders.

(d) A nail curving down at the tip often shows lung imbalance. White spots indicate trauma or illness.

(e) Beau's lines or horizontal lines may indicate trauma or illness. Where the line is gives you some idea when the trauma occurred. It takes approximately 9 months for a nail to grow from its bed.

(f) pitting of the nail is a clue to nutritional deficiencies or chronic infections.

Figure 6.3 (a–f) Nail problems

Dupuytren's contracture is permanent bending of the fingers because of fixation of the flexor tendons; in its early stages it can be treated with reflexology.

Deformities

The hand is subject to the same abnormalities as the feet. The terms are self-explanatory: claw hand, lobster hand, preacher's hand, etc. These can be caused by nerve or muscle damage.

Nails

Over the years, research has found that many endocrine disorders and glandular problems are shown in a malfunction of the growth of the fingernail. Just as in the foot, a normal healthy pink nail when pressed should have a quick return of colour. Figure 6.3 shows some nail defects.

The main signs are:

- Very ridged and fanning lines on nails – often indicate an overactive thyroid or myxoedema (figure 6.3a and b).
- Vertical ridges – may indicate shock or trauma (figure 6.3c).
- Horizontal ridges – may indicate acidity. Beau's lines (lots of ridged lines) often are related to a respiratory disorder (figure 6.3e).
- Pitted nails – indicate a skin disorder, either eczema or psoriasis (figure 6.3f).
- Concave nails – may indicate physical tension.

- Nails that curl at the base – often indicate lung problems (figure 6.3d and plate 14).
- Hippocratic nails (fingernails and toenails take on an exaggerated curvature) – often evident in people who have a respiratory disorder or a thyroid imbalance (*see* plate 14).
- Very arched and narrow nails – often indicate a serious lumbar problem (*see* plate 14).
- Malformed nails – often indicate a homeostatic imbalance in the pituitary function.
- Spoon-shaped or concaved nails – may indicate iron deficiency.
- White spots – may indicate weak constitution, or trauma (figure 6.3d).
- Very white nails – indicate a systemic disorder.
- Pale blue, eggshell-like, almost transparent nails – vitamin A deficiency.
- Blue or purple nails – often indicate poor circulation.
- Slightly detached and yellow nails – can be an infection (onchyomycosis).

Bacterial or fungus infections

The fingernails are subject to relatively few disorders, but they are prone to infection. If they are rough or disfigured in any way it could be caused by mycosis, a disorder caused by fungi, usually a form of ringworm. Candidiasis is found in the cutaneous areas, especially in moist sites between the fingers. Tinea unguium invades the nailplate, the keratinized tissues being particularly prone. This may also be an indication that there is an immune deficiency state. Reflexology has a direct influence on the body by increasing and strengthening the immune response. It is imperative to practise sound principles of health and hygiene to prevent cross infection.

Treatment procedure

Acupuncture is widely used on the hands in China. Those points between the fingertips and the elbow, and between the tips of the toes and the knee, are considered the most dominant and powerful points (*see* chapter 2).

The hand is also a common choice for acupressure and shiatsu from Japan, which is closely associated with acupressure. Both use fingertip pressure on specific points; however, in shiatsu the techniques often involve also the use of thumbs, palms, knees, feet; it also incorporates stretching techniques. Reflexology works in a similar fashion, but is less invasive and equally potent.

A full treatment session should be given to the hand at all times. Additional reflex points are also useful, however. These reflexes help a variety of disorders as extra target reflexes worked for specific problems and disorders; they can also be used for self-treatment and quick first aid, and are detailed after the treatment.

The hand sequence below is not a massage. Massages are often completed in 5–6 minutes per hand and forearm, and mainly consist of stroking and kneading movements.

Treatment sequence

Right hand

1 Stroke the right hand, with the left hand supporting. Work with your right hand pushing down into the palm of the hand and up to the wrist. Draw the hand back up to the thumb area.

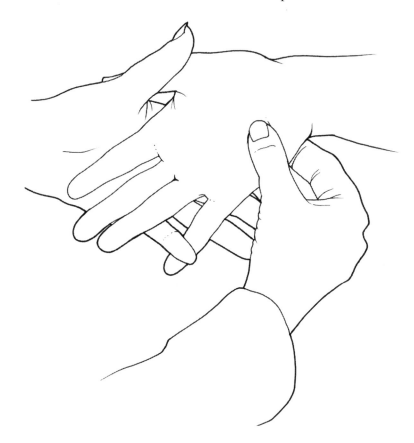

Figure 6.4 Sequence 2: applying deep pressure using circular rotational movements. Making sure that the hand is well supported, create deep pressure by applying palpation over the whole palmar surface.

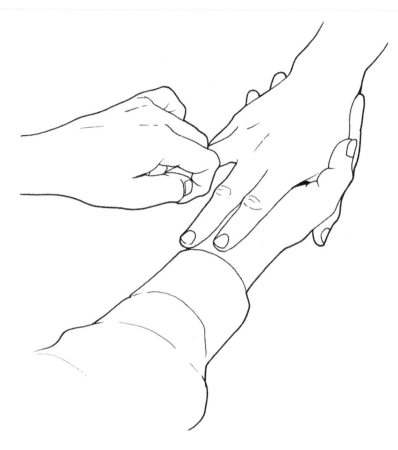

Figure 6.5 Sequence 6: using knuckles to stretch fingers and thumbs

Repeat this several times. (This helps to increase the blood flow and aids dispersal of any swelling due to oedema.)

2 Using deeper pressure and both thumbs (with the patient's palm facing upwards) make small circular movements over whole palmar surface and base of thumb (figure 6.4). This helps to improve the suppleness of the skin.

3 Support the hand as if you were going to shake hands, with your right hand to their right hand. With the hand of patient in the palm-down position, working from little finger side, pull each finger to stretch it. Apply only gentle traction, pulling along the whole length of the finger (*see* figure 6.5). Then rotate each finger, first one way and then the other. Work from the lateral edge of little finger to thumb on medial edge.

4 Return from the medial edge starting with thumb; this time, using firm pressure with the finger or thumb (whichever digit is most comfortable), palpate over whole area, covering the dorsal and palmar surface of each digit. Also cover the medial and

lateral side of each digit, going right down into webs, especially between the index finger and thumb and into the medial edge of thumb, following the line of the bone.

Note. Do not apply great pressure in the thumb web if the person is pregnant.

5 With the knuckle of the index finger, work on Shixuan points, supporting the fingers well (figure 6.8).
6 Return to the shaking hands position and, starting at little finger side, make a fist with your left hand and grip the patient's fingers between your knuckles at the proximal phalange. Pull each in turn up towards the distal joint, working from the lateral edge to the medial edge (figure 6.5).
7 Now, using both index fingers either side of the patient's fingers, rotate first on the eye reflex on the second digit, distal joint, and then on the ear reflex point on the third digit, dorsal joint (*see* plate 3).
8 Repeat this on the proximal interphalangeal joint palmar

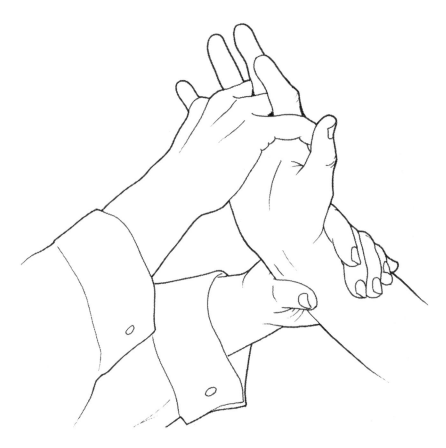

Figure 6.6 Sequence 10: palmarflexion and dorsiflexion. This movement will release any tension in the wrists.

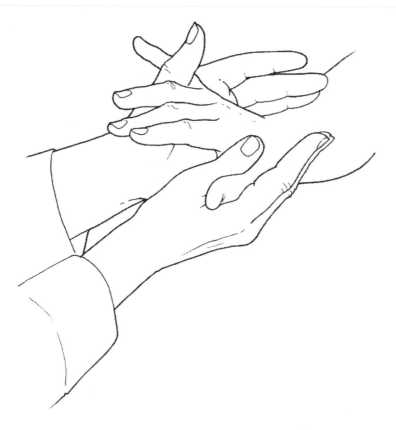

Figure 6.7 Sequence 13: stimulating blood flow. This action will stimulate blood flow to the muscles and ligaments of the hand.

surface only, but exclude the thumb (Sifeng points, on the four cracks of the knuckles). This helps to promote digestion.

9 Supporting the patient's right hand with your left hand palm upwards, work over the lung area (*see* plate 3). Work both ways, changing the support when needed. This is an important area as it aids the circulation and promotes relaxation.

10 Interlock your fingers with the patient's, palms together, right hand to right hand (figure 6.6). Your left hand supports the forearm. Do palmarflexion of the wrist then extend the wrist backwards. Repeat this two to three umes and then rotate the wrist, first to the medial edge then to the lateral edge. This loosens any adherent tissue and will soften and stretch the tendons and ligaments.

11 With the patient's palm facing upwards, link both your little fingers with the patient's thumb and little finger; support with your fingers underneath. Open up the patient's hands, stretching the palms as much as possible. (*See* figure 6.4 for holding technique.) Now, adapting your pressure accordingly, press and knead with your thumbs into the palmar surface, covering

the thenar eminence on the thumb side and the hypothenar eminence on the little finger side. This covers all the reflexes to the digestive and intestinal tract, also the bladder, ureters, kidneys and adrenals. Increase palpation gently on any sore spots. This is very stimulating; it will cause erythema but will also stimulate cellular activity generally.

12 Support the patient's hand with your fingers. Still working with your thumbs on palmar surface continue with circular movements up the wrist and forearm area, pressing and releasing over the whole area, working up the radial and ulnar bones to stimulate localized nerve endings and increase blood circulation. Then work up the middle of forearm, covering all the pressure points.

13 A relaxation technique can now be used, such as side to side relaxation, interlocking your thumbs with the patient's thumb and little finger, their palms facing towards you (figure 6.7). Repeat this procedure whenever necessary.

14 Support the patient's right hand with your left hand, their palm facing upwards. Make a knuckle with your index and third finger of your right hand. Work as deep as is comfortable for the patient, varying the pressure accordingly, over the whole palmar surface up the medial edge of the thumb and the lateral edge from the wrist up the little finger. This greatly increases the circulation to the area.

15 Turn the patient's hand into the palm-down position. Supporting with your fingers underneath, work with your thumbs in circular movements over the whole dorsum of the hand. If needed, get the patient to make a fist and do alternating pressure on the metacarpals and on the webs between them on the dorsal surface with the hands half clenched to find the points. Work the Baxie points firmly (*see* figure 6.8); this will relax the tendons of the hand. Continue up the wrist and forearm, working into the tendons of the forearm, covering all the pressure points.

16 Another relaxation technique is hand moulding. Interlock your thumb with the patient's thumb, palm to palm, fingers in an upright position. Mould and roll the patient's hands between your palms. Repeat this a few times.

17 Apply a little cream at this point (no bigger than a very small coin, like five pence piece) to dorsum and palmar surface. Repeat the first procedure on both sides.

18 Stroke the hand, both palmar and dorsal surface, of patient.

19 Sandwich the hand firmly and hold, pressing your hands together. Then release and slide off the fingers.

Left hand

Repeat all the above moves, changing support hand when necessary.

Finally, interlock both your hands with the patient's and gently shake the hands two to three times and gently release them.

Additional reflex and meridian points for first aid and self-help

There are many additional points that may be utilized for common disorders. They are also useful for quick first aid and self-help. Table 6.1 gives a list of these. Figure 6.8 shows the points on the hand surfaces.

These reflex points and meridian points indicate what a powerful and energetic area the hands are. With your hands you can self-work the reflexes daily without any undue side-effects. In the terminally ill, work all points gently, once a week to start with and increasing gradually to twice daily. This non-invasive therapy is extremely beneficial to everyone, but is particularly suitable for the elderly and children.

Hand exercises

1 Rotate the wrists both ways. Loosely shake the hands from the wrists.
2 Clench your fists, then fan your fingers out, stretching them as much as possible.
3 Point the thumb, then dorsiflex it.
4 Relax the hands by pressing them together and holding for at least 60 seconds.
5 For tired hands, clasp hands and press down into the webs.
6 Squeeze a squash ball, or put an elastic band around thumb and little finger and stretch it out; this increases the muscle tone of the thumb and palm.
7 Place the hands together in a praying position and press them together for 60 seconds.

Table 6.1 Additional target reflex and meridian points (see figure 6.8)

Problem	Indicated points
Abdominal discomfort	Hypochondrium down to abdominal area, PE-6, TB-4
Achilles tendon strain	Spinal area and sacral point, also SI-5 and 6
Acne	Endocrine glands, TB-6
Afterbirth pains	Abdominal area, LI-4*
Allergies	Reflex to problem, adrenal glands and lymphatic system, TB-6 and LI-4*
Alopecia	Thyroid area; rub fingernails together for 15 minutes daily
Angina	Heart and thyroid reflex, HE-5 and 7
Ankle or leg problems	Around wrist for ankles, SI-5 and 6
Anxiety	Pituitary, thyroid, adrenal glands, spinal area, HE-7, 8 and 9, PE-7 and 9
Arthritis	Reflex to problem area, thyroid, adrenal glands, HE-4, SI-6 and TB-5
Asthma	Respiratory areas, colon points, adrenal glands, upper lymphatic area, LU-7, 10 and 11
Autoimmune disorders	Spleen, upper and lower lymphatic areas, PE-8 and LU-9
Back problems	Spinal area, musculature, sacral point, adrenal glands, SI-3, 5 and 6
Blepharitis	Eye, facial reflex, trigeminal nerve, adrenal glands, SI-2
Bronchitis and other respiratory infections	Lungs, adrenal glands, upper lymphatic area, colon for mucus, LU-7, 8 and 10. Sifeng points
Bursitis	Area of problem, adrenal glands, SI-4 and 5
Colic (biliary or renal)	Area of problem, adrenal glands, upper hypochondrium, TB-3, LI-2 and 4*, SI-3
Colon problems	Intestinal areas, adrenal glands, spinal area, TB-4, LI-2 and 4*
Constipation	Ileocaecal valve, sigmoid colon, spinal area, LI-2 and 4*, LU-7
Cough	Lungs and bronchial, adrenal glands, LU-7 and 10, also Sifeng, second, third, fourth and fifth knuckles of the fingers
Cramp	Thyroid/parathyroid, adrenal glands, spinal area, SI-6
Cystitis	Bladder point, kidneys, pituitary, adrenal glands, groin lymphatics, spinal area, TB-4, LU-7, SI-2
Depression	Solar plexus, thyroid, adrenal glands, liver, PE-5, LI-6
Dermatological problems	Thyroid, liver, adrenal glands, LI-3 and 4*, TB-6, PE-4
Digestive disorders	Specific area of problem, liver/gall bladder, TB-3, 4 and 5, LI-4* and 5. Sifeng points (for indigestion)
Ear disorders	Ear reflex, trigeminal nerve, facial area, adrenal glands, TB-1 and 2, LI-4*

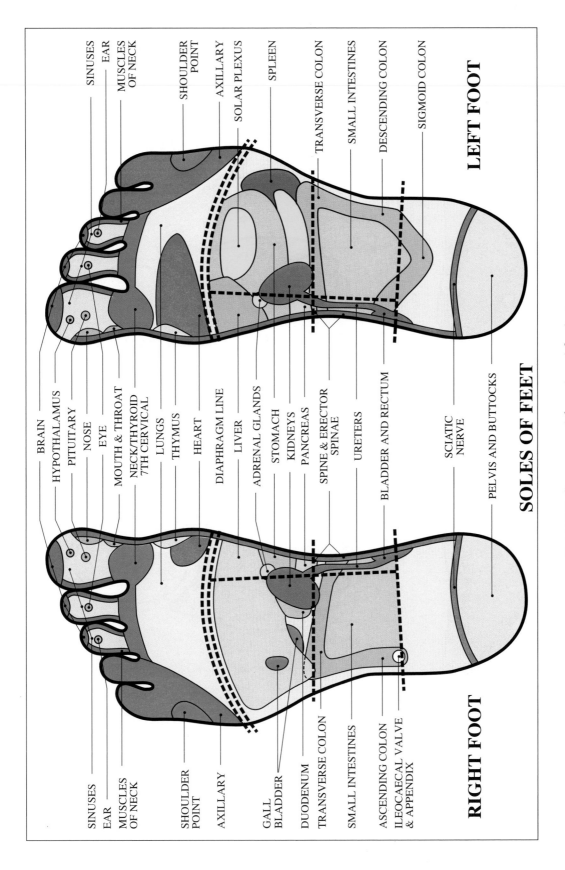

SINUSES
EAR
MUSCLES OF NECK

SHOULDER POINT
AXILLARY
SOLAR PLEXUS
SPLEEN

TRANSVERSE COLON
SMALL INTESTINES
DESCENDING COLON

SIGMOID COLON

LEFT FOOT

BRAIN
HYPOTHALAMUS
PITUITARY
NOSE
EYE
MOUTH & THROAT
NECK/THYROID 7TH CERVICAL
LUNGS
THYMUS
HEART

DIAPHRAGM LINE
ADRENAL GLANDS
STOMACH
KIDNEYS
PANCREAS
SPINE & ERECTOR SPINAE
URETERS

BLADDER AND RECTUM

SCIATIC NERVE

PELVIS AND BUTTOCKS

SOLES OF FEET

SINUSES
EAR
MUSCLES OF NECK

SHOULDER POINT

AXILLARY

GALL BLADDER

DUODENUM

TRANSVERSE COLON

SMALL INTESTINES

ASCENDING COLON
ILEOCAECAL VALVE & APPENDIX

RIGHT FOOT

PLATE 1 Reflex zones of the soles of the feet

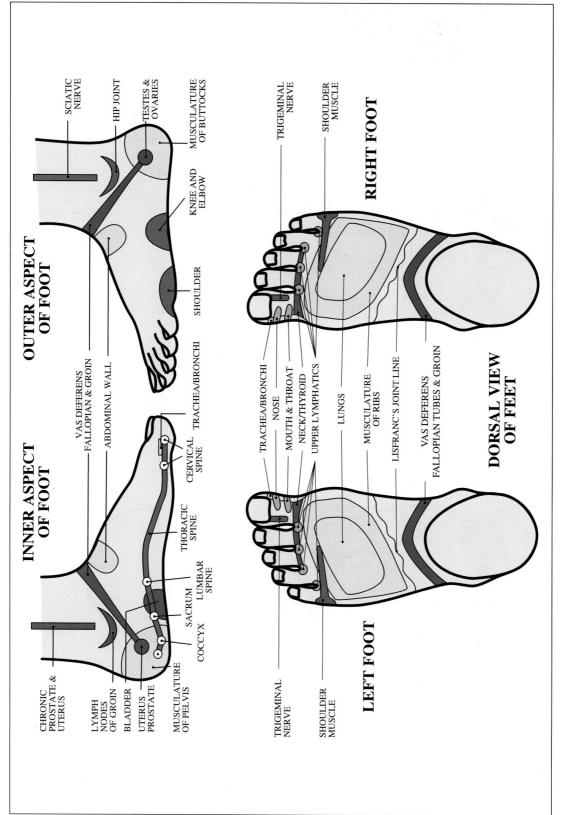

PLATE 2 Reflex zones of the inner and outer aspects of feet, and the dorsal surface

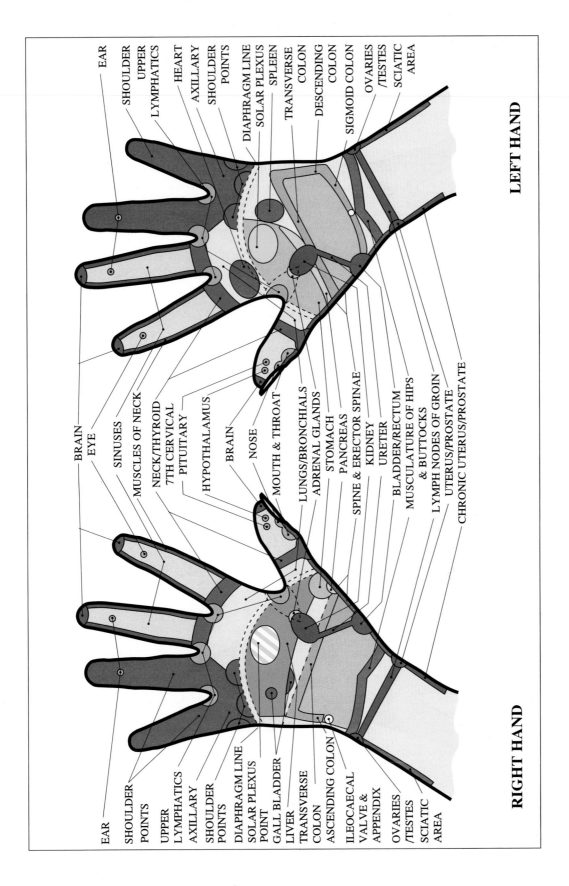

PLATE 3 Reflex zones of the palmar surface of the hand

LEFT HAND

EAR
SHOULDER
UPPER LYMPHATICS
HEART
AXILLARY
SHOULDER POINTS
DIAPHRAGM LINE
SOLAR PLEXUS
SPLEEN
TRANSVERSE COLON
DESCENDING COLON
SIGMOID COLON
OVARIES /TESTES
SCIATIC AREA

BRAIN
EYE
SINUSES
MUSCLES OF NECK
NECK/THYROID
7TH CERVICAL
PITUITARY
HYPOTHALAMUS
BRAIN
NOSE
MOUTH & THROAT
LUNGS/BRONCHIALS
ADRENAL GLANDS
STOMACH
PANCREAS
SPINE & ERECTOR SPINAE
KIDNEY
URETER
BLADDER/RECTUM
MUSCULATURE OF HIPS & BUTTOCKS
LYMPH NODES OF GROIN
UTERUS/PROSTATE
CHRONIC UTERUS/PROSTATE

RIGHT HAND

EAR
SHOULDER POINTS
UPPER LYMPHATICS
AXILLARY
SHOULDER POINTS
DIAPHRAGM LINE
SOLAR PLEXUS POINT
GALL BLADDER
LIVER
TRANSVERSE COLON
ASCENDING COLON
ILEOCAECAL VALVE & APPENDIX
OVARIES /TESTES
SCIATIC AREA

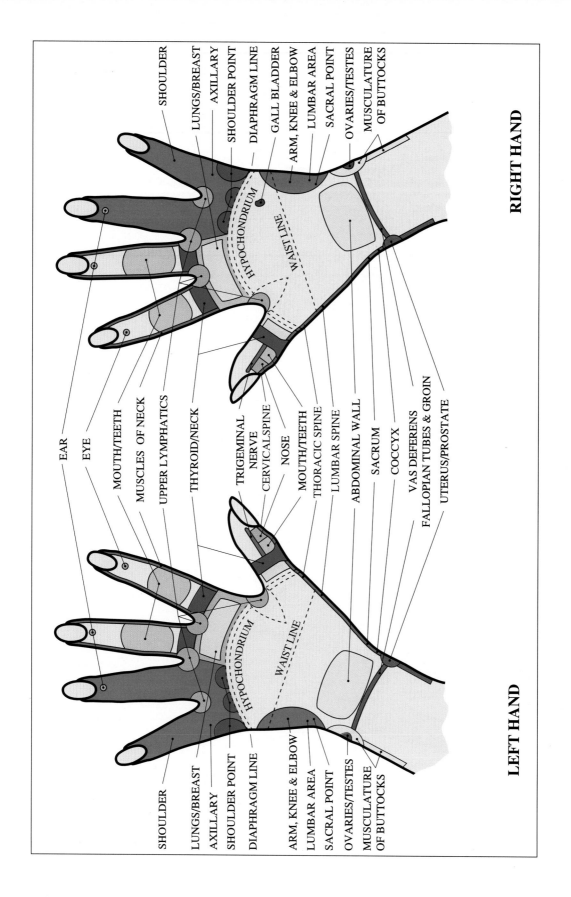

PLATE 4 Reflex zones of the dorsal surface of the hand

RIGHT HAND

LEFT HAND

SHOULDER
LUNGS/BREAST
AXILLARY
SHOULDER POINT
DIAPHRAGM LINE
GALL BLADDER
ARM, KNEE & ELBOW
LUMBAR AREA
SACRAL POINT
OVARIES/TESTES
MUSCULATURE OF BUTTOCKS

HYPOCHONDRIUM
WAIST LINE

EAR
EYE
MOUTH/TEETH
MUSCLES OF NECK
UPPER LYMPHATICS
THYROID/NECK
TRIGEMINAL NERVE
CERVICAL SPINE
NOSE
MOUTH/TEETH
THORACIC SPINE
LUMBAR SPINE
ABDOMINAL WALL
SACRUM
COCCYX
VAS DEFERENS
FALLOPIAN TUBES & GROIN
UTERUS/PROSTATE

SHOULDER
LUNGS/BREAST
AXILLARY
SHOULDER POINT
DIAPHRAGM LINE
ARM, KNEE & ELBOW
LUMBAR AREA
SACRAL POINT
OVARIES/TESTES
MUSCULATURE OF BUTTOCKS

HYPOCHONDRIUM
WAIST LINE

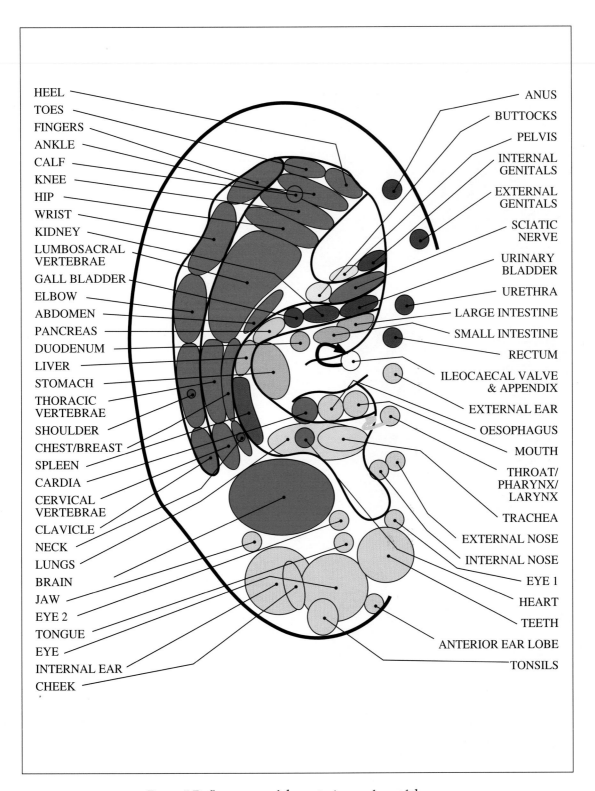

HEEL
TOES
FINGERS
ANKLE
CALF
KNEE
HIP
WRIST
KIDNEY
LUMBOSACRAL VERTEBRAE
GALL BLADDER
ELBOW
ABDOMEN
PANCREAS
DUODENUM
LIVER
STOMACH
THORACIC VERTEBRAE
SHOULDER
CHEST/BREAST
SPLEEN
CARDIA
CERVICAL VERTEBRAE
CLAVICLE
NECK
LUNGS
BRAIN
JAW
EYE 2
TONGUE
EYE
INTERNAL EAR
CHEEK

ANUS
BUTTOCKS
PELVIS
INTERNAL GENITALS
EXTERNAL GENITALS
SCIATIC NERVE
URINARY BLADDER
URETHRA
LARGE INTESTINE
SMALL INTESTINE
RECTUM
ILEOCAECAL VALVE & APPENDIX
EXTERNAL EAR
OESOPHAGUS
MOUTH
THROAT/ PHARYNX/ LARYNX
TRACHEA
EXTERNAL NOSE
INTERNAL NOSE
EYE 1
HEART
TEETH
ANTERIOR EAR LOBE
TONSILS

PLATE 5 Reflex zones of the anterior surface of the ear

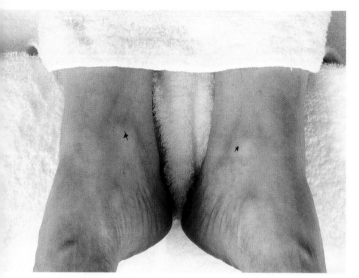

PLATE 6 Feet of a patient with low lumbar problems: these are the feet of a patient suffering from low lumbar problems on the right side. Observe how the medial mallelus is out of alignment; this gives a good guide to the side that is causing the trouble. The patient was complaining of discomfort in the left buttock and down the left leg. The problematic side is the right sacral area.

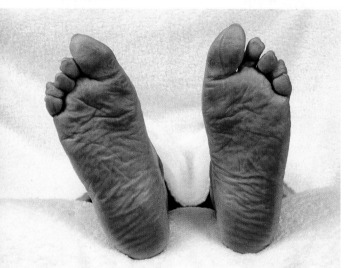

PLATE 7 Feet of the same patient as Plate 14, suffering from rheumatoid arthritis: the feet reveal extremely poor circulation. Note how rigid the foot appears; the spinal joints are very restricted. This patient has been given a very wide variety of drugs, so the liver is extremely tender.

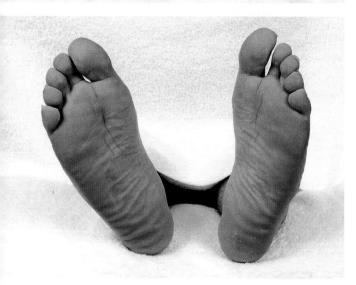

PLATE 8 Feet of patient suffering from chronic sinusitis / allergic rhinitis; this patient suffering from chronic sinusitis / allergic rhinitis has worked for many years as a sculptor using various materials, of which stone is one. However, he does not use a mask whilst working and the deep lines in the lung area show the amount of pressure that the lungs have been under. There is also a cornified area on the nose reflex. The left foot shows a great deviation: as the patient is left-handed he must adapt his manner of working in order to place less strain on his left side and thereby avert problems that will otherwise arise in the future.

PLATE 9 Feet of patient who has suffered from irritable bowel syndrome and wheat intolerance, and who has a history of smoking: note the cornified area of the lung zone; this patient has been a smoker for many years. There are also great striations on the intestinal area – in the patient's case history it was stated that she had suffered from irritable bowel syndrome and wheat intolerance. Smoking would also aggravate this area because of the resultant increased production of mucus. The patient complains of discomfort in left shoulder and pain from an injury to the arm; deviation of the left great toe indicates a neck and shoulder problem.

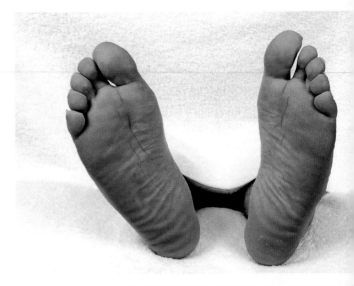

PLATE 10 Feet of patient who has had open heart surgery, and who has suffered from breathlessness: due to an impaired blood supply to the heart, this patient has had open heart surgery. He has also suffered greatly from breathlessness for many years. The deep vertical lines in the lung zones on both feet bear witness to the strain that has been put upon the lungs. The yellowing colour of the feet and some skin-shedding show that the liver is reacting against some form of toxin. The patient is on medication for hypertension; he also has elevated cholesterol levels, which are the result of a metabolic disorder rather than the wrong diet.

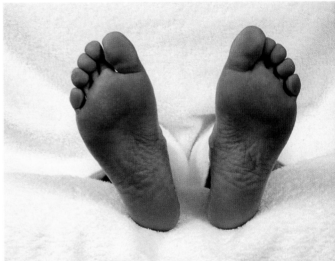

PLATE 11 Feet of patient suffering from chronic Gilbert's syndrome: note the deep crease in the liver area; this patient often complains of nausea and has suffered from great weight loss in previous years. Often her hands and feet are discoloured by mild jaundice. There is also a deviation of the right foot to the lateral edge, which reflects problems experienced by the patient in the areas of the right hip, calf and leg. Observe the area of pigmentation on the bowel area of the left foot: the patient has a tendency towards sluggish bowel movement. However, her general condition is much improved since having reflexology treatment.

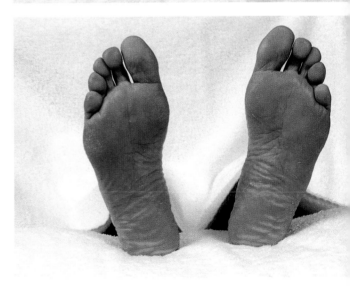

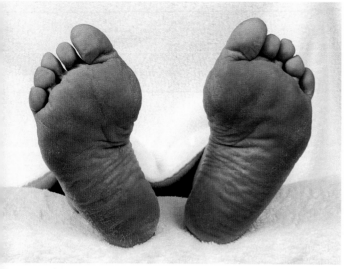

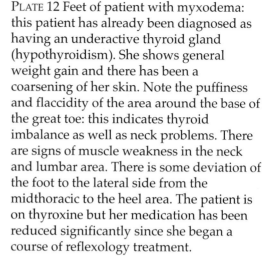

PLATE 12 Feet of patient with myxodema: this patient has already been diagnosed as having an underactive thyroid gland (hypothyroidism). She shows general weight gain and there has been a coarsening of her skin. Note the puffiness and flaccidity of the area around the base of the great toe: this indicates thyroid imbalance as well as neck problems. There are signs of muscle weakness in the neck and lumbar area. There is some deviation of the foot to the lateral side from the midthoracic to the heel area. The patient is on thyroxine but her medication has been reduced significantly since she began a course of reflexology treatment.

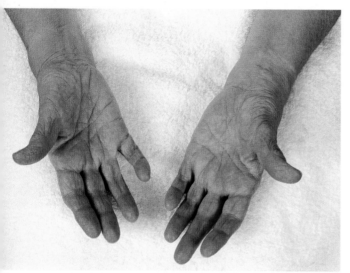

PLATE 13 Hands of a patient suffering from lethargy and anxiety: the hands of this 58-year-old patient reveal a great depletion of energy. Hot and dry skin indicate a lack of body fluid. The right thenar eminence shows low lumbar problems. The transverse lines on the tips of the thumbs and some fingers are indicative of a state of general anxiety.

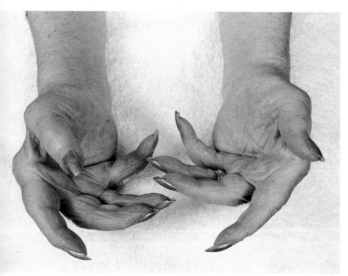

PLATE 14 Hands of a patient suffering from rheumatoid arthritis: the main devastating effect of rheumatoid arthritis upon this sufferer has been to the hands, although most of her joints have been affected in some way. This lady suffered from progressively worsening attacks, and was bedridden at the first home visit of her course of reflexology treatment. The vertical lines on her hands show a depletion of energy. By their curvature, the hippocratic nails indicate the presence of lumbar problems and a respiratory disorder (the patient suffers from pulmonary fibroses).

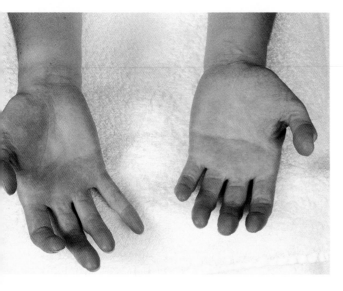

PLATE 15 Hands of a patient suffering from myasthenia gravis: problems in this case are worse on the right side of the body. Note the angle of the index finger. The patient suffers from drooping eyelids and double vision. Also note the position of the thumb; the patient suffers from facial muscle spasms and from muscular weakness in the cervical region.

PLATE 16 Pressure point to relieve headaches, the symptoms of glaucoma and trigeminal neuralgia: this pressure point is situated at the outer edge of the eyes.

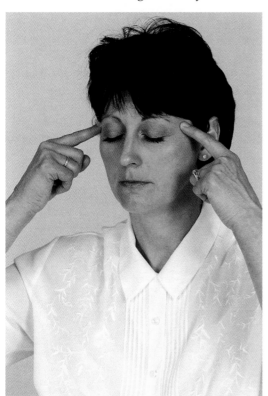

PLATE 17 The first point of the Bladder meridian: this point on the inner eye is known as eye bright. Apply pressure with finger and thumb to make the eyes feel rested, more animated and to give them sparkle.

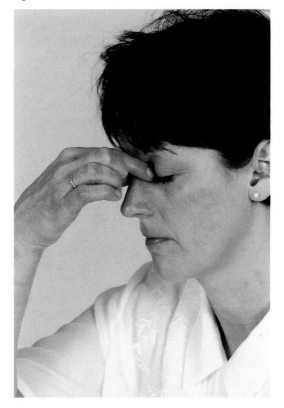

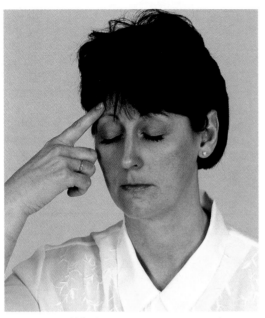

PLATE 18 Self-help pressure point to relieve headaches and insomnia: applying pressure to facial points is a good way to relieve any minor irritations.

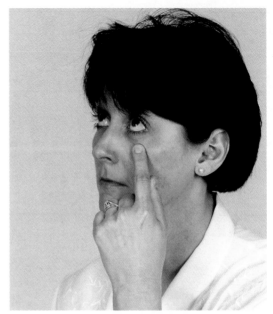

PLATE 19 The first point on the Stomach meridian: this point lies just below the centre of the eye. Pressure applied to it will aid all eye problems. Daily patting around this area is a wonderful first aid treatment for the eyes.

PLATE 20 The last point on the Small Intestine meridian: acupressure point SI-19 is the point of contact for the Gall Bladder and the Triple Burner channels. It lies in the depression formed at the sides of the face when opening the mouth. A division of the trigeminal nerve, the auriculotemporal and the facial nerve supply this area. The point is frequently used for relieving the symptoms of ear disorders, tinnitus, otitis media, deafness and toothache.

PLATE 21 The termination point of the Conception Vessel: this is an ideal point for treating constipation, all reproductive imbalances, fibroids, cancer of the womb and infertility. As the facial nerve serves this area, this point can also be used for treating xerostomia (dry mouth) and trigeminal neuralgia.

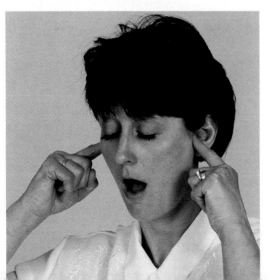

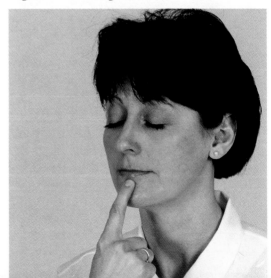

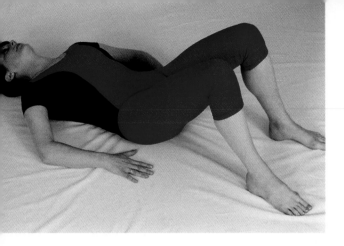

PLATE 22 Exercise 1 for lower back problems: this exercise is suitable for all lower back problems and can be accomplished quite easily whilst lying in bed before getting up for the day. The objective is to press the back into the surface area upon which you are lying. This action is sometimes referred to as the pelvic tilt as the pelvis rises when it is performed. This aids all the muscles of the back and has a relaxing action on all musculature of the spine.

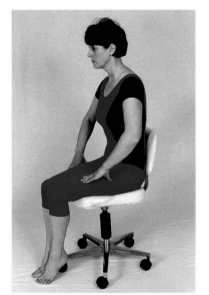

PLATE 23 Exercise 2 for lower back problems: this is a similar action to that in Exercise 1 but performed on a chair. This can be carried out at work, whilst travelling, or sitting at home. Keep the shoulders straight and try to push back into the chair. Repeat several times.

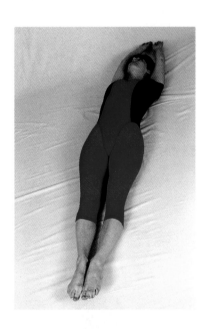

PLATE 24 Exercise 3 for the back: stretch out in bed and wriggle the fingers and toes.

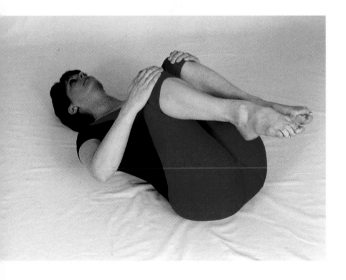

PLATE 25 Exercise 4 for the back: pull the knees up to the chest. To begin with, ease one leg up at a time. Take care not to lift the leg as this puts added strain on the back. Repeat with the other leg, then both legs at the same time. This stretches the spine and is a good exercise to perform before getting out of bed in the morning.

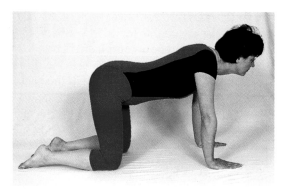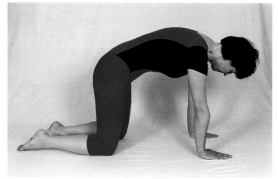

PLATE 26 Exercise 5 for the back: when you have completed exercises 1 and 4, perform exercise 5. This exercise is in two parts: (a. *left*) First take a deep breath through the nose as you lift your head and bottom upwards, whilst letting your back sink into a hollow. (b. *right*) Then breathe out through your mouth as you arch your back against your spine.

PLATE 27 Exercise 6 for the lumbar area: walk on your heels or tap your heels several times to aid the lumbar area.

PLATE 28 Exercise 7 for the lungs: walking on the balls of the feet will facilitate the whole breathing process and thereby aids the lungs.

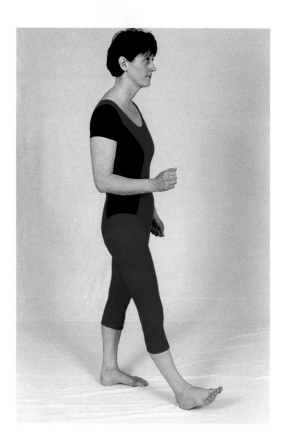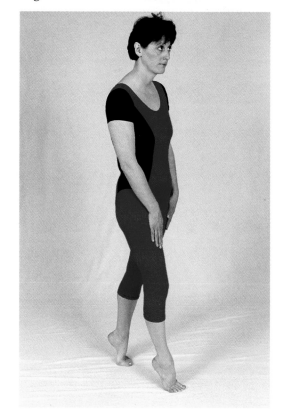

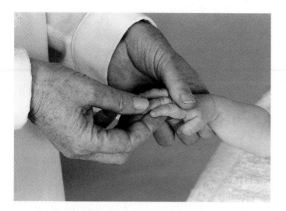

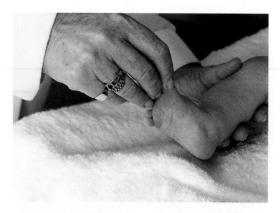

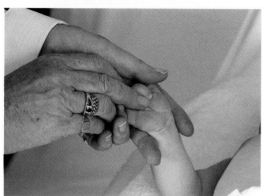

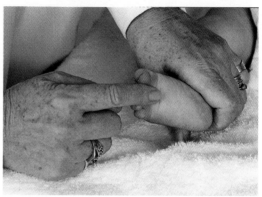

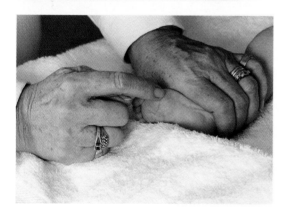

PLATE 29 (*top left*) 'This little piggy went to market' on the fingers: working all the fingers and toes will help to soothe a fretful baby. It will also help to calm the symptoms of little snuffles and coughs or colds.

PLATE 30 (*top right*)'This little piggy went to market' on the toes: working the toes will aid babies who are teething or have ear problems.

PLATE 31 (*centre left*)'Round and round the garden like a teddy bear': working the centre of the palm will help babies suffering from slight temperatures. It will also be of help if the baby is suffering from colic.

PLATE 32 (*centre right*)Calming baby: repeating 'round and round the garden' on the feet will have a general calming effect.

PLATE 33 (*below left*)A good point for soothing agitation: this picture shows a good point for soothing any agitation in the baby; it is also the thymus area so working it will benefit the entire immune system.

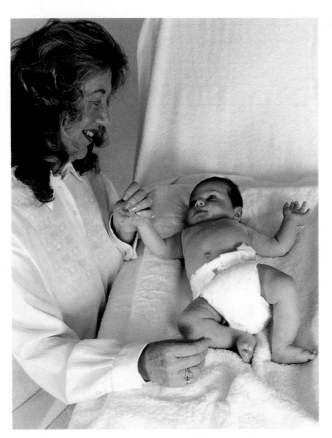

PLATE 34 (*left*) Working hands and feet at the same time: the baby is quite happy to have both feet worked at the same time.

PLATE 35 (*below*) Working the outer rim of the ear: this will help cure any respiratory disorders. Working the tip of the ear will have a soothing effect if the baby is fretful.

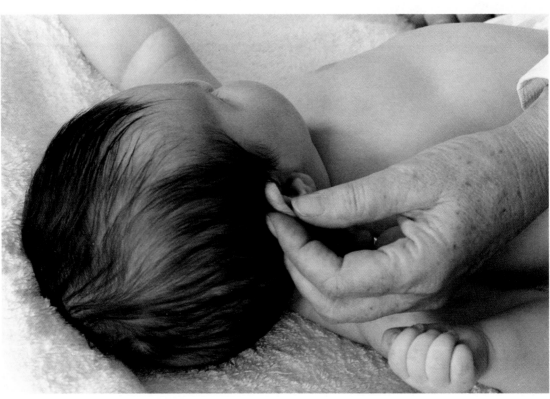

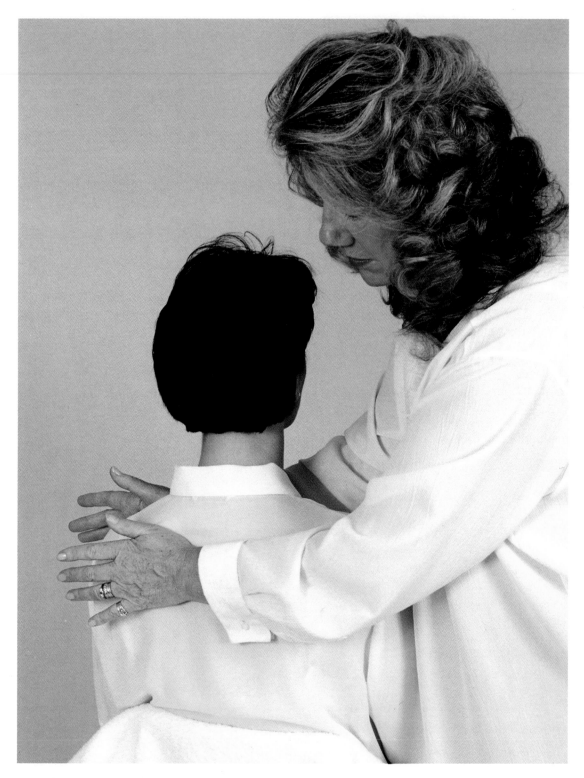

PLATE 36 Making small circular movements over the area of the shoulder and upper back: using the heel of one hand as a support, make small circular movements over the area of the shoulder and upper back. Repeat on the other shoulder. This will relax any tension in the area.

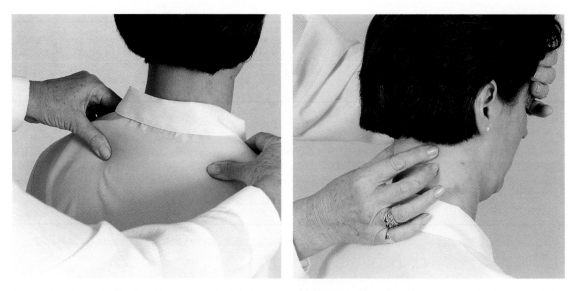

PLATE 37 Using both thumbs to apply friction over the same area: continue to apply friction right up into the nape of the neck (*see* pressure point for the head). This action will have a beneficial effect on everything from the cervical area to the lumbar region.

PLATE 38 Relaxing tension by applying pressure with your forearms: lean on the recipient's shoulders using your forearms. This will release any tension in the upper back.

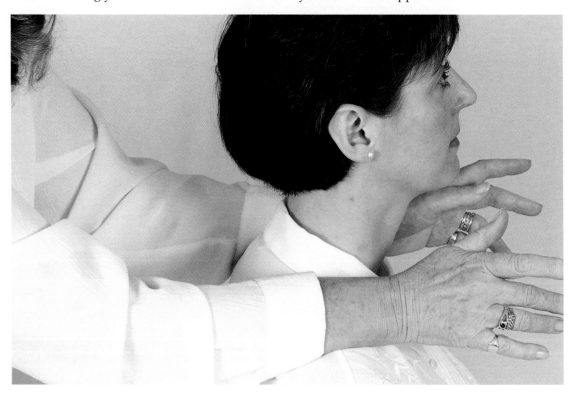

Table 6.1 continued

Problem	Indicated points
Epilepsy	Solar plexus, head-related areas, PE-8, HE-9, TB-1, Shixuan points. Also grip the elbows
Eye disorders	Eye reflex, trigeminal nerve, facial area, adrenal glands, SI-2, LI-1 and 4*
Facial neuralgia	Facial areas, adrenal glands, trigeminal nerve, SI-1, LI-4*
Fainting	Solar plexus reflexes, HE-9, PE-9
Fever	Hypothalamus, pituitary, spleen, PE-8, HE-7, SI-2 (always consult your doctor if it rises to 40°C or is raised for longer than 24 h)
Fibroids	Uterus and chronic uterus, pituitary, adrenal glands, lymph nodes of groin, PE-6, LU-6, LI-4*
Fibrositis	Area of problem, cross refex, adrenal glands, SI-5 and 6, TB-5, LI-4*, for arm or shoulder
Foot problems	Work corresponding area of hand, adrenal glands, spine, SI-4 and 5
Gall bladder problems	Gall bladder, liver, intestines, upper hypochondrium. SI-4, PE-6, TB-5 (also for cholecystitis)
Gastritis	Stomach, liver, upper hypochondrium, TB-3 and 4, LI-3 and 4*
Gout	Liver, kidneys, adrenal glands, related area of problem, TB-4
Haemorrhoids	Intestinal areas, lumbar spine, groin lymphatics, LI-2, 3 and 4*, TB-4
Headache	Liver, spine, head-related areas, LI-4*, SI-1, TB-2 and 5. Baxie points
Influenza	Liver, spleen, thyroid, LU-7 and 11, PE-8, TB-1 and 2
Insomnia	Solar plexus, thyroid, head-related areas, HE-6, PE-7, 8 and 9
Liver problems	Liver/gall bladder, PE-6, TB-3
Mastitis	Pituitary, adrenal glands, axillary areas, SI-1
Menstrual disorders	Uterus, ovaries, pituitary, thyroid, spine, LI-4*, TB-4, PE-6
Migraine	Liver, adrenal glands, head-related areas, SI-1
Nausea	Liver, kidneys, PE-5 and 6, TB-3 and 4, also scratch dorsal area of hand
Nervous disorders	Thyroid, pituitary, adrenal glands, solar plexus, HE-7, 8 and 9, PE-9
Oesophagitis	Stomach, liver/gall bladder, adrenal glands, TB-2, PE-6, LI-4*
Pain	Work related area, adrenal glands, pituitary, solar plexus points, PE-4, LI-4*
Parkinson's disease	Brain-related areas, spinal areas, HE-7 and 9
Pregnancy	General treatment (but *see* footnote)
Preventative treatment	General treatment daily
Prostate	Reproductive points, adrenal glands, LU-7
Urinary retention	Bladder, kidneys, pituitary, LU-7
Varicose veins	Colon, adrenal glands, liver, spleen, spine, SI-4, TB-4

* Do *not* work LI-4 during pregnancy

(a)

CHANNEL POINT	LOCATION	PROBLEMS TO HELP
HE-9	Inside of the little finger corner of nail, arises on dorsum	Anxiety, to restore consciousness, glossitis, palpitations
HE-8	In line with base of thumb web	Confused state, depression, dreams
HE-7	On heel of hand ulnar side	Irregular heart beat, angina, anxiety, stress; a calming point
HE-6	Half a thumb-width above crease of wrist	Insomnia, night sweating
HE-5	One thumb-width above wrist, ulnar side	Tonifies heart beat as a connecting channel; benefits intestines & bladder
HE-4	Two finger-widths above wrist crease, ulnar side	All muscular aches & pains in wrist & elbow, also forearm
PE-9	Off midpoint at tip of middle finger, arises on dorsum	Aneurysm, helps to restore consciousness, calms the mind
PE-8	In line with base of thumb web	Clears excess heat, for high fevers
PE-7	On wrist crease midpoint between tendons	Same function as HE-7, also conjunctivitis
PE-6	Two thumb-widths above wrist crease above forearm	*Vital point* for heart, liver, stomach, menstrual problems & nausea
PE-5	Four finger-widths above wrist crease	As PE-6, also depression
PE-4	One hand-width above wrist crease	All heart problems, any sudden pain
LU-11	Base of thumb nail, arises on dorsum	All throat problems & shortness of breath
LU-10	Two finger-widths below wrist crease on pad	Mucus in throat & lungs; regulates water passages
LU-9	On wrist crease, radial side	Contacting point for blood vessels
LU-8	Just above LU-9	Throat problems also connecting channel to large intestine
LU-7	Just above LU-8	All chest problems, asthma; opens passageways

Extra points
Shixuan
all acute problems

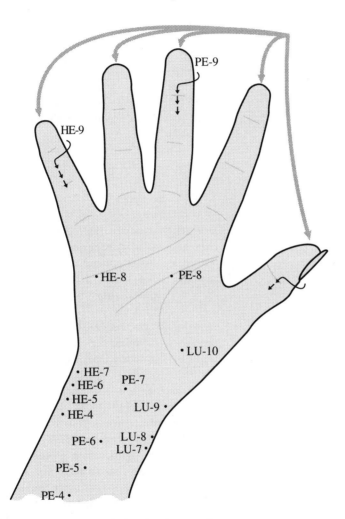

Figure 6.8(a) Pressure points on the hand: palmar surface;

(b)

CHANNEL POINT	LOCATION	PROBLEMS TO HELP
SI-1	Base nail bed of little finger corner of nail bed	Stiff neck, torticollis, headache
SI-2	Base of proximal phalange in line with TB-2 & LI-2	Problems with neck & eyes
SI-3	At start of metacarpals beneath little finger	Colic constipation, lower back pain, upper & lower spine
SI-4	Base of 5th metacarpal	Intestinal colic, wrist, arm, neck problems
SI-5	In hollow of wrist joint	As SI-4, also knee & lower back
SI-6	Two finger-widths above wrist crease	Neck & shoulder problems, tight tendons & ligaments
TB-1	Base of nail bed of ring finger, little finger side	Earache, painful stiff shoulders
TB-2	Just above web	Tinnitus, otitis media, headaches, pain in fingers
TB-3	Between 4th & 5th metacarpals	As TB-2, also upper hypochondrium & liver
TB-4	In depression of wrist in line with SI-4	Stomach problems; stimulates elimination of bladder & intestines
TB-5	Two thumb-widths above wrist crease	Arthritis of upper appendicular skeleton
TB-6	Four finger-widths above wrist crease	All skin eruptions, urticaria, hives, eczema
LI-1	Base of nail bed of index finger, thumb side	Sore throat, eyes; neck & shoulder problems; also calms the mind
LI-2	At base of proximal phalange	Constipation, abdominal pains
LI-3	At start of metacarpals	Throat problems, flatulence
LI-4	In web, highest point of mound	*Vital point. DO NOT USE DURING PREGNANCY.* Allergies, colds, constipation, diarrhoea, ear & eye problems, facial neuralgia, paralysis, hayfever, headaches, laryngitis, arm & shoulder problems; because this point has an antispasmodic effect on intestines & uterus *it must not be used during pregnancy*, but may be used for labour
LI-5	In depression of base of thumb	Similar function as LI-4 in all respiratory problems; for any mucus retention, etc
LI-6	Three finger-widths above wrist	

Extra points
Baxie
any hand or finger problems

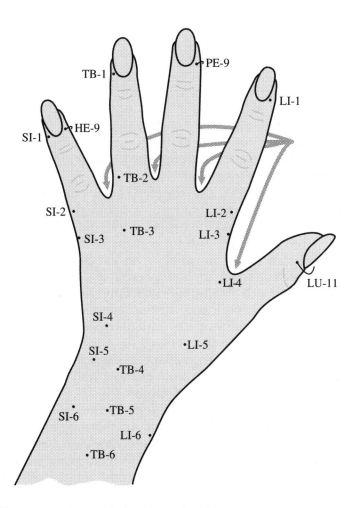

Figure 6.8 (b) Pressure points on the hand: dorsal surface

7   The ear, face and head

The ear

History and theory of auricular therapy

Ear acupuncture has been used for thousands of years. Auricular diagnostic and therapeutic methods were first documented around 200 BC. At one time there were over 230 different acupoints in the ear being used for treatment.

Dr Joe Shelby-Riley (*see* chapter 1) not only worked with the zones and their reflexes, but he also included the ear points. In his book he recommended the ear point for cold feet, paralysis, goitre and thyroid problems, also for earache or deafness. However, he never included any explanation of his ear chart.

A complete change in both theory and practice came about owing to a French practitioner, Dr Paul Nogier, who in the late 1950s introduced the theory of the inverted fetus shape and the corresponding pattern of the auricular points. He published his theories in 1972. Dr Nogier viewed the auricle as a homunculus of the human body, similar in shape to the inverted fetus, the head lying near the lower lobe and the feet and hands towards the upper rim, with the body in between.

Using a combination of Dr Nogier's theory and TCM theory, practitioners have developed auricular therapy. The diagnoses and treatment are mainly based on the meridian theory. Auricular therapy has over a period received increasing international recognition due to its positive results and because of its safety and simplicity of treatment.

Modern auricular therapy states that the ear shape resembles that of the internal organs. In TCM ears are closely linked with the kidneys, in both shape and development. Also, the cerebrum, with its deep convolutions, and its representative areas in the sensory and motor cortex, have a similar arrangement of body areas to that depicted on the auricle. Auricular therapy is now widely practised in many countries. In more recent years it has become more precise, and has always continued to be used with great success.

Anatomy

This organ is responsible for all auditory sensation and our sense of balance. It is divided into three parts. The outer ear is the outer flap of cartilage. The middle ear contains three tiny bones and two tiny muscles: the tensor tympana and the stapedius muscle, the latter being the smallest muscle in our body. The last compartment, the inner ear, is the delicate and extremely convoluted spiral chamber called the cochlea (after a snail's shell). The sensitive hair-containing cells here are responsible for maintaining our balance.

Sound waves that enter the external ear canal are channelled through the external auditory meatus and cause the tympanic membrane in the eardrum to vibrate. This vibration causes three tiny bones (called ossicles) to vibrate. These vibrations travel through the semicircular canals in the cochlea and activate the auditory nerve, the eighth cranial nerve (VIII), of which there are two branches, the vestibular nerve and the cochlear nerve. These then conduct the sound messages as electrical impulses to the brain. The eustachian tube allows the pressures on each side of the eardrum to remain equal.

The basic structure of the ear is shown in figure 7.1.

It is necessary to study the detailed anatomy of the ear in order to understand how the auricular points are named. The following terms are used:

- 'crus', meaning 'leg-like'
- 'fossa', meaning 'trench-like'
- 'tragus', meaning 'he goat' (used because of the hairy nature of the skin at that point)
- 'concha', meaning 'shell-like'
- 'incisura', meaning 'indentation or depression'.

The details of the ear's anatomy are as follows (see figures 7.1 and 7.3). The auricle or pinna is the part that is on the outside of the head. The helix is the prominent curved rim or roll of cartilage of the external ear. The scapha (or scaphoid fossa) is the long, narrow, curved furrow between the helix and the antihelix. The antihelix is the inner curvature of the ear, which forms part of the posterior rim of the concha (*see* figure 7.3). It splits superiorly into the two crura, or curved ridges, of the triangular fossa. The crus of the helix is the anterior continuation of the helix, a prominent ridge that divides the concha (the deepest cavity of the auricle) into two; it comes down to a point, which is the centre of the ear, making a double compartment. The crus of the antihelix is the

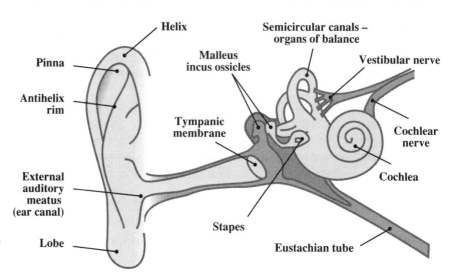

Figure 7.1 Structure of the ear

diverging ridged area that surrounds the triangular fossa. This is a subdivision of the antihelix. The triangular fossa lies between the two diverging crura (above) at its upper end; it is a triangular-shaped hollow. The concha has an upper hollow, known as the superior concha or the cymba concha, the lower, larger hollow being the inferior concha or the cavitas concha. The concha is partly surrounded by the antihelix, with the tragus and antitragus, the projecting tag of the auricular cartilage, overlapping it in front. The tragus is the projecting nodule or eminence, just below the crus of the helix and in front of the concha. The antitragus is the projecting nodule or eminence, which lies above the lobe of the auricle of the external ear. The intertragica incisura is the depression lying between the tragus and the antitragus, above the lobe of the auricle of the external ear. The lobe is the soft, rounded projection below the antitragus.

There are five principal nerves present in the auricle. This is probably why there is so much success with auricular therapy. The alternating palpation or consistent pressure, or any external stimulus, seems to bring about a rapid and beneficial response in the body. These nerves are as follows (figure 7.2):

1 The great auricular nerve – this stems from the second and third cervical nerves. This nerve arises and passes around the sterno-cleidomastoid muscle and ascends beneath the platysma to the parotid gland; it separates into two branches at the auricle, an anterior and posterior branch. The anterior branch distributes to the frontal and dorsal surfaces of the ear, covering

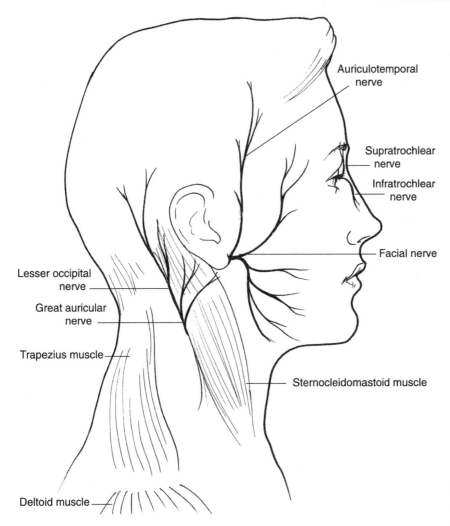

Figure 7.2 Superficial nerves and muscles of the head and neck

the scaphoid fossa, the helix and antihelix, the antitragus and triangular fossa, also the lateral borders of the superior and inferior concha. The posterior branch covers the skin over the mastoid process, the back of the auricle, and ear lobe, going primarily to the lower two-thirds of the dorsal surface of the auricle, the helix, the antihelix and the triangular fossa.

2 The auriculotemporal nerve – this is a sensory branch from the mandibular branch of the trigeminal nerve and further separates into three branches: (a) to the external auditory canal, the drum membrane, the crus of the helix and the superior concha, (b) anterior auricular branches to the tragus and the temporo-mandibular joint, (c) temporal branches to the temple and scalp.

3 The lesser occipital nerve – this stems from the second cervical nerve and separates into three branches, supplying the scalp between the territories of the great auricular nerves, and the skin over the cranial surface of the upper third of the pinna, the superior border of the helix, the triangular fossa, the superior and inferior crura of the antihelix, and the upper part of the scaphoid fossa.

4 A combined branch of the facial nerve, the glossopharyngeal nerve and the vagus nerve – this separates into two branches: (a) the anterior branch, bearing sensory and parasympathetic preganglionic fibres, traverses the internal acoustic meatus and enters the facial canal; the vagus branch supplies sensory fibres to the ear; (b) the posterior branch leaves at the stylomastoid foramen and distributes to the muscles of the auricle and the superior and inferior concha.

5 The sympathetic nerve – this stems from the sympathetic plexus, and is also composed of two branches: (a) the caroticus internus, a fine nerve passing upwards from the superior cervical sympathetic ganglion to join the internal carotid plexus; it accompanies the carotid arteries; (b) the caroticotympanic, two tiny filaments that leave the internal carotid sympathetic plexus to pass through openings of the carotid canal and enter the middle ear.

So we see that nerves that distribute to the auricle include both spinal and cranial nerves. Nearly all nerves send branches to the triangular fossa. Internally there are the deep petrosal nerves, vestibulocochlear nerve and the stapedius nerve. The blood supply to the auricle is very rich, all arteries stemming from the external carotid artery, the temporal artery and the posterior auricular artery. There is also an abundant supply of lymphatic vessels that drain the lymph into the venous system, the main ones being the preauricular lymph nodes.

Auricular points

In 1982 the World Health Organization (WHO) felt that, because of its safety and effectiveness in treating so many varied disorders, there ought to be set standards of points. Together with the Chinese Acupuncture and Moxibustion Association a number of standard points were formulated; these are known as ISAP. Most auricular maps show about 60 areas. Each area is then subdivided into points that are thought to correspond to the body. There are

90 points listed in the ISAP and these are classified as being of four types:

- The majority of points are named according to the different anatomical areas of the body, using their anatomical name or function. These also include the TCM organ systems, named fu (*see* chapter 1). They are outlined in plate 5. (The colour coding enables this diagram to be used in conjunction with the other zone charts (plates 1–4).)
- A number of points are named according to the auricular anatomy. These points are on the anterior surface, but shown separately from the auricular pressure points; they include points on the dorsal surface. These are shown in figures 7.3 and 7.4.
- A few points are named according to orthodox medicine.
- A few points are named according to TCM.

Points named according to auricular anatomy

The following points are named according to auricular anatomy (figure 7.3).

- Apex of ear – ideal for any inflammatory condition, and any fever; it has a soothing and analgesic effect on the body.
- Helix 1–6 – for all upper respiratory tract infections, tonsillitis, pharyngitis and fevers.
- Centre of ear – or Zero Point; it is used for any neurosis. The vagus nerve passes through the ear at this point, and it can be used as a stimulating or sedation point for the parasympathetic system; it is excellent for neurosis, and also an ideal point for hiccups.

The triangular fossa – a vital area that is divided into four parts.

- The superior triangular fossa – known as the hypertension point, marvellous for lowering blood pressure.
- The middle triangular fossa – also called the asthma point; this has an antiallergic and antirheumatic action, and it is used as an hepatitis point.
- The lower triangular fossa – is divided into two parts: (1) the ear Shenmen, used extensively for relieving pain, and has strong analgesic properties; (2) the pelvis, ideal for low lumbar disorders, as it corresponds to the areas within that region; thus it can be used for hip, or sacral problems. (*See* 'Points named in accordance with Traditional Chinese Medicine', for more information on these two points.)
- Apex of tragus – an all-inclusive point beneficial for all

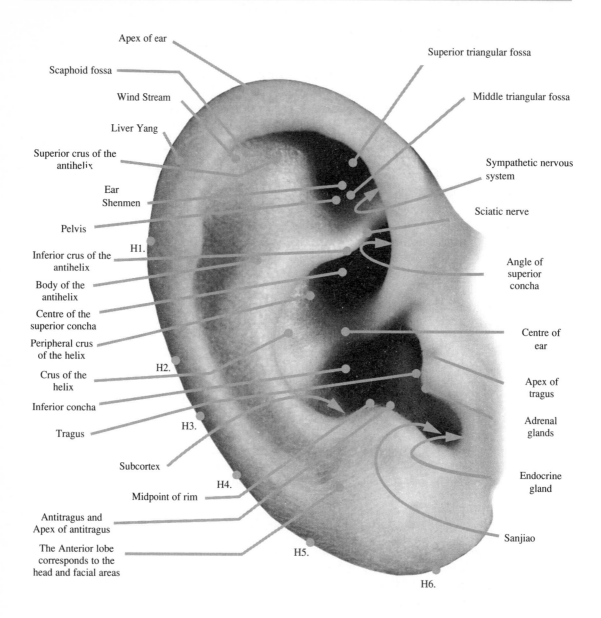

Figure 7.3 Anatomy of the ear and auricular pressure points (anterior surface)

inflammatory disorders, useful for disorders where fever is indicated and helpful as a thirst point. Used extensively to relieve pain.

- Antitragus – corresponds to the head and brain. Also contains midpoint of rim, which is the brain point, and has a stimulatory or inhibitory effect on the cerebral cortex, ideal for any diseases of the nervous, digestive, endocrine or genitourinary systems. Also a suitable point for haemorrhage and Ménière's syndrome. Subcortex is for any functional disturbance in the autonomic nervous system.

- Apex of antitragus – for inflammatory problems, anything ending in 'itis', and useful as an asthma-relieving point.
- Angle of superior concha – prostate and urethritis point and for any infections of the urinary tract.
- Centre of superior concha – any abdominal pain or distension, and circulatory disorders.
- Anterior lobe of the ear – corresponds to the head and facial areas; this also acts as an anaesthetic point for tooth extraction.
- Scaphoid fossa – corresponds to the upper limbs.
- Superior crus of the antihelix – corresponds to the lower limbs.
- Inferior crus of the helix – corresponds to buttocks.
- Body of the antihelix – corresponds to the trunk.
- Peripheral crus of the helix – corresponds to the digestive tract.
- Crus of the helix – corresponds to the diaphragm.
- Inferior concha – corresponds to the thoracic cavity.
- Tragus – corresponds to the throat and internal nose, external ear and adrenal glands.

Points on the dorsal surface

The points on the dorsal surface include the following (*see* figure 7.4).

- Upper ear root – corresponds to the spinal cord; used for hemiplegia and lateral sclerosis.
- Lower ear root – used for hypotension; the same as upper ear root.
- Root of vagus nerve – this nerve conveys both afferent and efferent fibres; this is a point to contact the vagovagal reflex. Stimulation here of the sensory receptors slows the heart down, and helps with any visceral disorders or abdominal pain. This also includes the 5 Zang (but not the pericardium) and 6 Fu organs (see chapter 1, page 6).

The vagus nerve, or pneumogastric nerve, is known as the wanderer. It leaves the lateral aspect of the medulla oblongata and descends through the neck and thorax into the abdomen. There are some offshoots that form major branches to the laryngeal nerves, the meningeal nerves, the auricular nerves, the pharyngeal nerves, and the bronchial plexus and cardiac plexus. Finally it

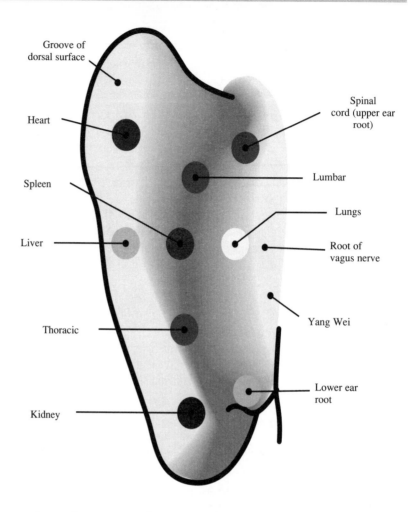

Figure 7.4 Auricular pressure points (dorsal surface)

descends to the gastric, hepatic, coeliac and renal rami. So we see sensory fibres extending to the ear, tongue, pharynx, larynx and oesophagus, with the parasympathetic and visceral afferents going to the abdominal region as far down as the splenic flexure.

- Groove of dorsal surface – for lowering blood pressure.
- Heart of dorsal surface – for insomnia, nightmares, palpitations.
- Lung of dorsal surface – for all bronchial problems.
- Spleen of dorsal surface – for indigestion, gastric pain; it stimulates the appetite.
- Liver of dorsal surface – for any pain in the hypochondrium area.
- Kidney of dorsal surface – for neurosis, dizziness, headaches.
- Yang Wei – the tinnitus point.
- Lumbar point of dorsal surface – connects with the anterior surface lumbar point; for lower back pain.

- Thoracic point of dorsal surface – connects with the anterior surface thoracic point; for upper back pain.

Points named in accordance with orthodox medicine

Five points are named according to Western medicine. These are as follows (*see* figure 7.3).

- Adrenal glands (tragus) – this point has marvellous anti-inflammatory and antiallergic properties and is also suitable for rheumatic disorders. It is a widely used point as it regulates vasoconstriction as well as vasodilation, as in hypertension and hypotension.
- Endocrine point (inferior concha) – for all menstrual problems, diabetes, obesity, and extremely good for aiding urogenital problems in the male and female. This is another point with anti-inflammatory properties.
- Sciatic nerve (antihelix) – for any problems of the hip and all sciatic disorders.
- Subcortex (antitragus) – this point also has an analgesic action on the nervous system. It should be used for all nervous problems, insomnia and for any circulatory or functional disorder   of the autonomic nervous system. It also contains powerful analgesic properties.
- Sympathetic nervous system (antihelix) – this point's main function is to alleviate any visceral pain (eg biliary colic) or cramps. However, any heavy pressure or auricular taping should not be used in acute abdominal distension and pain as it may mask the symptoms and prevent the correct diagnosis and treatment. This point will also help in coronary heart disease, angina, spasm or constriction of arteries or veins. It also inhibits glandular secretion, so it can be used for hyperhidrosis and seborrhoeic dermatitis.

Points named in accordance with Traditional Chinese Medicine

Points named according to TCM are as follows (*see* figure 7.3). The lower triangular fossa is divided into the two remaining parts:

- Ear Shenmen – this point is used very extensively to relieve pain as it acts as an extremely good analgesic. It also possesses antiallergic properties. It functions on the cerebral cortex to regulate overexcitation or to act as an inhibitor; it is therefore a regulatory point, and calms the mind. It is useful for nightmares and insomnia.

- Pelvis – this can be used for all gynaecological disorders, so is ideal for any pelvic inflammation. At the lowest point of this region is the Guguan point (lumbago point), which is frequently used for aching in the joints of the lower limbs.
- Liver Yang (helix) – this point is for headaches, dizziness or hypertension.
- Sanjiao (Triple Burner) – three major nerves pass through this point: the glossopharyngeal, the facial and the vagus nerve. It is used for any problems in the facial area: paralysis, spasms, Bell's palsy, trigeminal neuralgia and toothache. It is also used for abdominal disorders.
- Wind Stream (scaphoid fossa) – this is used for any allergic disorders (it is also called the allergy point) and is suitable for skin disorders such as eczema, urticaria, or cutaneous pruritus, and allergic rhinitis and rheumatoid arthritis.

Inspection

Auricular diagnosis is an important aspect of auricular therapy. Any problem in the body is diagnosed by a sign or mark in the corresponding area of the auricle, indicating that the area may be out of balance.

The auricle should be carefully examined in a good light. Look from the top to the bottom, inside and outside; examination of these tiny manifestations needs to be carried out particularly carefully. If a positive sign or mark is found, stretch the skin so that you can distinguish the size and shape, also the colour. When any blemish, however small, is found, check the other auricle to see whether this is a positive sign. When any eminence is found, determine whether there is any tenderness when it is palpated with the fingers or a probe. Often the area may feel puffy and tight.

When examining check particularly for any of the following:

- colour variations and broken capillaries
- deformities
- desquamation (flaking skin)
- spots and pimples (any slight inflamed swelling)
- enlarged pores
- abnormal sacs, or cyst-like areas
- tenderness on palpation.

Colour variations may take a number of forms. Areas may be

spotty or patchy. Redness indicates an acute disorder. Light red indicates a chronic disorder. Whiteness indicates a chronic or deficient disorder (respiratory, cardiac or rheumatic). Dark brown areas, resembling freckles, indicate chronic disorders.

Pimples indicate chronic inflammatory disorders.

Desquamation indicates chronic inflammatory skin disorders, or a disorder in the corresponding area of the body.

Pain on palpation is often classified in three grades. It is imperative to try and ascertain whether an area shows only mild tenderness, whereby you would get a slight reaction, moderate tenderness, where the patient may frown or blink, or severe tenderness, in which the patient often flinches.

Palpate all points with even pressure, and compare points with adjacent points. Always observe the patient's reactions. However, by comparing ears you can often feel the area that feels different as there is a change of texture when there is a problem.

Note. Remember that individuals' pain thresholds may differ.

Massage procedure

Auricular massage can achieve a wonderful therapeutic effect on the body, alleviating pain and stiffness from the muscles and joints generally. Massage and palpation on specific points can also activate the meridians, regulate the Qi (energy), and stimulate the functions of the Zangfu organs. Massage also stimulates the brain, brightens the eyes and benefits the ears. It aids the circulation in general, and improves the movement of lymph. Auricular massage is simple and safe and has proved to be effective in the treatment of many disorders. The results are obvious and rapid. There are no contraindications at all to this treatment; it can be performed on the very young to the elderly or the infirm.

Note. Do not work on any area where there is any broken skin.

Sequence

Rub your palms together until they are warm, and massage both the frontal and dorsal auricular surfaces between your palms. Then, using the thumb and finger, apply little circles or palpate on the dorsal surface and the anterior surface. Pressure should be only as much as the person can bear comfortably. Use the index finger in all the hollows, as this is the most sensitive of all the fingers.

It is always advisable to have a plan of working. The precise arrangement of movements can be changed at any time, but the following order of areas (*see* figure 7.2) is a suggestion.

1 The helix
2 The peripheral crus of helix
3 The scaphoid fossa
4 The triangular fossa
5 The antihelix
6 The concha
7 The tragus and antitragus
8 The lobe; also work up the area where the ear joins the facial area
9 The whole surface of the dorsal area, with particular attention to the vagus nerve for any cardiac irregularities, which may be stress related
10 Always end with deep stroking of whole ear.

These procedures should be repeated several times until the auricle is quite hot. Increased stimulation is very effective for relieving pain in any part of the body (*see* plate 5). When the session has finished, the client should have a wonderful sense of well-being, and feel agreeable and profoundly relaxed. This sequence can also incorporate the facial pressure points in the following section.

Auricular taping using a seed or small bean is common practice in China, and is widely used to treat many disorders. It should preferably be an organic bean, and this can be located according to the specific problem and also the area of assistance. It is advisable that this is not undertaken by the novice as only a trained and experienced professional practitioner who has skill in the subject should do so. When the seed has been attached, there may be heat or slight discomfort. It is pressed periodically throughout the day, and left on for between 4 and 7 days. When it is removed, clean the area thoroughly, before any subsequent seed or bean is applied.

Self-help tip. Use a flannel daily to apply firm pressure all over the ear surface – anterior and dorsal.

The face and head

Pressure points on the face and head

The facial and head points can be used for both diagnosis and treatment. These points include the 'Ah Shi' TCM points. The theory of the Ah Shi points was first developed by Sun Si Miao during the Tang dynasty (AD 581–682). This theory stated that, wherever there was a sore spot on palpation or pressure, it did not matter whether or not it lay on a meridian channel, but was nevertheless indicated as a point to work. The hypothesis was that the channel network was so dense that the channels or meridians traversing through the body often merged, so that more than one organ system could be reached. Dull soreness or tenderness on palpation or pressure indicated an empty condition, and the practitioner would refer to the channel or meridian nearest to the sore point. However, if the point when pressed or palpated gave a sharp sensation and pain was elicited, this often implied an acute problem; again the channel or meridian nearest to it would be used.

Acupressure can be used on all areas of the face and head with very beneficial results. Perhaps this is why facial massage is so rejuvenating, as many of these points are contacted during facial massage. The advantage of facial pressure rather than massage is that there is no need to use cleansers to remove make-up, and it still gives as much boost to the circulation by improving the lymphatic flow, and thus the complexion in general. Eyes become brighter and vision is improved.

It is a particularly good and easy way of relieving the many physical symptoms of stress, including tension headaches. It also eases flatulence or indigestion. A full treatment of the face and head acts as a mood enhancer, and the client is less likely to feel depressed or tearful and have mood swings, and is better able to concentrate. Indeed most parts of the body are stimulated bringing about a much healthier constitution and correcting impaired sleep patterns, jaded appetite and any sluggish bowel action.

We often use head acupressure unknowingly; here are several examples.

- A common habit of many people is to press the sides of their temples when they have a headache or migraine (*see* plate 16). This is the Taiyang point, a point not on the meridians (called Extra Point 5, or EX-5). The temporal nerve is evident at this point.
- How often when concentrating do you put your index finger in the middle of the eyebrows? This is EX-2, called Yintang; it is for calming the mind.
- The inner edges of the eyes are often squeezed together when we remove our glasses or when our eyes are tired (*see* plate 17). This is the first point on the Bladder meridian, called Jingming; the ophthalmic nerve passes through at this point.

- If a person is hysterical how often do we grab them at their wrists? This is the point HE-7, known as Shenmen.
- If your shoulders are stiff, you may press or massage the shoulder muscle because of tension or tightness in this area. You are working the Jianjing point, GB-21. This point is marvellous for all shoulder and neck problems. It is a meeting point for the Triple Burner and Gall Bladder meridians. It is also an empirical point for any problems related to childbirth or threatened miscarriage. At this meeting point it connects with the Conception Vessel (*see* 7.6), a meridian that originates in the uterus of the female, hence its usage for the conditions above. It is also an empirical point to promote lactation. As the Gall Bladder meridian descends in the chest, it passes the first point on the Pericardium channel just lateral to the nipple; this point (PE-1) is used for mammitis and insufficient milk.

The reason the points on the face are so well used is that they incorporate all six Yang meridians. The three Yang meridians of the hands ascend from the fingertips to the face: these are the Large Intestine, the Small Intestine and the Triple Burner (*see* chapter 1, page 7).

The three Yang meridians of the foot descend from the face: these are the Stomach, Gall Bladder and Bladder (*see* chapter 1,

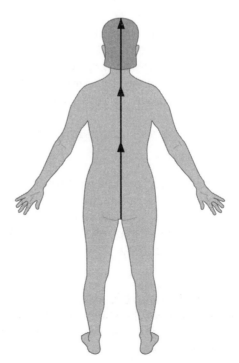

Figure 7.5 The Governing Vessel

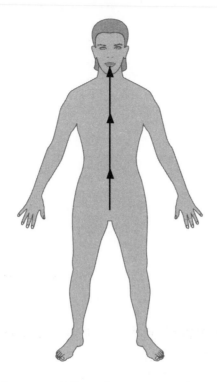

Figure 7.6 The Conception Vessel

page 7). These three meridians have two points each that can be used on the face.

There are two other important body meridians that terminate on the face, the Conception Vessel, which arises from the perineum and terminates on the lower lip, and the Governing Vessel, which arises from the coccyx and runs up the length of the spine, contouring the head to complete its circuit on the upper lip (figures 7.5 and 7.6).

So the face is an area that has both terminating points and originating points. Many of these points pass over or near major nerves of that area. These points on the meridians of the head and neck, together with the extra points shown, make up a daily pressure point exercise. This practice, if performed regularly, will aid the body with many minor everyday problems and calm the mind when stressed or tense.

Self-help tips

Pressure points on the face and head for daily use include points both on the front of the head and face and on the back of the head and neck. The points are shown in figure 7.7a and b.

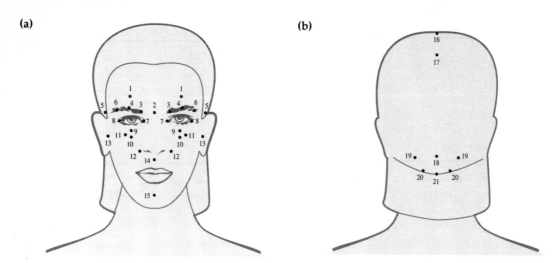

Figure 7.7 (a) Pressure points of the face; (b) pressure points of the head (see text for point names and explanations)

On the anterior aspect of the head and face (figure 7.7a)

1 **Yangbai** (GB-14) (*see* plate 18) – this point lies on the Gall Bladder meridian, a Yang vessel about one finger-breadth above the midline of the eyebrow. The largest branch of the frontalis nerve and the supraorbital nerve supply this area, with offshoots serving the frontal sinus, the conjunctiva, the eyelid, the pericranium and the scalp. It is used for all types of headaches, and trigeminal neuralgia.

2 **Yintang** (EX-2) – point lies on the midpoint between both of the eyebrows, and contacts the seventh cranial nerve, the facial nerve, which has sensory and parasympathetic fibres, of which there are branches to the scalp, auricle and the face. It is used for all headaches, insomnia, vertigo, or nasal problems.

3 **Zanzhu** (BL-2) – a Yang vessel, this point lies on the Bladder meridian on each of the medial edges of the eyebrows. Branches of the frontalis nerve and the facial nerve supply this area. It is ideal for 'floaters' in the eyes, glaucoma, headache and trigeminal neuralgia.

4 **Yuyao** (EX-3) – this lies right on the middle of the eyebrow, immediately beneath GB-14 (Yangbai). The supraorbital nerve and the facial nerve serve this area. This is used for myopia, conjunctivitis, also ideal for just relaxing and brightening the eyes.

5 **Taiyang** (EX-5) (*see* plate 16) – this point lies one finger-breadth behind the lateral edge of the eyebrow, in the

depression. The auriculotemporal nerve serves this area, also branches of the mandibular nerve, the largest division of the trigeminal nerve, which supplies the auricle and the tragus, the lower lip, the tongue, teeth and gums. There are also branches of the facial nerve at this point. This point is used for all facial problems, headaches, migraine, trigeminal neuralgia and toothache.

6 **Sizhukong** (TB-23) – is the last point on the Triple Burner meridian, a Yang vessel; it lies on the lateral side of the eyebrow. Branches of the frontalis nerve and the facial nerve serve this area. It is used for headaches, facial problems and conjunctivitis.

7 **Jingming** (BL-1) (*see* plate 17) – this is the first point on the Bladder meridian. It contacts the third cranial nerve, the oculomotor nerve and one of the divisions of the trigeminal nerve supplying the eyes, the orbit and the nasal cavity. It lies in the depression just above the inner canthus of the eye. This point is known as 'eye brightness'; it is suitable for many eye disorders, such as conjunctivitis, myopia, glaucoma and retinitis.

8 **Tongziliao** (GB-1) – this point is the first point on the Gall Bladder meridian. It contacts branches of the trigeminal nerve, the fifth cranial nerve, and the largest of the cranial nerves. There are three major divisions of this nerve: the ophthalmic nerve, the upper maxillary nerve and the lower mandibular nerve. Also the facial nerve supplies this area. This point is known as the 'pupil crevice' and it lies on the outer canthus of the eye. It is again suitable for all eye disorders (as above) and migraine.

9 **Chengqi** (ST-1) (*see* plate 19) – this is the first point on the Stomach meridian, a Yang vessel, and it lies just below the eye, in line with the pupil, on the bone of the orbit. It contacts branches of the oculomotor nerve, the third cranial nerve, and the seventh cranial nerve supplying the facial area. It is an ideal point for all eye problems, such as tired eyes, any degeneration of vision such as myopia (shortsightedness) and any redness. This point is very near the surface and is rich in blood vessels so light tapping is all that is needed.

10 **Sibai** (ST-2) – this point lies on the Stomach meridian, immediately below Chengqi point. It contacts the infraorbital nerve, which is a continuation of the maxillary nerve, supplying all the lower eyelid, the nose, cheek and upper lip. The facial nerve also supplies this region, making it a good point for all eye disorders, and ideal for any facial spasms or trigeminal neuralgia. In conjunctivitis (pink eye), it eases the pain and discomfort.

11 **Qiuhou** (EX-6) – this point lies almost in line with the above

point laterally and in line with the outer canthus of the eye (where the upper and lower lids meet). It contacts the zygomatic nerve, a branch of the fifth cranial nerve, supplying the temple and the cheek. It is ideal for all eye problems.

12 **Yingxiang** (LI-20) – this is the last point on the Large Intestine meridian, a Yang vessel. It lies in the crease as you smile, as near to the nose as possible. It contacts the infraorbital nerve and the facial nerve supplying this region. It is a good point for all nasal problems, sinusitis, allergic rhinitis and loss of the sense of smell, and is an ideal point to stem a nosebleed. Trigeminal neuralgia can also be relieved.

13 **Tinggong** (SI-19) (*see* plate 20) – this is the last point on the Small Intestine meridian, a Yang vessel. It is an important point because it also contacts the Gall Bladder and the Triple Burner channels. It lies in the depression that occurs when you open your mouth. Both the auriculotemporal and the facial nerve supply this area. It is frequently used for all ear disorders, tinnitus, otitis media, deafness and toothache.

14 **Rhenzhong** (GV-26) – this is the last point on the Governing Vessel. It lies directly under the nose (push up on the midline of the depression). It is known as the 'middle person' as it ascends the centre line from the coccyx. It is a major point and is excellent for fainting, shock or for anyone in a state of coma, and also a good point for any mental disorder and epilepsy. It is also used as an empirical point for any acute lumbar problems, but only if it is on the vertebrae itself; this will aid movement when standing and arching the back as pressure is applied on the point.

15 **Chengjiang** (CV-24) (*see* plate 21) – this is the last point on the Conception Vessel, which commences from the vaginal opening of the perineum in females and terminates directly beneath the lower lip. The Conception Vessel is a regulating channel for all Yin channels. The point is ideal for constipation, all reproductive imbalances, also fibroids, cancer of the womb and infertility. It can also be used for xerostomia (dry mouth) and trigeminal neuralgia as the facial nerve serves this area.

Note. Dr Joe Shelby-Riley advocated the use of CV-24 for constipation; he stated 'press with fingertips into chin for 7 or 8 minutes'.

On the posterior aspect of the head and neck (figure 7.7b)

16 **Baihui** (GV-20) – the Yang channels meet at this point. It lies in the centre of the head, drawing a direct line between the apex

of each ear, on the vertex of the midsagittal line of the head, and contacts the branches of the occipital nerve that supply the scalp in this region. This is ideal for headaches, dizziness or any vertigo. This point aids in clarifying the mind and uplifting our life force, so it is an ideal point to use when a person is depressed. It can also be used for a prolapsed uterus or rectum.

17 **Houding** (GV-19) – this point lies two finger-breadths below the above point. The branches of the occipital nerve serve this area. Use both the index and middle fingers of both hands on each point and move the scalp gently several times. It is a good point for headaches, or any cerebral congestion, vertigo and migraine, and a powerful calming point for any anxieties.

18 **Fengfu** (GV-16) – this point lies on the midline in the depression at the base of the occiput, just at the edge of the hair line. The occipital nerve also supplies this region. It is a good point for headaches, or any mental disorder. It also clears the mind and clarifies the thoughts.

19 **Fengchi** (GB-20) – the occipital nerve again supplies this region; it passes through the trapezius muscle and the sterno-cleidomastoid muscle. It is used for all pains in the neck or any stiffness, eye disorders, rhinitis, tinnitus and hypertension, and is a helpful point for the common cold.

20 **Tianzhu** (BL-10) – this point can be found on the posterior surface of the nape of the neck, lateral to the trapezius muscle. It contacts the third cervical nerve (the eight cervical nerves form the cervical plexus; these communicate with the tenth, eleventh and twelfth cranial nerves). This is a vital point for headaches, stiff necks, and is also one of the major points to use for lower back problems. It has even been known to help a sore throat.

21 **Yamen** (GV-15) – as with the point above, the third cervical nerve supplies the region. It is a good point for ear disorders, and all mental disorders such as epilepsy, as there is a direct connection with the medulla oblongata.

All the points above may be palpated for at least 30 seconds; if there is any undue discomfort discontinue immediately.

8   A–Z of disorders of the body

How to use this chapter

It is essential that a full professional clinical treatment is given at all times on either the hands, feet or ears. However, synthesizing pressure points on legs, hands and ears makes a very powerful combination treatment when using certain reflex points and acupressure points together. Hence references are made to the most active pressure points to use for each disorder, to create a much greater sense of well-being in the patient. In addition to the main reflex, it is essential also to know which additional reflexes can be worked in a treatment session, as many areas of assistance have an anatomical link. Reference is therefore made to these and to cross reflexes that can be used. Finally, it is essential to be aware of the contraindications and cautionary warnings that are highlighted on each chart; these are mentioned where relevant. In general, self-treatment should never be applied when you are pregnant or if you are taking regular medication. Also any long-term chronic disorders should be referred to the patient's medical practitioner prior to seeking treatment.

Abbreviations

The following abbreviations are used throughout this chapter:
M/R – main reflex to work on feet or hands. This refers to the organ or structure that may be out of balance.
A/A – areas of assistance. This refers to an organ or a structure that has an anatomical link.
C/R – cross reflex. This refers to an organ or a structure that has a direct connection through the zonal pathway as follows: hands–feet; fingers–toes; wrists–ankles; elbows–knees; forearm–foreleg; eyes–kidneys; throat–bladder; cervical vertebrae–coccyx; shoulder–hip.
P/Hs – pressure points of the hands. This indicates which pressure points to use on the six meridians that either arise or terminate in the hands. They are illustrated in figure 6.8 on pages 209, 211.

P/LL – pressure points of the lower limbs. This indicates which pressure points to use on the six meridians that either arise or terminate in the feet. They are illustrated in figure 5.41 on page 180.

The following indicates which pressure points to use on the ear. They are illustrated in figures 7.3 and 7.4 on pages 218 and 220.

P/AS – pressure points of the anterior surface of the ear, according to the corresponding organ

P/AA – pressure points in accordance with auricular anatomy

P/OM – pressure points in accordance with orthodox medicine

P/TCM – pressure points in accordance with Traditional Chinese Medicine

P/HF – pressure points of the head and facial areas – this indicates which pressure points to use on the head and face. They are illustrated in figure 7.7, page 228. Self-help tips are also listed throughout.

Abdominalgia

Symptoms

This spasmodic pain can occur any time; distension in the abdomen and cramping pains in the lower abdomen often have a simple explanation and most problems respond. Relief is gained from a general treatment. The abdominal area contains many of the organs of digestion: the liver, gall bladder, stomach, pancreas and intestines, and also the organs of excretion, kidneys, bladder and, in the female, the reproductive organs. It is important to be aware of any sudden change in bowel habits and any pain that is experienced. The site of the pain, intensity and length of time give some indication of the problem. If pain persists for more than a few hours and other symptoms such as vomiting, diarrhoea, or blood from any orifice are present, it is essential to contact your medical practitioner immediately.

Areas to work

M/R. This should correspond to where the pain is felt and to the organs of digestion. Work all areas of elimination to ensure that toxins from waste material do not accumulate as this may upset the overall balance of the body (*see* Acid–base balance, page 237).

A/A. Extra pressure and hold on the adrenal glands point on hands or feet as this will help reduce any slight inflammation. Work the abdominal wall on the dorsal aspect of hands and feet.

P/Hs. Self-help tip: scratch and rake the back of the hand. Also PE-6 and LI-4 are very useful for any pain in the abdomen. (Warning! LI-4 must not be used if you are pregnant.) TB-4 for stomach problems.

P/LL. B-63 for bladder and abdominal pain. ST-35 and 36 for all abdominal problems.

   Warning! ST-36 must not be used on young children.

P/AS. Work stomach point and the liver.

P/AA. Ear point and centre of superior concha for abdominal pain and distension, also the point corresponding to the anatomical area of problem.

P/OM. Sympathetic nervous system point for gastrointestinal spasms.

P/TCM. Shenmen for pain relief, Sanjiao for abdominal distension and constipation. However, no acute pain in the abdomen should be ignored. Consult the GP if pain continues in case of something more serious such as appendicitis, perforated or peptic ulcers or rupture, as these need urgent treatment from a medically qualified person.

   (*See also* Bowel disorders, Indigestion, pages 260 and 300.)

Abscess

Symptoms

A tender inflamed area on the skin or anywhere in the body. Often there is a localized collection of pus due to a local build-up of bacterial infection such as the common staphylococci, as it is the body's immune system that fails to overcome the invading bacteria. This common species of microorganism can enter a hair follicle on the skin causing boils. If an abscess invades the deeper tissues or the internal organs and a fever is present it is essential to seek medical advice.

Areas to work

M/R. The area directly affected, ie teeth or mouth, facial area, trigeminal nerve or breast.

A/A. The upper lymphatics to help reduce any swelling and combat the infection. The spleen will aid the general constitution as it filters the blood and removes any foreign bodies from the bloodstream. The adrenals are a vital area to work for any inflammation; the naturally occurring corticosteroids have a very powerful anti-inflammatory effect. The brain and pituitary gland with their naturally occurring encephalins relieve pain; these peptides have an effect similar to the opiates. The liver cleanses the body of toxins as it plays a vital role in detoxification of any poisonous or unwanted substance. The kidneys filter the blood so aiding drainage. The thyroid helps the skin in general. A total treatment aids the whole body as every organ or gland plays a part in the overall healthy maintenance of the skin. Reflexology seems to stimulate the abscess to burst and drain spontaneously. Again balance is the key word. The liver and spleen exercise a certain control of blood composition and maintain the chemical stability of blood.

P/Hs. LI-4 is very useful for any pain or swelling in the body. TB-6 for any skin eruptions.

Warning! LI-4 must not be used if you are pregnant.

P/LL. ST-45 and GB-44 for any mouth problems. GB-42 stimulates the axillary area and breast if this is the area of problem.

P/AS. Work the area of problem ie mouth, teeth, breast etc.

P/AA. Apex of ear for any inflammation; it also has an analgesic effect. Apex of antitragus for inflammation.

P/OM. Adrenal glands for the powerful anti-inflammatory properties.

P/TCM. Wind Stream, which helps to dissipate any heat.

P/HF. For facial problems, Yangbai GB-14 on the midpoint above the brow.

Achilles tendon strain

Symptoms

Pain in the back of the heel and up to the calf when walking. A strain or inflammation of the main tendon of the muscle in the calf of the leg. If there is any general bursitis around the heel insertion it could be due to pressure from ill-fitting shoes or boots. The Achilles tendon is often involved with the other two muscles, so one must be aware of the anatomical relationship (*see* figure 5.9a, page 153) and action of the other muscles such as the gastrocnemius, which forms the greater part of the calf, helping to flex the knees and foot thus helping the toes to point. Also important is the broad flat soleus muscle in the calf of the leg beneath the gastrocnemius; this has a similar action of flexing the foot and aiding the toes to point downwards. This muscle complex is involved in many sporting activities; even stepping off a kerb suddenly can cause problems.

Areas to work

M/R. Spinal area as all the nerves that feed the area arise from the lumbosacral plexus. Work hip- and leg-related area.

A/A. The adrenal glands for their powerful anti-inflammatory properties. A full treatment session will relax tight muscles and any muscle spasm; this helps reduce any joint stiffness. Many of the passive relaxation techniques help mobility very quickly. The spinal reflex for any leg problems is the lumbar region of the spine; L4–S3 supply the posterior aspect of the leg.

C/R. Self-help tip: work all corresponding area on the arm, following the same line as the Achilles tendon.

P/Hs SI-5 for knee and lower back, for the spinal nerves from the lumbar and sacral areas.

P/LL. GB-40 and 41 for any pain or leg problems. GB-36 for leg problems. Also B-58 for leg disorders in general.

P/AS. *See* calf point specific.

P/AA. Apex of ear for pain relief.

P/OM. Adrenal glands for their powerful anti-inflammatory properties.

P/TCM. Shenmen for instant pain relief.

(*See also* Sports injuries, page 339, Leg and foot problems, page 303.)

Acidosis

Symptoms

A disturbance in the acid–base balance. After excessive vomiting or severe diarrhoea there is a loss of bicarbonate, which is an alkali that the body needs in the right quantities. Diabetics often suffer with loss of vital salts in their urine (*see* Diabetes mellitus, page 278).

Acidosis is often due to a high rise of acid in the body fluids and there is a failure of the body's chemistry to maintain a balance between acids and alkalis. The body should be more alkaline than acid for good health; an acid body is often associated with ill-health. However, the acid–base balance must be maintained. A large proportion of the body is water in which many other substances are suspended or dissolved. The acid–base balance must be maintained at equilibrium (homeostasis); if this balance is upset it leads to acidic or overalkaline conditions.

Areas to work

M/R. A general treatment helps the whole homeostasis of the body to return to normal. The main points are lungs and kidneys and the pancreas.

A/A. Also work the liver/gall bladder, pancreas and intestines together with the kidneys/adrenals. The first three have a quantity of sodium bicarbonate in their fluids to act as buffers to the acidity of chyme, helping to neutralize and balance the whole system. Stimuli to the three reflexes need to be very thorough, using minute alternating steps.

P/HS. PE-6, LI-2, TB-3 and 4 all help the digestive tract.

P/LL. ST-36. Work the whole meridian through from the lateral side of the second toe to the knee.

P/AS. Lung and kidney points.

P/AA. Centre of superior concha, for any abdominal distension.

P/OM. Subcortex for any functional disorder of the autonomic nervous system.

P/TCM. Shenmen for pain relief.

Acid–base balance

This is the maintenance in the blood and tissues of correct levels of chemical substances such as bicarbonate and carbonic acid; the plasma should maintain a neutral point of pH 7.4. (The pH scale is from 0 to 14. Values below 7.4 show increased acidity; values above 7.4 show increased alkalinity.) Any slight changes in pH values may lead to acidosis or alkalosis. Three organs of the body are involved in the acid–base balance: the pancreas, with its strong alkaline buffers (sodium bicarbonate), the lungs and kidneys (*see also* chapter 11).

Acne

Symptoms

Inflammation of the follicles and skin eruptions. This is a skin disorder where the sebaceous glands can become blocked and inflamed. In adolescents this can be a very distressing condition; the sebaceous glands are most active at the time of puberty as a result of androgenic stimulation. Hygiene is of the utmost importance; it is no good applying creams and other substances to the surface area until the inside of the body has been successfully treated. Eliminate all processed foods as they are often high in salt content and hidden sugars; drink lots of water (at least one and a half litres per day) – water is of vital importance to the skin as it fills out the skin cells, and is also a valuable aid in eliminating metabolites and other toxins from the system through the eliminating organs, the liver and kidneys. Eat fresh fruit and vegetables. Psychological factors need to be taken into account as the person becomes further distressed because of the physical scarring.

Areas to work

M/R. All the endocrine glands as this will calm the sebaceous glands that produce the oil and sebum. Hormonal imbalance often causes this distressing problem.

A/A. Liver area and spleen; both are involved with the quality of blood. Also large intestine for removal of excess waste matter and kidneys to refine the end product of filtration. The adrenal glands produce their own corticosteroid, which has a powerful anti-inflammatory effect; extra pressure or rotation on this reflex point for 1 minute has a direct effect on the inflamed areas.

P/Hs. TB-6 for all skin eruptions.

P/LL. GB-41 for any general pain or discomfort.

P/AS. Liver and endocrine points to regulate functions.

P/AA. Apex of ear for any inflammatory disorder.

P/TCM. Shenmen for pain relief.

Addiction

Symptoms

This is a state of dependence on a certain substance such as food, smoking, alcohol, medicines or drugs. Often people are unaware how habit forming substances such as nicotine, caffeine, chocolate and alcohol can be. Most are used as a crutch; for example, the continual coffee drinker cannot cope with a situation under stress; the same can be said for tea, which contains caffeine and tannin, again a stimulant. These substances stimulate the nervous system, often temporarily, making you more alert and less tired, but too much caffeine can have an adverse effect on the system in general, often causing headaches, insomnia, general restlessness and ringing in the ears. These products can also cause more acid release in the stomach, which can aggravate stomach disorders. Most stimulants that have an effect on the brain will often do more harm than good. One should find the reason why a person is using a crutch; is he or she determined to help themselves? It is down to the individual patient to be motivated to discontinue the use of whatever substance is causing the problem. Reflexology is of enormous value as it relaxes the person, relieving the stress and anxiety states that are often linked to dependence. Muscular tension is released, and the person feels less weary and weak. Reflexology also restores the immune system and helps in detoxifying the liver. However, no treatment should be a complete support; aim at a gradual withdrawal if the person is on drugs or dependent on alcohol. Always work closely with their GP; give nutritional advice and advise the patient to seek counselling if necessary.

Areas to work

M/R. A full treatment session, at first one a week in case there are too many toxins released. If there is a gentle reaction to the healing process increase to two or three times per week. Again it must be stressed this is only a support to enable the patient to withdraw gradually from whatever has become an excess or a craving. This holistic therapy will aid any tremors or further anxiety. Make sure you refer the patient to a higher authority if you are in doubt.
A/A. Self-help tip: a daily auricular massage will be beneficial.
P/Hs. HE-7 and PE-7 are good calming points.
P/LL. KI-1 for all acute problems.
   Self-help tip: this can be accomplished by putting a squash ball under the ball of the foot and rolling it for 5 minutes on each foot daily.
P/AS. Liver and brain.
P/AA. Centre of ear. This a vital calming point.
P/OM. Subcortex for aiding the autonomic nervous system, which helps the whole digestive tract.
P/TCM. Shenmen for pain relief; this point has a tranquillizing effect on the body.

Alkalosis

Symptoms

A disturbance in the acid–base balance where there is an accumulation of alkali. Overuse of antacids or overuse of bicarbonate in cystitis can do this. Overexertion and excessive exercise can lead to respiratory alkalosis, which in turn can cause muscular cramps. Panic attacks, whereby the patient hyperventilates, can also upset the overall acid–base balance of the body.

Areas to work

M/R. Pancreas, liver and gall bladder to calm the flow of pancreatic fluid and the production of the alkaline bile from the liver; do very gentle circular movements over whole area.
A/A. Pancreas, liver and gall bladder. A daily foot or hand massage will benefit.
P/Hs. PE-6, LI-2, TB-3 and 4. All points help the digestive tract.
P/LL. ST-36. Work the whole meridian through from the lateral tip of the second toe to the knee.
   Warning! ST-36 is not to be used on young children.
P/AS. Lung and kidney points.
P/AA. Centre of superior concha, for any abdominal distension.
P/OM. Subcortex for any functional disorder of the autonomic nervous system.
P/TCM. Shenmen for pain relief.

Allergies

Symptoms

This is a hypersensitivity state that can often be caused by food colourings, additives and preservatives from processed foods. (*See* appropriate condition for individual exaggerated conditions such as asthma, hay fever or rhinitis.) People are now much more aware that they may have a hypersensitivity reaction to certain things, and most people take the necessary steps to avoid these allergens. The following areas are for all allergies, and then refer to the specific condition. (*See also* chapter 11, page 386.)

Areas to work

M/R. Regular treatment with a professional practitioner helps to strengthen the body's immune system. Work the area of problem.
A/A. Adrenal glands, first and foremost, for any allergy, then the liver specifically to remove excess toxins.
P/Hs. LI-4 for all allergies.

Warning! LI-4 must not be used if you are pregnant.

P/LL. SP-1 and KI-1 are two general calming points in all acute conditions.

P/AS. Adrenal glands and the liver.

P/AA. Apex of ear has a soothing analgesic effect.

P/OM. Adrenal glands (tragus). This point has antiallergic properties.

P/TCM. Shenmen for pain relief.

Alopecia (baldness)

Symptoms

An absence of hair can be a progressive loss due to age or an hereditary factor. It can sometimes be due to illness, an injury or the use of chemical substances for treatment of some diseases; this can also be partly hereditary.

Areas to work

M/R. Regular treatment with a professional practitioner helps to strengthen the body's immune system. The patient is usually very tense regarding the problem, which can only make matters worse. The holistic concept is to calm the anxieties and encourage the person to relax.

Self-help tip: William Fitzgerald spoke of rubbing the nails together for 15 minutes per day; this can be done at intervals, eg 5 minutes in the morning, lunchtime and evenings. This seems to stimulate hair growth in some, with new tufts appearing in about 3 months.

A/A. Stimulate the liver for release of the B vitamins (*see* chapter 11, pages 378, 387). Good sources of these are: liver, milk, eggs and fish. Work the thyroid reflex to help hair, skin and nails; also a general treatment will stimulate the blood supply to the dermis (this is the layer of skin that feeds the capillaries that supply the hair papilla, the bulb and root of the hair).

P/Hs. Liver and thyroid areas.

P/LL. SP-1 and KI-1 are good calming points.

P/AS. Liver and thyroid areas.

P/AA. Apex of ear has a soothing effect on the body.

P/OM. Endocrine point.

P/TCM. Shenmen for pain relief, and this point has a tranquillizing effect on the body.

Alzheimer's disease

Symptoms

This is a degenerative disorder of the cerebral cortex where there is a great loss of the neurones. The causes of this disorder are still not fully known as many hypotheses have been put forward. One thing is very evident and that is that the very confused state creates even more anxieties. The aim is to give a good general treatment of either the hands or feet, combining one of them with a full ear massage, and working specific points.

Areas to work

M/R. A full treatment session to alleviate many of the minor irritating problems and create a relaxed state. The brain and spinal pathways can be worked many times, as this can only stimulate blood to the brain area, and may even act as a vasodilator and widen the healthy blood vessels that are undamaged. Stimulation of the digestive system helps any of the other problems that may cause concern to the patient, for indigestion or constipation. Work the liver area if the person is on drugs as this helps the toxin release. The hands can be worked daily, and so can the ears. On the day that a full foot treatment is given, just work the areas below.

A/A. Thyroid for the general metabolism of the body.

P/Hs. HE-7, 8 and 9 for any confused state.

P/LL. KI-1 and SP-1 for acute problems but are also calming points. BL-64 is a good point for cerebral congestion. ST-45 can also be worked for dementia.

P/AS. Liver, kidneys, brain and spinal areas. According to TCM the liver and kidneys tonify the blood, which helps the brain.

P/AA. Centre of ear is a good calming point for any neurosis.

P/OM. Subcortex contacts the cerebral area of the brain.

P/TCM. Shenmen for pain relief; this point has a tranquillizing effect on the body.

Self-help tip: get the person to clasp their hands firmly, for 10–15 minutes daily. Stroke the back of the auricle on the dorsal surface for the vagus nerve direct, a great calming point.

(*See also* Nervous disorders, page 312.)

Anger

Symptoms

Emotions need to be put into perspective, and anger and tension are part of our everyday lives and human existence. Even grief has a part to play occasionally. We all get angry or sad at some time or another; it is only when this anger gets out of control or is in excess that we need to worry.

Anger is natural at certain times, but suppressing it is dangerous, as if anger is directed inwardly it can lead to many different health problems manifesting. Eating disorders are thought to stem from internal conflict; alcoholism and drug taking are thought to be due to suppressed anger which could stem from even early childhood and early unhappy relationships.

Anger is a strong feeling of hostility and displeasure often leading to the desire to hurt or stop the person or the thing that is causing this anger. No two people respond to anger in the same way. The consequence of anger can be widespread; if the person expresses their anger behaviourally they may bang or break something, or shout and swear or cry; this a normal response to anger so long as it is not in excess or leads to violence or damage to other people's property. However, anger can create fatigue, frustration, hunger, stress, thirst and many other physical reactions. When great anger overtakes you, a response known as the 'fight or flight' reaction occurs: you may feel hot, your heart could pound, you may feel as though you want to go to the toilet, your mouth even may feel dry. This is all because there has been a huge release of adrenaline and this activates your body, causing these physical reactions. It is at this time that it essential to have an outlet to get it out of the system.

One should never vent one's anger in an uncontrolled way. Being assertive is a good way to start if something irritates you over a period of time. Psychologists recommend many rituals that may help, but simply banging something to make a noise is a marvellous release, pummelling a cushion and stating what made you angry is most satisfying. Stamping your feet as you would in childlike anger is another good release. Competitive sports where you are using lots of energy help enormously, such as tennis, squash, badminton, which all involve hitting something. Some people find relaxation and release of tensions in loud music; others need peace and quiet to sort their troubled emotions out.

Reflexology gives the individual the attention many people need. Identifying the patient's disharmony is an important part of the holistic differential diagnoses of reflexology, as often the problem presenting itself is only part of the symptoms, just one of the expressions of the real disharmony within the body. This can be shown in loose stools, tiredness, headaches and many other signs that are often a warning that all is not well within. A reflexologist looks at the many ways that a person can help themselves. Just like any stress disorder, symptoms are the body's response to negative and psychological factors.

Areas to work

M/R. As mentioned with regard to alopecia, regular treatment with a professional practitioner helps to strengthen the body's immune system. The client is usually very tense regarding the problem, which can only make matters worse. The holistic concept is to calm the anxieties and encourage the person to relax.

A/A. Treatment sessions will include work on the brain reflexes, mainly the hypothalamus for mood swings, to balance the hormones and lift depression. Also stimulation on the brain reflex releases the endorphins or encephalins that naturally occur in the brain; these have similar properties to those of the opiates, but are natural relievers of pain, and are often needed if neck or back muscles are stiff. (The old expression you are a pain in the neck, or a pain in the backside is very true.) The solar plexus is a reflex that may be very tender in many stress-related disorders; it is an area rich in nerves.

P/Hs. The tips of the fingers; Shixuan helps all acute problems – apply pressure on each fingertip with the other knuckle, working as close to the nail tip as possible. Also work on the points HE-9 and PE-9; press on the base of the nail beds then on the pads of these fingers. Work LI-1 around nail bed to calm the mind.

P/LL. KI-1 on the plantar aspect of the foot for all acute problems. The Chinese refer to this point as the 'Bubbling Spring' or 'Bubbling Well'. KI-1 is the first point of the Kidney channel, and an essential point for all acute and major problems as it is extremely calming and will help to relieve tension. Hold pressure on both KI-1 points for 1 minute.

P/AS. Direct pressure on brain area; this will give relief for all excess anger of sudden onset. Palpation on all the endocrine glands balances the hormones as an imbalance can effect the whole body.

P/AA. Centre of ear is the main point. Stroking behind both of the ears contacts the vagus nerve and will calm the heart. Repeat these moves several times.

P/OM. Subcortex (cerebral area).

P/TCM. Shenmen to tranquillize the mind.

P/HF. In the centre of the two eyebrows, Yintang (EX-2) is a good calming point that will also assist disturbed sleeping patterns.

Self-help tip: knowing how to help yourself is most important; patients should work their own hands daily as this is of marvellous benefit (*see* chapter 6, pages 200, 205). Patients should clasp their hands firmly on a daily basis for 10–15 minutes. Stroke the back of the auricle on the dorsal surface for contacting the vagus nerve direct, a great calming point.

Arthritis

Symptoms

Any abnormality of a joint with heat, pain and inflammation. Arthritis puts stress on the body, which is often in a highly acidic state. Disorders such as rheumatism, fibrositis, lumbago, gout or synovitis may involve inflammation, stiffness and pain in a joint. Most of these problems are due to large quantities of acid waste material (uric acid); this affects the bony structure of the body because it has not been eliminated properly from the system, and there is often a build-up in the body. Acid waste material seems to have a natural affinity for joints, often making these bony structures swell and in some cases can even cause complete calcification and deformity because of the erosive action. It is essential that all organs of elimination are stimulated. By working on the liver area we help detoxify an acidic system; also working the lymphatic system will help remove more waste thus enhancing the immune system. It is vital that the fourth zone on both hands and feet are worked thoroughly as this contacts the right lymphatic duct and the thoracic duct; these ducts return the lymph back into the bloodstream preventing any accumulation of lymph being retained in the tissues and producing swelling.

Fasting is one of nature's ways of healing, in which waste products and impurities are removed from the system. However, one should never embark on a fasting programme before consulting one's GP. Fasting is a therapeutic method of releasing toxins from the body; most animals when unwell will stop eating instinctively and will drink only water. This allows the body to recuperate and the internal organs to have a well-earned rest. The value of fasting in the treatment of many systemic disorders has been demonstrated many times in naturopathic practice.

Areas to work

M/R. A general treatment paying particular attention to the area of problem: knee, shoulder, hip, legs, low back, etc.

C/R. *See* explanation at front of this chapter.

A/A. The area of assistance would be the thyroid/parathyroid to balance calcium and potassium. T_3 and T_4 substances found in the thyroid are associated with growth and development of tissue, especially that of the nervous system; this also regulates the metabolism of the body. Calcitonin is secreted by the C cells in the thyroid and this acts directly on bone and kidneys; this hormone encourages the bone to reabsorb calcium and then stimulates the kidneys to release it, thus reducing blood calcium levels. Stimulation to the adrenal glands helps to reduce any inflammation because it releases corticosteroids having an anti-inflammatory effect. A general treatment over several weeks will alleviate many of the distressing symptoms; stiffness in the muscles and joints is reduced, and mobility is gradually maintained. Even patients with severe rheumatoid arthritis respond; the joints seem to be less swollen and stiff. The deformity once formed will not change but there can be relief even in the first few treatments. Regular reflexology will help to prevent further bone deformity.

P/Hs. HE-4 for all muscular aches and pains in wrist and elbows, and also the forearm. TB-1 and 5 for arthritis of the upper appendicular skeleton and shoulder pain.

P/LL. ST-38 helps all shoulder problems. LIV-8 helps all four limbs. SP-3 strengthens the spine.

P/AS. Area of problem; applying firm pressure gives almost instant relief from even the most chronic problems.

P/AA. Apex of ear for all inflammatory disorders.

P/OM. Adrenal glands (tragus). Because this point has anti-inflammatory and antiallergic properties it is suitable for all rheumatic disorders.

P/TCM. Shenmen for pain relief.

P/HF. Acupoint Rhenzhong (GV-26) is ideal to strengthen all the spinal areas.

A case history of rheumatoid arthritis is given in box 8.1. (*See also* plates 7 and 14.)

Box 8.1   CASE HISTORY: Rheumatoid arthritis

Female, aged 72 years, very happily married with a grown-up family. I had known her over many years and she was cheerful and outgoing.

Psychological state. I was asked to attend this lady by another patient, who was a friend and a neighbour of hers. On the first visit I had to struggle not to show my shock at her appearance; she was like a little crumpled-up child lying on top of the bed in her dressing gown, and appeared to be in a great deal of discomfort. She looked very sorry for herself, and she was constantly licking her lips, which were extremely sore and red for a good inch around the lips. She appeared in a state of total despair.

Clinical problems presented at first treatment. This lady was in great pain and had difficulty moving; her hands were so deformed with her disorder that she used her arms or elbows to move. She complained of having no appetite, and she had been unable to eat solids for many weeks. She had not left the house for several weeks, and her husband did the shopping and was attentive to her needs.

Background medical history. This lady suffered rheumatoid arthritis, which had affected her lungs in earlier years, and her joints of the fingers, wrists and ankles were also affected.

Medication. She was taking seven different drugs when I first visited her. One of these was a narcotic analgesic for pain; a side-effect of this was nausea, the very thing that was causing her so much trouble. She was also taking three over-the-counter preparations for relief of her low backache.

Observation of the hands, feet and general evaluation. Every joint was stiff and rigid. There was very poor colour in the feet, a bluish discoloration, and they were cold. She had very poor mobility, and poor general health. She weighed about 6 stone (38kg), and had no appetite and difficulty swallowing anything due to the state of her mouth.

On the first treatment I worked only one way on the feet, and did lots of relaxation techniques as best as I could in the circumstances. I massaged her ears and applied two beans – one for pain relief on the Shenmen point, one on the apex of ear; both are soothing and have an analgesic effect. I explained that the medication that was making her sick was only a palliative and would only give temporary relief from the pain; it would not cure it. I asked her to contact her doctor to see if he could prescribe an alternative drug. I left with the promise to return in a few days' time as I was travelling abroad to lecture and would be away for 2 weeks. The second treatment took place on the morning of the day I was leaving.

On my return 2 weeks later, I visited her again, and was pleasantly surprised at the slight improvement. She was dressed but still very stiff, but her colour was much better in her face and extremities. There was no improvement to her mouth or her appetite, although she did say she thought that she was not quite so stiff. Her whole demeanour over the next few visits improved considerably. On week five I worked yet again on the reflexes to the mouth and brain area; I also worked on her hands, which had seemed to open up a little bit. I applied four beans on her ears – two as all other visits and one on the Sanjiao and one on the adrenal glands point. After working on these points for a few minutes, we were both surprised that she had some moisture in her mouth; she commented that she was looking forward to having some toast, something she had not been able to have for a considerable time.

Current health status. PATIENT'S COMMENTS. I started having reflexology in the spring of 1996, and have to say that I knew very little about it. I weighed only six and a half stone and was unable to eat any solid food. I suffer from rheumatoid arthritis, and am prone to anaemia. Over the years I have tried numerous forms of treatment. I had been taking a course of tablets in May 1995, from which I had terrible side-effects. I was left feeling physically ill, weak and suffering from a very sore dry mouth. I was unable to eat properly and consequently lost a lot of weight. Having experienced these side-effects using conventional medicines, when reflexology was recommended by a friend I decided to try it.

I started with six weekly treatments at home. At first I did not notice a great deal of difference in my condition, but I did find it very relaxing. After a few sessions, my back felt more mobile and I was able to straighten it. I decided to have further treatments during the rest of 1996.

At one of the earlier sessions the reflexologist addressed the problem I was having with my dry mouth: I was told to lick my lips. I was surprised and pleased to find I now had moisture in my mouth; it was wonderful. The condition of my mouth has continued to improve. I now have more movement in my body, and my general health has also improved. My appetite has returned and my taste buds are almost back to normal, it is a joy to even fancy food. I am still taking some conventional medicines, but have halved the daily dosage of the tablets I take for pain relief. I do still attend regular hospital visits. My reflexologist has been kind, sympathetic and helpful.

At my last visit, my consultant was so pleased; not only had my blood count risen, I had also weighed in at 8 stone exactly.

I have now reduced my treatments to once every 2 weeks, and later on will reduce it again to once a month. I am hopeful that during this time I will be able to strengthen and straighten my back more, and that my general health will continue to improve, something I had not thought possible in early 1996.

Asthma

Symptoms

Muscle spasm in the small passages. The mucous membrane becomes thick and sticky, constricting airways and making breathing difficult. The mucous membrane then becomes a breeding ground for bacteria. Asthma can be exacerbated by allergies, excitement, overexertion and stress.

Asthma is caused by a narrowing of the bronchi due to muscular contractions in response to some hypersensitivity or stimulation of the bronchial tubes. The person can usually inhale air into the lungs but is unable to exhale fully and wheezes because there is a restriction of the trachea and bronchi. The usual treatment is the use of a bronchodilator in the form of an inhaler, or in a severe case a corticosteroid is used to reduce the inflammation of the mucous lining of the bronchial passages. However, persistent use of these medications can cause hoarseness, high doses can affect the heart rate, and sometimes they can induce fine muscular tremors, head-aches and cause nervous tension.

A qualified holistic practitioner looks at the whole person, not specifically the disease. A reflexologist can aid asthma by enabling the person to breathe more easily and freely, and preventing tension in the diaphragm area. Most asthmatics have problems because of excess mucus, which could become a breeding ground for bacteria, so diet and lifestyle are addressed. Asthmatics and people with breathing problems need to be aware of the foods that can aggravate their problem. Excessive consumption of dairy products such as milk, cheese, butter and chocolate all increase mucus levels. Smoking and drinking alcohol, particularly at night, irritates the mucous membrane lining of the epiglottis, making the tissue swell at the laryngeal entrance, which may impair the air flow to and from the lungs, again diminishing the amount of oxygen taken in.

Areas to work

M/R. Trachea/bronchi. The adrenal glands for the relaxation of the airways; it seems to calm the mucous membranes – they become less sticky and clogging. The stimulation helps the bronchial smooth muscle. Also work the lungs, as this aids the whole breathing process.

A/A. Work the liver reflex in case of infection to clear toxins. Stimulate the upper lymphatics so that filtration is improved; work the spleen to filter out bacteria and produce lymphocytes. This all helps in the general defence against any microbial infection.

P/Hs. LU-7, 11 and 10 help remove any mucus in the throat and lungs thus aiding any shortness of breath.

P/LL. ST-40 is a helpful point in asthma.

P/AS. Lungs, throat, pharynx, larynx.

P/AA. Middle triangular fossa is a good asthma point. Helix 1–6 will help in the case of any upper respiratory tract infections.

P/OM. Adrenal glands (tragus); if there is an allergic cause this point will also be beneficial.

P/TCM. Shenmen to help tranquillize and for pain relief.

P/HF. Chengjiang (CV-24) in the depression below the bottom lip. This area helps to regulate all the Yin channels, Lungs, Spleen, Heart, Kidneys, Pericardium and the Liver, which all assist in this disorder.

Self-help tips

A good reflexologist will recommend some treatment on the hands. Here the reflex points are a powerful and energetic area to work on. The hands can have the reflexes worked daily without any undue side-effects, and obtaining great benefit. They are a marvellous aid to any respiratory disorder, which includes coughs, colds, asthma, bronchitis and emphysema. Apply pressure on the thumb on the base of the nail bed and on the palmar surface with the hand facing you; press all around the thumb and down to the base of the palm (the thenar eminence). Continue pressing down to the wrist area for about 7cm (3"), still on the thumb side; this will aid the removal of phlegm and excess mucus. You can then continue on the dorsal area, from the web between the thumb and index finger; LI-4 can be worked quite firmly. (*Warning!* Use LI-4 only if the person is not pregnant, as it is an empirical point to promote delivery during labour.) This vital area will aid and relieve many problems such as allergic rhinitis, hay fever, sneezing, runny itchy eyes; also it has a stimulating dispersing effect on the lungs. It also has a strong calming influence on the mind and helps to relieve any anxiety. ST-40, a major point on the legs, six finger-breadths below the knee in between the tibia and fibula, helps asthmatics as it helps to eliminate phlegm. These points aid all respiratory problems such as nasal obstruction, runny nose, loss of smell in smokers, and a stiff neck, and some headaches also respond to these simple pressures. The tip of the great toe, SP-1, for a blocked nose.

People who are tense or anxious often have a diminished ability to take in sufficient oxygen. This is often because of tension on the diaphragm muscle, which frequently goes into spasm and then the lungs do not expand enough. Press all over the great toe and thumb, at the tips and the base of the digits; this will help facilitate the breathing process and because the vagus nerve is stimulated also helps slow the breathing and heart rate. It also stimulates the smooth muscle of the bronchial tree and the phrenic nerve, which helps to bring about regular contractions of the diaphragm during breathing. Also stroking the back of the ear on the dorsal surface contacts the vagus nerve directly; this has an immediate effect on the organs of the chest cavity.

Asthmatics can aid their breathing by standing on the tips of their toes; this will also apply pressure on the ball of the foot (the lung area). Also press the upper palms of the hands together (the lung area). Splay fingers and toes as much as possible (this helps the sinuses). Then tap the sternum; this contacts the thymus, which will stimulate energy and strengthen the immune system.

These are all self-help tips for all sufferers with respiratory problems but they will also benefit from regular professional clinical reflexology treatments. As a person ages the lungs tend to lose their natural elasticity; regular sessions of reflexology enable the respiratory process to function better, so breath is not so restrained.

(*See also* Respiratory problems, page 333. Also look at the breathing exercises for stress in chapter 10, page 375.)

This non-invasive natural therapy is extremely beneficial to everyone, young and old alike. In the terminally ill you would work the points more gently. Each practitioner adapts their pressure accordingly, the patient's response is the best guide, over a period treatment should be comfortable but firm.

Warning! Reflexology is not to be used instead of professional medical advice; for any acute breathlessness one should see a doctor immediately.

A case history of asthma is given in box 8.2.

Box 8.2 **CASE HISTORY: Asthma**

Female, aged 28 years, manageress of a fashion store.

Psychological state.   The husband had his own building business and his office was run from home. They had a woman who did secretarial work a few mornings a week and a bookkeeper who came in twice a month to get invoices out and do the accounts. She was responsible for all other duties when she returned home in the evenings from business and at weekends. She was a farmer's daughter and loved horses, and often rode in her spare time.

Clinical problems presented at first treatment.   Asthma, hayfever and eczema-type rash on feet and constant sinus problems since a young age. Very overweight and with a stressful work and home environment. She had a poor diet, eating lots of refined foods, and snacks at regular intervals.

Background medical history.   Had attended her GP over many years for the above problems and also lower back problems. Many topical applications were tried for the skin disorder but without success. Her asthma had become an accepted disorder, with daily use of Ventolin. The patient had no history of asthma in the family, but her mother had a tendency to a chronic rash on the feet.

Medication.   Ventolin and Beconase; she also took over-the-counter preparations such as Otrivine and Sinutab.

Observation of the hands, feet and general evaluation.   The feet were extremely red and itchy with little blisters, and she picked the skin of her feet. She also had rashes on the elbows and knees. At the first treatment I worked on the hands in order to ensure that not too many toxins were released. There were a few areas I could not work on because of splits in the skin. For the next few treatments I used water jets on the reflexes of the feet. On week six I decided to apply pressure on the direct reflex points of the feet, mainly the liver, adrenal glands, kidneys and thyroid for the skin problems. Over the next 2 weeks we saw such a remarkable improvement; the patient's bad back improved and new skin was being formed on the feet and hands. I also applied taping to the ear points on the middle triangular fossa. I would often work the acupoint LU-7 on her wrist. She was able to work this point herself when she had any slight problem with breathing. Over the first 2 months she noted a distinct drop in the amounts of Ventolin that she was using.

Her diet was examined and all mucus-forming foods were restricted. We also looked at her hobby of horse riding and she was asked to be aware of her problems to see if this exacerbated her condition. We found that when she came into contact with the hay and horse feed this seemed to make her breathing problem worse.

Current health status.   At the conclusion of ten treatments, the hands and feet were totally free of any eruptions. Her hayfever and asthma had improved considerably. She felt much less stressed and more able to cope. She now has regular reflexology sessions and has not encountered any return of her original problems, except for when she was pregnant and then she had to return for a few more treatment sessions. She is generally much more relaxed and has more energy. This patient was the subject of an article in a leading magazine on complementary medicine, not only because of the success of the treatment but also because I treated three generations within this family.

Back chat

Symptoms

Lower backache or difficulty when moving or pain in the region of the lower back of any description. This can happen quite suddenly and may be caused by twisting, bending or overstretching. Even getting up and sitting down can create a problem, as the force of any activity is passed down the spine through to the feet. Stress can affect the spine. The spine can never rest – every time we breathe our thoracic vertebrae move. Even our heads weigh 2 per cent of our body weight, so even too much movement of the head and neck when we exercise can create stress on the spine. Postural deficits are one of the chief culprits, so it is important to address lifestyle (*see* chapter 3) as sedentary habits can compromise our posture. Many disabling conditions are directly related to incorrect movements such as walking, lying, sitting, bending or lifting incorrectly. These incorrect movements pull the spine out of alignment, and often involve more than one part of the spine, not only the musculature, but the area from the cervical down to the pelvis may also be affected.

The medical term for a stiff painful back is lumbago. A slipped disc is the colloquial term for a prolapsed intervertebral disc (PID). This may involve the sciatica nerve because there has been a displacement of the inner substance of the intervertebral disc; this may cause compression on adjacent nerves and ligaments, which may lead to loss of sensation throughout the nerve pathway as the sciatic nerve is the major nerve of the leg and arises from spinal segments L4 to S3. This nerve runs down the back of the thigh passing through the buttock; just above the knee it divides into two branches to become the tibial nerve on the medial edge, which stimulates the tibial muscles, inverting the foot. The peroneal nerve feeds the outer muscles on the fibular side of the leg; these muscles are involved in everting the foot. There is a definite connection between the foot and the spine (*see also* Biomechanics of the foot, chapter 5, page 121). The standing posture is so important to the stability of the spine. If the foot is pronated in any way this can lead to an imbalance in the kinetic energy (the balance of motion). Reflexology, together with the combination points, acts as a powerful pain reliever.

Areas to work

M/R. Spinal area and musculature of corresponding area. The sciatic nerve is the major nerve in the leg; work this area for all back problems, and work the cross reflex.

A/A. The adrenal glands reflex helps to relieve any inflammation; this powerful anti-inflammatory area also gives pain relief. You need to rotate for 1 minute on this reflex area. Also work on all brain reflexes as this helps the body produce its own natural endorphins, which have pain-relieving properties but do not suppress the central nervous system. Reflexology has a similar action on the nervous system of pain relief, giving a sense of euphoria but without the side-effects of diminished mental activity.

P/Hs. SI-3, 4 and 5 for all back problems.

P/LL. SP-3 strengthens the spine. Also KI-1 (Bubbling Spring or Bubbling Well point) on the plantar aspect of the foot, for all acute problems. KI-1 is an essential point for all acute and major problems, so for a sudden onset of lumbago it is extremely calming and will help to relieve pain. Hold pressure on both KI-1 points for 1 minute. Also KI-3, B-56, 57 and 59, and B-62 for all lumbar problems. A vital point is BL-60 in alleviating severe discomfort in the lumbar region, but this must not be used during pregnancy. GB-41 acts a pain reliever.

P/AS. Direct pressure on the lumbar area can help to relieve most back pain.

P/AA. Apex of ear has a soothing effect on the whole body.

P/OM. Sciatic nerve point on the antihelix.

P/TCM. Shenmen for pain relief.

P/HF. Acupoint Rhenzhong (GV-26) is ideal to strengthen all the spinal areas.

The prognosis is very poor with back problems. Most medical practitioners suggest an anti-inflammatory combined with an analgesic, and bed rest. These do provide pain relief in most cases; however, they do not address the cause. Reflexology would look at many factors to see what possible explanation could be found of cause and onset; this includes looking at lifestyle and behaviour patterns, which all involve posture. Stress can affect the spine very quickly, tightening up the muscles of the spinal area. Professional reflexology treatment over a period of time actually helps to strengthen the back with less likelihood of a further problem arising. Bed rest is not actually needed, so patients do not have to take time off work.

(*See also* the simple exercises for back problems (plates 22–28); these help to keep the back more supple and they aid in strengthening the back. Also foot analysis, chapter 5 page 126, and plate 6.)

Case histories of lower and upper back problems are given in boxes 8.3 and 8.4.

Box 8.3 CASE HISTORY: Lower back problem

Female, aged 65 years, spinster, lived alone. Had been a magistrate and also held a high administration post at her local hospital.

Psychological state. A very tense abrupt woman who lived alone but travelled to and from Scotland and Bristol regularly to see relatives, mainly cousins. She was also the chairperson for an old people's home in the private sector. She walked her dog daily; she loved the animal but treated it very firmly, and often spoke of how she had punished it if it had misbehaved. This usually consisted of a smack or no treats, as she put it. I was unable to find out about diet because she was very reluctant to discuss this.

Clinical problems presented at first treatment. Lower back pain and pain in left rib cage, also problems with kidneys, but she would not discuss this in detail.

Background medical history. Ongoing back problem was the only information given.

Medication. Would only comment 'painkillers, as and when needed'.

Observation of the hands, feet and general evaluation. She was covered over the whole dorsum area of her feet with a rash and small vesicles. The plantar area of the foot was clear but the upper part was so bad I could not hold the foot. She had pes planus, which indicated a back problem, and a red area on the left foot around the fifth metatarsal notch relating to her waist line. Her first treatment was on the hands and ears. Over a period of 4 weeks I suggested daily lukewarm water footbaths with three drops of tea tree oil. Together with the reflexology the rash began to clear, but one week it would be less inflamed and the next it would have broken out again. At about week six I decided to work on the feet. I had to wear a surgical glove on one hand to hold the foot as there was broken skin but I was able to work on the plantar area. The liver reflex was very tender so I again requested to know what medication was being taken but to no avail; questions regarding diet also achieved very little response. I did some intensive work on the adrenal and thyroid reflex.

When she arrived on week seven I could not believe my eyes; the area on the dorsum was not red and angry, the eruptions had scabbed and a few had fallen away. There was new skin forming, red and shiny. This was proof that the extra work on the liver and adrenal and thyroid area had helped enormously.

This lady attended every 6–8 weeks; she has never been bothered by any other skin problems. The lower back improved greatly but the pain in her left midwaist comes and goes. I pick up the left kidney point and suspect this is related, but again she will not discuss this. When I look back I can see that this lady's whole demeanour has changed; she is much softer and will smile, but still does not talk a lot. She had never commented that she enjoyed the treatments until the last one, when she had presented herself with severe bruising to the foot and leg after a fall from a chair. There were so many ruptured blood vessels in both legs, the dorsum of the feet and around the heel that I stressed she should have sought medical advice. I informed her that I could not work on her feet owing to so many broken blood vessels and so I worked on her hands. She cancelled the next appointment the morning before attending, saying that she so enjoyed having her feet done and felt so much better she would wait until her legs and feet had healed and then she would return for treatment. Praise indeed after so long!

Current health status and foot observation. Very few problems in the lower back region; the red area on foot (in line with waist) is no longer evident. Occasionally she will comment about her kidneys but she is very pleased that the mysterious rash she had for so long has completely cleared.

Box 8.4 CASE HISTORY: Upper back problem

Male, aged 63 years old. He runs his own plumbing business.

Psychological state. Patient had his own business for many years. He had a large family of five children, three sons and two daughters; only one was married and all the rest were still at home. The wife loved to have family gatherings. Two of the sons helped in the family business and the wife did all the office and clerical work. The youngest son (20 years old) seemed to cause a lot of friction between the husband and wife; the patient felt that the wife spoilt the son and waited on him hand and foot. At the time of his first visit he had not spoken to this son for many weeks owing to some minor misunderstanding about the son's music (he played the guitar at home). He was in such a state physically he thought that he would have to relinquish his business to one of the sons. The medical profession had suggested a brace and he attended a back pain clinic but without much success. He was a heavy wine drinker, often consuming a bottle and a half of red wine per night.

Clinical problems presented at first treatment. Pain in upper back, rib cage and hip. He could walk only short distances and then was in extreme pain. He also became breathless.

Background medical history. The patient had an extreme kyphosis of the spine, which I felt was due to his work patterns, and he had suffered over many years. He also had a hip problem and was limited as to the amount of walking he could do. He also had high blood pressure.

Medication. Prescribed analgesics and non-steroidal anti-inflammatory drugs (NSAIDs); the latter caused him to have severe indigestion. He also took Moduretic for the high blood pressure.

Observation of the hands, feet and general evaluation. The feet were very hot, red and scaling over the whole plantar aspect. They were so bad that I worked on his hands and used the water spray on his feet. I also worked on his ear points. His ears were also red and flaky. He said he could not remember a time when his feet had not been uncomfortable. He had ten treatments. Within the first two treatments the first thing he noticed was that he could walk further, had less pain in his back (upper and lower) and he felt his breathing was easier. The feet cleared within four treatments. I had also suggested a daily footbath using tea tree oil. By week six his statement when he arrived was 'it's as if you have got into my brain and changed my mind'. He could not understand why he was not irritated by his youngest son any more and was delighted that his long-standing foot rash had cleared.

Current health status. This patient is an ongoing case. He attends regularly on a 3–4 week basis, and often states that he feels he could not survive without his reflexology. On this gentleman's 40th wedding anniversary, to which I was invited, he danced the night away, a thing he could not have done in the past. The feet are now completely healed, with new skin forming about week four to five. He was advised on footwear and foot hygiene. All the family have now left home; two are in the course of getting married, the others have all moved into their own homes. There is less stress in his daily life and this shows in the healthy state of his feet. I treat his wife and one of their sons also on a regular basis; at one time I was treating five members of this family, who are now friends as well as patients.

Bladder problems

Symptoms

Any pain or discomfort while urinating. The bladder's weakness is mainly due to infections causing inflammation of the inner lining of the urinary epithelium. Calculi (stones) are hard masses that may form anywhere in the urinary tract; they are commonly composed of calcium oxalate, limestone and other inorganic salts. People with an acidic constitution are prone to stones and this may lead to deposition of urates around the joints or other parts of the body. Calcium phosphate calculus may also form in the urinary tract; this calcareous material may form in the prostate gland of the male. The correct diet is essential so that other stones do not form (*see* chapter 11).

Areas to work

M/R. Kidney and bladder reflex to balance the urinary pH.

A/A. The adrenal glands produce their own corticosteroid that has a powerful anti-inflammatory effect; extra pressure or rotation on this reflex point for 1 minute has a direct effect on the inflamed areas. Work all spinal areas as this helps the nerve supply to the pelvic viscera.

P/Hs. LU-10 helps to regulate all the water passages.

P/LL. BL-63 and 66 are major points for all bladder problems.

P/AS. Urinary bladder, urethra and kidney areas.

P/AA. Apex of ear for inflammatory disorders.

P/OM. Adrenal glands (tragus): hold on the adrenal gland reflex for 1 or 2 minutes and then rotate with firm pressure, as this point exhibits an anti-inflammatory action.

P/TCM. Shenmen for pain relief.

For females *see also* Cystitis, page 274; for males *see also* Prostate problems (which includes urethritis), page 328.

Blood pressure

Symptoms

High levels can indicate hypertension. Never self-treat this condition; always check with your GP that you can receive treatment. It could be due to kidney disease, or endocrine imbalance. It is often known as the silent killer because the person is unaware of it until complications set in. Stress can cause many problems; check the work lifestyle, particularly working too hard and too long. Being under constant pressure is depleting to the system in general. Address diet and everyday lifestyle; relaxation and the right kind of exercise are important. Often the cause is unknown and it is essential that it is treated. With high blood pressure the kidneys have to work twice as hard to pump blood around the body. They release renin in response to stress; this reacts with a substance from the liver to produce angiotensin, which may cause constriction of blood vessels. Angiotensin is a protein that can cause an increase in output of aldosterone from the adrenal cortex; this regulates the kidneys' salt and water balance and overproduction may cause hypertension. Thus an increase in blood pressure can lead to hypertension. By maintaining equilibrium in the body this balances all the internal environment. Some books on reflexology state that you should not work on the adrenal reflex for hypertension; this is incorrect as treatment is aimed at balancing and normalizing function.

Areas to work

M/R. This is a combination of different imbalances that may be causing the problem. Working the endocrine system balances hormones, heart and lungs, strengthening the whole cardiovascular function and regulating blood flow, and kidney/adrenals helps to normalize any water retention and the mineral corticosteroids also help to balance the potassium and sodium levels.

A/A. Pituitary for hormonal control and balance. Diaphragm relaxation facilitates breathing process. Also put extra pressure on the solar plexus reflex.

P/Hs. LU-9, PE-9 and HE-9 all benefit the blood vessels. HE-7 is a good calming point.

P/LL. KI-1 on the plantar aspect of the foot is for all acute problems; it is the first point of the Kidney channel, and a vital point for hypertension.

P/AS. Kidney and endocrine point.

P/AA. Superior triangular fossa for lowering blood pressure.

P/TCM. Shenmen to act as a tranquillizer.

P/HF. The Fengchi point (GB-20) on the Gall Bladder meridian is found at the back of the neck in the depression; it is a very potent point to lower blood pressure. If the neck is stiff this can exacerbate the disorder.

Bowel disorders

Symptoms

Any change in bowel habits should be checked out. If there is a loose passage of faeces followed by constipation it is often referred to as irritable bowel syndrome; this can have many causes, and it may be due to diet, eg allergy to some particular food. However, stress seems to be the major cause with other factors exacerbating the problem. Most forms of bowel disorder are due to a build-up of waste materials, which block and invade the human system. All dietary indiscretions make these products accumulate at an alarming rate so the eliminating organs cannot deal with the excesses and this starts the clogging process, which is the prime cause of ill-health. Most drugs do not address the problem and they do not cure; their aim is to calm the afflicted area so that self-healing takes place. Many drugs cause other side-effects, often creating unpleasant flatulence; the bulk-forming agents often create a greater problem in the early stages.

The reflexologist practitioner can apply stimulation to the general surface senses or reflex points. Reflexology ensures that muscular activity is improved by increasing peristalsis when needed, and generally controlling the speed of passage of food and the rate of digestion. When we think how the alimentary canal has to deal with some of the food we eat often in excess to our needs, we can see why there is such a great prevalence of diseases of the bowels. It does not only have to contend with poor eating habits but smoking, viruses or even an immunological disorder, and stress and anxiety as stated all play a part. The inevitable result is that the intestines are perpetually at a great disadvantage from the strains imposed on them; colon disorders are now very common.

Distension of the abdomen can be caused by many things such as inflammation of the diverticula (diverticulitis); these small pouches often form at weak points causing lots of lower abdominal pain, followed by either diarrhoea or constipation. Irritable bowel syndrome, mucous colitis and spastic colon and constipation are common conditions now experienced; the cause is often unknown. One modern-day problem is Crohn's disease affecting all ages and any part of the digestive tract from the mouth to the anus. Irritation of the lining of the bowel, causing long-term inflammation, may lead to anal abscesses and narrowing or long-term problems. Treatment is often one of palliation and no real attempt is made to find the real cause. Embracing the holistic theory, clients are encouraged to take part in their healing process, by applying themselves to a change in dietary habits.

Areas to work

M/R. Firm extra pressure on the ileocaecal valve and colon area because the contents have to move against gravity and this pressure seems to stimulate the strong rhythmic, muscular contractions of the large intestine so the contents are propelled forwards. By palpation and percussion on all colon reflex areas one can then detect or distinguish any deposits on areas that may be out of balance. You often get a hot spot if the nervous system is overactive. If the area feels cold it could indicate a poor circulation to the region. Anyone who has had reflexology will attest to its benefits in improving bowel action.

A/A. For all sluggish bowel conditions work on toes for

stimulation to the cranial nerves, mainly the vagus nerve because it increases activity, even though we know that there is not as much peristaltic action in the large intestine as in other parts of the digestive tract. Apply stimulation also to the liver/gall bladder area because bile helps peristalsis in the duodenum. If there is any diarrhoea or inflammatory disease of the mucosa and infection is present where inflamed areas have ulcerated, we have three vital areas needing extra stimulation. (1) Stimulation to the adrenal gland area encourages production of the gluco-corticosteroids, which have a very powerful anti-inflammatory effect; this also helps regulation of salt and water balance. There is loss of vital electrolytes with excessive diarrhoea. It also allows the inflamed tissue to heal itself. (2) Stimulation of the spinal area contacts the sympathetic nervous system; this calms the activity in the bowels. The combination of working the whole spinal area helps to balance the stimuli from the vagus nerve and the coeliac plexus that serve the whole abdominal viscera. (3) The spleen is a vital area for both of these problems; this adjusts the quality and quantity of blood in the circulation; we know according to Chinese medicine it is responsible for peristalsis in the colon and it helps remove foreign bodies from the bloodstream. Extra stimulation to this area helps contraction, thus squeezing every little bit of reserve of nutrient-rich blood into the general circulation. Working the whole system correctly enables the eliminating organs to function normally; detoxification then takes place enhancing the immune system and balancing homeostasis.

P/Hs. LI-2 and 4, and TB-4 are all very effective for constipation. For intestinal colic, SI-3 and 4.

Warning! LI-4 can be used only providing the person is not pregnant, as it is an empirical point to promote delivery during labour.

P/LL. SP-5 and LIV-1 are good for constipation. ST-35 and 36 are ideal for gastritis or diarrhoea.

Warning! ST-36 must not be used on young children.

P/AS. Both large and small intestine points, also the ileocaecal valve.

P/AA. Apex of ear for any inflammatory problem. Centre point for abdominal pain and any distension.

P/OM. Sympathetic nervous system (antihelix) is a powerful point for all gastrointestinal spasms.

P/TCM. Shenmen for pain relief and also a calming point.

P/HF. For constipation or diarrhoea a good point on the face is Chengjiang (CV-24) in the depression below the bottom lip. The CV meridian starts in the perineum.

(*See also* Colon problems, page 272.)

Breast problems

Symptoms

Most breast discomforts are due to hormonal imbalances. Any lumps that appear should be investigated immediately, especially if there is any discharge from the nipple. In cystic mastitis, little lumps develop. All breast problems should be investigated; the GP should be contacted to ensure that there is no malignancy or invading tumours.

Areas to work

M/R. A general treatment, paying particular attention to the axillary and breast area zone halfway between the second and third toes, making sure the upper lymphatics and zone 4 are used as this is an elimination point.

A/A. For general inflammation work the adrenal and endocrine glands. Because the breasts contain many lymphatic vessels they respond very quickly to treatment. They are also influenced by hormonal activity, hence the need to work all glands of the system thoroughly. The uterus is an area of assistance.

P/Hs. LI-4 this helps the whole axillary area.

   Warning! LI-4 can be used only providing the person is not pregnant, as it is an empirical point to promote delivery during labour.

P/LL. GB-42 and ST-36: the former helps in mastitis and the axillary area, while the latter helps to strengthen the whole body.

P/AS. Breast and endocrine point.

P/AA. Apex of antitragus good point for general inflammation.

P/OM. Endocrine point has anti-inflammatory properties.

P/TCM. Shenmen for pain relief.

Candida

Symptoms

Candida is a very complex problem of the twentieth century; this yeast-like fungus can cause many problems in the mucous membranes of the body such as the mouth, vagina and respiratory tract. Allergic reactions have been blamed in some cases as often the body responds after antibiotics. Diet also plays an important part. It is only when there are unexplained symptoms that it comes to light.

Candida can act as a trigger affecting the autonomic nervous system, creating muddled thinking, altered sleep patterns, exhaustion syndrome and general malaise. It causes a reaction in the immune system and what starts out as a small problem becomes magnified out of all proportion. Be aware of diet; anything containing yeast or anything that a fungi can form on must be eliminated from the diet, and only fresh foods with no hidden sugars or sweeteners should be eaten. Cut out fresh fruit for a few weeks then reintroduce them slowly. It can take up to a year for the body to normalize and be free of the *Candida*. The drugs often used by the medical profession do not kill the fungus but they stop its further growth. Check the feet to see whether the skin is affected; it is often found to be present elsewhere in the body.

Areas to work

M/R. A good general treatment. For both male and female, work the whole system paying particular attention to lymphatic spleen and intestines.
A/A. Endocrine system to balance hormones.
P/Hs. PE-6 aids the body in general; it also contacts the Triple Burner channel, which contacts all the related viscera.
P/LL. SP-6 is a vital point and will help any lower abdominal pain.
   Warning! SP-6 can be used only providing the person is not pregnant, as it is an empirical point to promote delivery.
P/AS. A good general massage will strengthen the whole body.
P/AA. Apex of antitragus for any inflammation.
P/OM. Endocrine point has anti-inflammatory properties.
P/TCM. Shenmen for pain relief.

Cerebral palsy

Symptoms

Because this is an abnormality of the brain it can affect the general development of the child. Sometimes there is spasticity and lack of balance; in some cases speech may be affected also.

Areas to work

M/R. Reflexology is aimed at helping all functions of the body. A light general treatment daily is a must; no one area alone is out of balance as it is a homeostatic imbalance and functional disorder of the nervous system.

A/A. Extra work on the brain and spinal reflexes, then the specific area that is out of balance.

P/Hs. A daily hand treatment, alternating it with the feet; or the hands can be worked whenever there is a particular problem.

P/LL. KI-1 on the plantar aspect of the foot, the first point of the Kidney channel, being an essential point for all acute and major problems.

P/AS. Gentle pressure on the brain point.

P/AA. Brain point.

P/OM. Subcortex for all nerve-related problems.

P/TCM. Shenmen for pain relief.

P/HF. For constipation or diarrhoea Chengjiang (CV-24) in the depression below the bottom lip.

(*See also* Nervous disorders, page 312.)

Children's ailments

Any undue pain or abnormal disturbance should be referred to your local medical practitioner prior to seeking treatment, to ensure that your doctor is agreeable for your child to receive this remarkable therapy.

I often wonder if there is more to the games we play with little children. Playing the game of 'This little piggy went to market' on all the toes and fingers of even the youngest child will benefit them enormously; gently stretch and rotate each finger and toe, as this will contact all the 10 zones and the 12 meridians. Also the rhyme game of 'Round and round the garden like a teddy bear' on the hands or feet will have a calming action on the whole body; if a child is fretful or may have a slight temperature this little exercise will reduce it quite quickly. Work the thymus area for any agitation in the youngest child; this point is particularly beneficial as it is also such a vital part of the whole immunological system. **Remember to barely caress the surface**. (*See* plates 29–35 for some baby exercises.)

When they are a little older, for all childhood illnesses a general but gentle treatment will often lower high temperature and ease any fretfulness. Work the reflex area of problem; stimulation to the whole skeletal area will disperse lymphocytes into the circulation. Working over the diaphragm relaxes the breathing; also work the cervical reflex as the phrenic nerve that arises from

C3–C5 from the cervical plexus innervates the diaphragm and the pericardium and coeliac plexus.

The pad of the great toe is a good point to work for the hypothalamus/pituitary point; this reflex controls the autonomic functions and regulation of the body temperature, and gentle rotation on this point will help lower temperature. Also stimulation to the back of the ear will trigger the vagus nerve into action; it is known as the pneumogastric nerve because it innervates the respiratory processes; also parasympathetic and visceral afferent fibres to the thoracic and abdominal viscera as far as the splenic flexure are stimulated.

Spleen.   This secondary lymphoid organ processes all incoming blood, filters out damaged cells and destroys foreign substances; it also helps in the production of antibodies. Like other lymphoid tissue it is an aid to immunity. Working on the foot on the point SP-2 almost at the base of the great toe helps any agitation in children.

Thymus.   This will help the whole immune response as the thymus is the primary organ of the lymphoid system and defence mechanism. Gently rotate from the neck reflex down to the diaphragm line on hands and feet. As children get older this area can be worked several times when there are any infections.

Thyroid.   Barely caress this reflex as it needs to be soothed; it speeds up or slows down body processes and maintains the metabolic rate. It covers the surface of the second, third and fourth areas of the trachea, in line with the fifth, sixth and seventh cervical and first thoracic vertebrae. There is a complex connection between the thyroid, the nervous system, and the regulation of metabolism, as the thyroid hormones affect the sensitivity of the anterior lobe of the pituitary gland.

It is essential that diet is addressed as this can often cause problems throughout the early years; eating processed foods, or foods that are high in hidden sugars, often leads to a clogged state and creates excess mucus. Children can also be subject to great emotional trauma when they start school; any unhappiness should always be explored.

Specific points for certain problems

P/Hs. For convulsions LI-4. For dreams or night-time disturbances HE-8 and PE-8. In digestive disorders PE-6 balances the liver and any little tummy problem.

P/LL. KI-1 on the little toe as this point also arises there; these are both good balancing points to use in any fretfulness. As they get older, SP-6 can also be worked. ST-44 and 45 for troublesome teething problems.

P/AS. On the medial edge of the lobe, gently apply pressure on the point for the teeth (perhaps this is why young children pull their ears when they are teething).

P/AA. For respiratory disorders work all around the helix (*see* plate 34); this helps tonsillitis, and any fever.

P/HF. If the child is constipated, apply gentle pressure at the base of the lower lip in the upper cleft of the chin.

Note. For any disorder of young children it is imperative to seek medical advice prior to giving a full treatment.

Chronic fatigue syndrome or ME

Symptoms

Total physical exhaustion is quite common in this disorder; it is thought that it is the end result of a viral infection. Severe depression may arise, adding further to the problem of recovery. General muscle weakness and joint pain are experienced, which make even light exercise impossible as the person is left in a state of fatigue. Headaches and changes in sleep patterns are quite common in sufferers. The cause is still not fully understood, but the mind and body need sympathetic understanding and care. Reflexology provides the means whereby the system is stimulated into normalization. By stimulating all the excretory organs the body gets rid of all the unwanted substances. Prior to treatment the patient may lead a sedentary lifestyle owing to the disorder; this often causes shallow breathing. The lungs are able to function better as reflexology facilitates and improves this process ensuring the removal of unwanted carbon dioxide. The kidneys are stimulated so that excess urea and salts are excreted; this also helps the blood to remain at a steady concentration so that osmosis (regulation of water content) takes place. Filtration in the kidneys also functions more efficiently, and absorption of the required substances is stimulated; the unwanted substances are encouraged to be excreted. The liver is stimulated to improve its detoxification of unwanted substances to rid the body of excess toxins. All these organs, the lungs, kidneys, liver and the skin, are involved in the homeostasis of the internal environment; these are maintained at equilibrium, despite external conditions.

Areas to work

M/R. Reflexology is aimed at helping all functions of the body. A light general treatment of hands and ears daily is a must; no one area is out of balance as it is a homeostatic imbalance and maybe there is a functional disorder within the nervous system. A full clinical reflexology treatment can be given once or twice a week, to help normalize the body.

(*See also* Nervous disorders, page 312.) A case history of chronic fatigue syndrome is given in box 8.5.

Box 8.5   CASE HISTORY: ME/CFS

Female, aged 46 years. Patient had to travel some considerable distance to attend for treatment.

Clinical problems presented at first treatment. Myalgic encephalomyelitis (ME) or chronic fatigue syndrome (CFS). All movement was extremely painful. She complained of muddled thinking and poor concentration, together with great fatigue, and she often felt depressed. She complained of frequent night cramps and snoring. She felt that she was completely flustered and disorganized.

Diet. Patient had a good diet, and was quite health conscious.

Observation of feet and hands. The feet and hands were very moist, with poor colour in lower part of feet but very red on the balls of the feet, and the toes were very red. The feet felt as though they were lacking in vitality and there were lots of cold areas. The nails were well manicured.

Background medical history. This patient has suffered over the last 2 years and had to give up all employment. Doctors had divided views on whether she had ME and one felt that she may be suffering from neurosis. She had been married twice and the second marriage was experiencing problems due to ill-health. She had suffered in her early years from a very bullying father and in both marriages she had chosen dominating men. Over a period she had been treated with antianxiety drugs and muscle relaxants, which seemed to be making the problem worse as she was becoming more and more tense.

On the first treatment, her toes were so painful that only the lightest of pressures could be used. The brain and spinal areas and shoulders were also very tender to touch. The liver area was excruciatingly tender in a small area, as was the kidney reflex. Spleen area appeared cold and empty. Over a period of the next few months, with treatments each week, the areas of tenderness were reduced considerably. By week six, her movement had improved so much that she resumed her swimming, which she enjoyed greatly, the snoring stopped and her whole demeanour changed towards her husband. Her depression lifted dramatically, also her outward appearance improved. Treatments commenced from 2 week intervals to 3 and so on until she was attending only every 6 weeks with no relapse and no medication. To date this lady has resumed most of her daily activities and is now undergoing a training scheme to become a reflexologist. She feels much better and attended for treatments every 4 weeks for a very long time. Her comment then was reflexology is 'as necessary to me as going to the dentist or having my eyes checked'.

Observation of feet at end of treatment. Her feet showed good health and a much better colour, and were quite even in temperature.

Circadian rhythms

The study of biological rhythms, technically known as chronobiology, is the study of the effect of time on living systems. Circadian rhythms, sometimes referred to as biological rhythms or diurnal rhythms, are biological patterns that are based on a daily cycle. The word 'circadian' is taken from 'circa', meaning around or about, and 'dian' meaning to a day. Biorhythms determine how our whole being behaves – that is the mind, the body and the emotions. It is thought that the light/dark cycle plays its part and this may entrain the rhythms. We are all aware that we have good and bad days, and weather plays a vital role in how our emotions are easily upset. Everyone is uplifted on a bright sunny day, whereas on a dull wet day people are often depressed and tense. We all know how our temperature rises as the day goes on, reaching its high point in evening and then dropping in the early hours of the morning. Pulse rate and blood pressure follow a similar pattern; maybe this is why heart attacks are more common in the early morning or late evening. There are more births in the early hours of the morning also. Depression, especially in shift workers who do not adjust to time changes, and jet lag are two of the disorders that researchers are looking at.

Body rhythms are affected by the release of a hormone called melatonin from the pineal gland (*see* The zones of the endocrine system, chapter 5, page 140). A great deal of research has been undertaken over the last 20 years as to the benefits of taking melatonin to alleviate these problems, but a lot of research still needs to be done on long-term usage (*see* Nervous disorders, page 312 and SAD, page 334).

Circulatory disorders

Symptoms

Homeostatic imbalances can affect every part of the body. Reflexology helps direct the free flow of energy and improves the nerve supply throughout the body, thus encouraging normalization of all bodily functions. The autonomic nervous system supplies the muscle fibres within the tunica media of the blood vessels; these nerves arise from the vasomotor centre in the medulla oblongata, and stimulation to the great toe and lesser toes will help the circulation and the whole cardiac cycle. The liver, lungs and kidneys are of particular importance because of their anatomical connections in the pulmonary and systemic circulations. The nerve and blood supply work together, transporting an immense variety of different substances around the body; these nutritive elements are in the blood plasma which reaches all organs and tissues of the body. It is imperative that some exercise is undertaken to strengthen the heart, even walking for approximately 20 minutes per day will stimulate the cardiac output. No intense exercise programme should ever commence without a health check first.

Areas to work

M/R. A good general treatment, with emphasis on area that is problematic; *see also* above.
A/A. According to Chinese medicine the spleen is the most important organ in relation to the blood. It is responsible for the origin of blood because it produces the necessary elements for its formation, and responsible for removing foreign bodies from the bloodstream. The spleen stores extra blood for release when shortages occur. Peristalsis helps contraction of the spleen, squeezing reserves of nutrient-rich blood into the general circulatory system. Energy or Qi is the activating force for the movement of blood.

P/Hs. Work the Heart meridian, from the tips of the fingers (HE-9) to just above the wrist (HE-4).

P/LL. SP-4 helps the spleen and any cardiac inflammation. KI-1 on the plantar aspect of the foot, the first point of the Kidney channel, for all acute and major problems.

P/AS. Spleen and cardia points.

P/AA. Centre of superior concha for any circulatory disorder.

P/OM. Subcortex for any functional disturbance of the autonomic nervous system.

P/TCM. Sanjiao (Triple Burner) helps all functional disturbances.

P/HF. Self-help tip: the point on the upper lip is a vital point; push up towards the nose for a few minutes daily.

(*See also* Heart disorders, page 297.)

Colds

Symptoms

Inflammation of any of the mucous membranes of the upper respiratory tract. Sinus infections often spread from the nose, which can involve the nasopharynx, and in turn the pharynx, larynx or tonsils. All organs of the respiratory tract are subject to the same viral and bacterial infection; also colds are nature's way of getting rid of surplus toxic waste. The four structures most often involved are eyes, ears, throat and nose; the common factor is the mucous membrane. No one who is perfectly clean inside should ever catch a cold. Nutrition is a most important factor; refined demineralized foods lead to a clogged state and toxins are generated. Foods that are high in refined starches are lacking in freshness. The intestinal area is always an area of assistance for any excess mucus. Toxins in the blood are normally eliminated by the lungs, kidneys and colon; a toxic state within these tissues produces large amounts of mucus to protect the mucous membrane. Improving the general elimination processes to remove these excess toxins is most important.

Areas to work

The common cold usually lasts about 4–5 days regardless of any patent medicines taken. A general treatment will aid a sore throat and runny nose and relieve any general malaise and other physical discomforts. Work the areas of any problem. Extra work on the adrenals will aid breathing, also the spleen to stimulate the reticuloendothelial system, which acts as a defence against microbial infection and helps against secondary infection.

P/Hs. LI-4 helps all head-related areas and is ideal for relieving the many symptoms allied to the common cold.

Warning! LI-4 can be used only providing the person is not pregnant, as it is an empirical point to promote delivery during labour.

Colon problems

These include Crohn's disease, digestive disorders, diverticulitis, ulcerative colitis and IBS (*see also* Bowel disorders, page 260 and Ulcerative colitis, page 349).

Symptoms

Persistent colicky abdominal pain (this should never be ignored, consult your GP if problems persist); any continuous episodes of diarrhoea with blood or mucus.

Crohn's disease.   This disorder can take place in any part of the digestive tract. The section between the small and large bowel, the terminal ileum, is often affected, or the bowel; in severe cases both are involved, which may lead to deep ulceration and granulation of the tissue. There is a chronic inflammation, which can become widespread throughout the alimentary tract; it is thought there may be an immunological abnormality present in some individuals; there is also sometimes a hereditary factor.

Digestive disorders   and most colon problems. These are due to catarrhal conditions of the stomach and intestinal areas. This can create excessive secretion of acid and uric acid. The intestines become distended, especially in the caecum, ascending colon, descending colon, sigmoid and rectum, owing to an accumulation of waste, food material and faeces. Inflammation of the large intestine is often due to constipation or sluggish bowel action. Faecal deposits accumulate in the walls of the colon. It is essential that the colon receives the right amount of natural roughage, as the colon draws water and recycled fluids out from the food we eat to hydrate the body and transfer vital electrolytes back into the system. We are what we eat, so poor diet may be the culprit. Apples, oranges, grapefruits, grapes (red ones), broccoli and carrots are good for maintaining a healthy bowel, or the juices from these products. A full reflexology treatment acts like a colonic cleanse. Faulty assimilation within the intestines is a common trigger to abdominal discomforts. (*See also* Digestive disorders, page 279.)

Diverticulitis.   This is small pouches within the mucosa blown out or protruding into the peritoneal cavity; this often occurs at the weakest points, and faeces then become impacted causing inflammation and oedema.

Irritable bowel syndrome or IBS   is recurrent abdominal pain with constipation or diarrhoea. This condition is often stress related, but the wrong diet can also aggravate the problem.

Ulcerative colitis.   This is a condition in which the lining of the colon (the mucosa of the large intestine) and the rectum may become chronically inflamed.

Areas to work

M/R. Stimulation to the parasympathetic and sympathetic nervous systems is required, mainly on the great toe as the vagus nerves are responsible for peristalsis in the duodenum. This stimulates other abdominal organs of the alimentary tract as it contains motor, secretory, sensory and vasodilator fibres. The vagus nerve is known as the great wanderer as its fibres stray downwards reaching right down to the spleen, and stimulation helps all these muscles contract and improves secretion of digestive juices. Stimulation directly to intestinal reflexes helps normal absorption and assimilation. Extra work on the rectum and anus helps normalize elimination of the terminal part of the large intestine.

A/A. Also work the lower part of the spine for the sacral nerves, which serve the distal parts of the intestines, mainly the descending colon. Working either side of the spine area will contact the sympathetic nervous system reflexes, reducing muscle contraction and glandular secretion. We do not need to decide whether extra stimulation to one area will cause any imbalance as these two systems work closely together. In a treatment one influence may compensate the other according to the needs of the body. The adrenal glands will aid any inflammatory disorder. Every reflexologist will attest to how a thorough treatment will improve bowel function, reducing any inflammation.

P/Hs. LI-4 helps all intestinal-related areas and is ideal for relieving the many symptoms allied to bowel problems.

Warning! LI-4 can be used only providing the person is not pregnant, as it is an empirical point to promote delivery during labour.

P/LL. SP-5 and 6 will help any lower abdominal pain. LIV-5 is good for colic and any spasms of the abdomen. ST-35 and 36 are ideal for gastritis or diarrhoea.

Warning! SP-6 can be used only providing the person is not pregnant, as it is an empirical point to promote delivery during labour. ST-36 must not be used on young children.

P/AS. Both large and small intestine points, also the ileocaecal valve.

P/AA. Apex of ear for any inflammatory problem. Centre point for abdominal pain and any distension.

P/OM. Sympathetic nervous system (antihelix) is a powerful point for all gastrointestinal spasms.

P/TCM. Shenmen for pain relief and also a calming point.

P/HF. For constipation or diarrhoea a good point on the face is Chengjiang (CV-24) in the depression below the bottom lip.

Cystitis

Symptoms

Pain and discomfort in the bladder, and the desire to pass urine more frequently, with discomfort in varying degrees from mild to severe pain. Inflammation of the bladder is often due to *E. coli* bacteria sticking to the bladder tissues, which can cause problems in the whole urinogenital tract. Personal hygiene is essential after passing a motion and after intercourse. To safeguard, always wipe from front to back and do not use flannels. Wear cotton under-wear, not synthetic. Drink copious amounts of water. Cranberry juice and boiled beetroot juice are very helpful in maintaining a healthy lining of the bladder and these help prevent the bacteria from sticking to the bladder wall.

Areas to work

M/R. The whole pelvic area because so many other organs can be affected such as the uterus and the upper part of the vagina, also the small intestine. The bladder point is often red, raised and puffy when there is a problem. The bladder is a mass of blood and lymphatic vessels with a strong nerve supply.

A/A. The kidneys are always an area to assist the bladder in any disorder. These are also paired organs in the meridian theory. Work all spinal reflexes from L2 down to sacral point as this helps relax the pelvic visceral nerves; also work the adrenal glands for inflammation.

P/Hs. LI-4/LU-10 opens up the water passages; this is the same line as for bladder and kidneys in reflex zone of the hands (*see* figure 6.8a and b, pages 209 and 211).

Warning! LI-4 can be used only providing the person is not pregnant, as it is an empirical point to promote delivery during labour.

P/LL. SP-1 and 6, LIV-4 and 5, BL-66 and 39, and KI-2 are helpful points to relieve discomfort. These points aid quickly if pressure is applied directly on the area after a full treatment session.

Warning! SP-6 can be used only providing the person is not pregnant, as it is an empirical point to promote delivery during labour.

P/AS. Bladder, urethra and kidney point.

P/AA. Angle of superior concha for infections of the tract.

P/OM. Adrenal glands (tragus) for the marvellous anti-inflammatory properties.

P/TCM. Shenmen for pain relief.

Depression

Symptoms

A deep feeling of sadness and complete hopelessness, agitation and a general feeling of anxiety prevails regardless of what the person does. There are many stress-related causes to this problem (*see* chapter 10).

Areas to work

M/R. A good general treatment, with emphasis on any area that may be a problem.

A/A. Brain and spinal area, also the solar plexus and all the endocrine glands.

P/Hs. HE-9, 8 and 7, also PE-9 and 5 and LI-1 are major points worked together with a full treatment session or applied by themselves. They are excellent for reducing any confused state and they have a calming action on the body.

P/LL. KI-1 on the plantar aspect of the foot, the first point of the Kidney channel, is an essential point for all acute and major problems.

P/AS. Brain area.

P/AA. Midpoint of rim; this relates to the cerebral cortex.

P/OM. Subcortex for all cerebral disorders.

P/TCM. Ear Shenmen has a wonderful calming action.

A case history of depression is given in box 8.6.

***Box 8.6* CASE HISTORY: Depression**

Female, aged 42 years, housewife with two teenage daughters, and a very supportive husband.

Clinical problems presented at first treatment. Depression. Headaches, feeling of a tight band around head, painful periods, disturbed sleep, general feeling of anxiety and panic attacks.

Diet. She felt it was good when she could eat. Her appetite was poor and she had no inclination for food generally. When she did cook for the family she enjoyed it.

Background medical history. Had experienced problems before; periods of depression were short, but they had always lifted. This episode had lasted for about a year. She had been suffering with feelings of depression, she was weepy and she would not go out, she suffered sleepless nights and low energy levels and loss of libido. She also complained of pains in her chest and she had terrible thoughts thinking she was going mad. Her GP prescribed Prozac for her and for a brief time she felt better, even though she had a marked reaction to the drug and the most annoying intestinal fluctuations. When she came to see me she had been on the drug for 9 months; she complained of headaches and feelings of nervousness. She could not sleep and her bowels were still causing a problem. The main problem was that she felt as though she had a tight band around her head. Her GP had said this was due to fibrositis of the head, and nothing to do with the medication. She was also seeing a psychologist and she felt she was getting worse instead of better and she found that attending a clinic within the same hospital that her father was in most alarming and upsetting.

History of patient. Her parents had a history of nervous disorders. Her mother had had a nervous breakdown in her mid thirties and the daughter had remembered this time with horror. Her father had a brain tumour and was now hospitalized with some diminished functions of the brain, and this all added to her general stress levels.

Observation of the feet and general evaluation. The tips of her toes very red and feet in general felt hot and clammy. The feet felt lifeless. Liver area very red and a patch of dry skin just below balls of both feet solar plexus area.

When she presented herself on the first day, the general feeling was of poor muscle tone; generally the foot was very tender to the touch, with great sensitivity on all toes when palpation was given, also the liver area was very tender. I gave this lady a full treatment and she was very, very tender in most areas. I repeated these treatments on a weekly basis over the next 4 weeks; she gradually reduced her medication over this period, a thing she felt she was unable to do before. She had consulted her doctor and told him she was having reflexology and would like to wean herself off the medication gradually. She had tried this twice before but her GP had taken a firm line and had instructed her not to do so. She said she felt she was very much more positive now and could stand up to her GP and consultant, who also had been firm in her attendance at the hospital and continuing her medication.

By week five, she had had no headaches for 10 days. She was much more alert-looking, fresh and radiant and more full of energy. She remarked on her alertness and vitality – where had this come from? This gave me room for thought. Do we stimulate more adrenaline and dopamine production, the excitatory transmitters that can promote this state. Why was she sleeping so soundly after months of sleepless nights? Had the stimulation to the brain area and central nervous system produced the right levels of serotonin to help the process of sleep?

Current health status. This lady now attends on a monthly basis just to ensure that she does not have a relapse. Her comment on her last visit was: 'I have never felt so well and full of life, I can visit my father in hospital without it upsetting me too much. I have started employment 3 days a week, and it seems that I can cope with all of this. Thank you for the reflexology – it is wonderful.' I assured her it was her own healing that had taken place, and we were just practitioners who aided this. After 4 months' treatment, her toes are pink and warm, her feet are firm and strong, and the dry patch on solar plexus is no longer evident.

Diabetes mellitus

Symptoms

This is a disorder of the pancreas in which there is quite simply more sugar in the blood than there should be. There is a homeostatic imbalance causing a derangement in the carbohydrate metabolism and the sugars are not oxidized sufficiently, which is due to a lack of or too little insulin, the pancreatic hormone. This hormone is important to the body as it acts as a regulator of the sugar levels. An imbalance can lead to many other complications, even to a disturbance in the acid–balance. If a person is born with an existing imbalance due to a hereditary factor or it develops in early childhood the prognosis is not quite so good for achieving a swift response. However, if this disorder is of late onset due to any severe stress, which then affects the whole body clock and totally disorientates all the systems of the body creating a homeostatic imbalance, then reflexology can help enormously. The patient is encouraged to lead as normal a life as possible. Dietary habits must be addressed together with lifestyle.

Reflexology will help balance all the systems of the body and make the person relax completely. Professional treatment is essential as glucose levels cannot be controlled by diet on its own and it is imperative to prevent hyperglycaemia developing, which could lead to other serious long-term problems.

Note. The patient should closely monitor the levels of blood glucose to ensure there is not too great a change of insulin levels. Patients should check with their medical practitioners to make sure they are happy about them receiving reflexology.

Areas to work

M/R. A good general treatment, with emphasis on the pancreas area. This helps to stimulate any remaining insulin secretory cells.
A/A. The liver is the area to work to ensure functioning of its many metabolic functions such as: conversion and synthesis of fats, proteins and all the carbohydrates. The liver has the advantage of having an active detoxification process. Also work the immune system, the thymus and spleen to help to trigger the body's defence system.
P/Hs. PE-6 is a vital point for the liver and stomach and the epigastrium (the upper central region of the abdomen). Also use LI-4.
Warning! LI-4 can be used only providing the person is not

pregnant, as it is an empirical point to promote delivery during labour.

P/LL. ST-35 and 36 are ideal for balancing points.

Warning! ST-36 must not be used on young children.

P/AS. Pancreas point as the main area of problem.

P/AA. Apex of antitragus, if there is any pancreatitis.

P/OM. Subcortex and sympathetic nervous system (antihelix) as they both help any functional disturbance of the autonomic nervous system.

P/TCM. Shenmen for pain relief and as an overall calming point.

Digestive disorders

Symptoms

From simple indigestion to abdominal pains. Digestive disorders can be due to many causes such as eating under emotional stress, tension and anxiety, eating hurriedly; even inactivity can create a sluggish digestive system. Poor diet is often the cause of toxic congestion, which can result in the body lacking in vitality causing constant tiredness. We should work the entire digestive system, mouth to anus. Remember as practitioners we must think of the holistic approach, which entails looking at lifestyle and eating patterns.

All secretions of the digestive tract depend upon a very complex relationship between the autonomic nervous system and the hormones that are produced locally within each of the organs. Smokers often have digestive problems because of the inhibition of their smell reflex; the first cranial nerve may be activated to help in this process. Or the alkaline secretions of the pancreas, which neutralize the acids, are inhibited and cannot fulfil their function of acting as a buffer.

Gall bladder stimulation helps emulsify fats so that they are more digestible by the pancreatic lipase. Bile has an aperient action on the bowel, increasing peristalsis in the duodenum. The duodenum is often tender as it has a lot of work to do, releasing enzymes like succus entericus, the necessary enzymes to help the food to be broken down; working the small intestine, the jejunum and ilium, helps in the efficient absorption of food. This is a vital area as most of the digestion and absorption of food takes place here. This stimulation further assists in eradicating any infection as the mass of lymphatics in the small intestine, the peyer's patches, become more efficient in engulfing any bacteria.

Many people suffer from a slight liver imbalance and may feel a little bilious. Gilbert's syndrome is quite common, affecting over 2 per cent of the population. One of the chief constituents of bile is bilirubin; this is derived from haemoglobin, the red pigment of the red blood corpuscles. In this syndrome for some reason this is not processed correctly by the liver. Symptoms are mild jaundice, with a general malaise, abdominal pain, nausea and anorexia (loss of appetite). As there is no treatment for this disorder, life can be quite troublesome to a sufferer; diet must be addressed as certain foods exacerbate the disorder. Together with reflexology this calms the whole system and restores homeostasis to the liver quite quickly.

(*See* plate 11 of a patient's foot with this disorder; also refer to The zones of the digestive (gastrointestinal) system, chapter 5, page 143.)

Areas to work

M/R. Stimulating the tenth cranial nerve, the vagus nerve, the reflex which lies on the great toe in the brain area, has an action of stimulating many of the natural reflex actions such as salivation, the sensations of taste from the mouth, and some gastric secretions. The vagus nerve supplies the stomach, liver, small bowel, large bowel, and regulates acid and pepsin release. It increases peristalsis in the duodenum. Also stimulation of sacral nerves helps sacral outflow of parasympathetic fibres to the terminal parts of the colon to aid defecation.

The sympathetic nervous system (SNS) also needs to be balanced. Work the main area of problem, and then down the spine from T1 to L2 approximately; it is here that the sympathetic ganglia ends in organs or tissues, serving all the blood vessels of the various regions. Disorders like irritable bowel syndrome, diarrhoea and colon diseases are very common. Refer to first causes which are often stress related, incorrect diet or over-working. If the SNS is overactive, motility is often decreased and digestion is poor. Disorders like candida can cause great problems, and may be related to diet and stress. Working the liver lowers the levels of toxins in the system. We aim to stimulate all eliminating organs in a fine and precise way.

A/A. Work the adrenals to help improve any inflammatory process. Stimulation helps the whole process of the immune system, working the lymph in the groin, thymus and spleen. Diet must be looked at. Remember immune function is a key factor in many health problems.

P/Hs. PE-6 is a vital point for the liver and stomach and the epigastrium (the upper central region of the abdomen). TB-3 and 4 stimulate elimination and help the stomach.

P/LL. ST-35 and 36 are ideal for a balancing point. SP-2 aids digestion in general. SP-7 helps flatulence. LIV-5 aids any flatulence.

Warning! ST-36 must not be used on young children.

P/AA. Apex of antitragus, if there is any inflammation.

P/OM. Subcortex and sympathetic nervous system (antihelix), as they both help any functional disturbance of the autonomic nervous system.

P/TCM. Shenmen for pain relief and as an overall calming point.

P/HF. For constipation or diarrhoea a good point on the face is Chengjiang (CV-24) in the depression below the bottom lip.

Ear disorders

Symptoms

Any problem of the ear should never be neglected. Earache is often caused by infection; this can come from the nose, throat or from the teeth. Otitis media is a common disorder of young children; many times this is a secondary infection as infection travels from the nose or throat up the eustachian tube to the ear. Treatment to all areas of the upper respiratory system is essential. The aim is to relieve the congested state by breaking down any excess mucus or catarrh.

Areas to work

M/R. Ear points, facial and head-related areas. Reflexology is a marvellous way to detoxify the body, working on the liver reflex as this will help to eliminate any excess toxins from the body. Also work the upper cervical C1–C4, as these areas also connect with some of the cranial nerves, mainly the vagus nerve that serves the ear.

A/A. Stimulation to the adrenal glands with its powerful anti-inflammatory properties will calm and relieve any tendency to inflammation, also any wheeziness, breaking up any stubborn congestion, facilitating the whole breathing process, from the nose through to the throat and nasopharynx. This will help the ear.

P/Hs. TB-1 and 2 are ideal points for otitis media and general ear problems.

P/OM. Adrenal glands (tragus) for the powerful anti-inflammatory properties.

P/LL. GB-43 and 44 are good points for ear problems.

P/AS. Adrenal glands point as the corticosteroids aid in calming even the most inflamed area.

P/AA. Apex of ear and apex of antitragus help in all inflammatory disorders.

P/TCM. Shenmen for pain relief and calming point. Wind Stream, an allergy point.

(*See also* Sinusitis and Tinnitus, pages 336 and 345.)

P/HF. Tinggong (SI-19) is ideal for all ear problems.

Eczema

Symptoms

Any superficial inflammation of the skin. Eczema is taken from the Greek word (*Ek Zeein*) meaning to boil, seethe, or anything thrown off or out by an internal reaction. All of these definitions imply excess heat or excess turmoil within. Eczema is often exacerbated by stress-related problems. Skin disorders often manifest owing to poor function and activity within the internal organs; this malfunction is often manifested as the large amounts of toxic waste that the skin will try and eliminate when it cannot excrete it by other means. Patients with skin problems often have tender liver, spleen, kidney and lung reflexes; this indicates an imbalance within the organs involved in the homeostatic functions of the body. Many sufferers of eczema also have asthma or breathing problems. A reflexologist sees these disorders as neither solely allergic in origin, nor particularly as an inherited tendency, because manifestataions of these conditions have so many variable causes. A proficient practitioner will embrace the total holistic concept, including nutrition and lifestyle; stress also causes an inhibition of the normal flow of energy and an interruption in nerve impulses or electric signals throughout the body.

As stated, the manifestation of this condition has so many variable causes: it is not solely allergic in origin as we know stress can play a part in this disorder, which, in turn, is exacerbated by the very problem the patient is suffering from. Eczema is an attempt by the body to throw off the unwanted accumulation of toxins from the system through the skin. Many foods that contain additives are often the culprit. Applying substances or salves to the skin may force the problem deeper. It must be tackled at its source. Reflexology and diet help enormously. A fast is advised for 2 to 3 days, with lots of water, then a restricted diet for about 2 weeks. This should consist of lots of raw salads, lightly cooked vegetables, and dressings made with olive oil and lemon. Quantity does not matter; let hunger be the guide of the amounts to eat. Then a bland diet should follow until all eruptions have completely healed and disappeared. It is important to check to see whether there are any stomach problems, flatulence, or acid regurgitation; this is often a sign that there may be an allergy, which may be a lactose intolerance, and dairy products could be making the problem worse.

Areas to work

M/R. All digestive areas. Reflexology is a marvellous way to detoxify the body; working on the liver reflex will help to eliminate any excess heat in the body. The skin is related to the lungs according to the Chinese theory; it is amazing how many sufferers of eczema also have asthma or breathing problems, so work this reflex.

A/A. Stimulation to the adrenal glands with its powerful anti-inflammatory properties will calm the most persistent itching, and relieve any tendency to wheeziness, breaking up any stubborn congestion, and facilitating the whole breathing process.

P/Hs. TB-6 for all skin eruptions, urticaria, hives and eczema.

P/LL. ST-35 and 36 are ideal for a balancing point.

   Warning! ST-36 must not be used on young children.

P/AS. Adrenal glands point as the corticosteroids aid in calming even the most inflamed area.

P/AA. Apex of ear helps in all inflammatory disorders.

P/OM. Adrenal glands (tragus) for its powerful anti-inflammatory and anti-allergic properties.

P/TCM. Wind Stream, an allergy point. Shenmen for pain relief and as a calming point.

   (*See also* chapter 9.)

Eye disorders

Most general disorders can be helped enormously with reflexology. The majority of minor inflammation can be greatly eased. With the ageing process other problems can also occur; even medication can create imbalances in the eyes. All the 'itis' disorders can be helped.

Symptoms

Any sudden change in vision should always be investigated; however, there are many points to help in everyday irritating problems.

Areas to work

M/R. Eye area, on the distal phalanges of hands and feet, in zones 2 and 3. The neck and cervical area will stimulate the nerve pathways, also the brain area for the optic nerve, the second cranial nerve.
A/A. The kidneys have a zonal link.
P/Hs. SI-2, LI-1 and 4 for all eye problems.
  Warning! LI-4 can be used only providing the person is not pregnant, as it is an empirical point to promote delivery during labour.
P/LL. GB-44 for any eye disorder. GB-37 is a distal point for any optic atrophy and is known as the eye-brightening point.
P/AS. All the eye points. Eye 1 is ideal for glaucoma, or shortsightedness. Eye 2 is mainly for any astigmatism.
P/AA. Apex of antitragus for all the 'itis' disorders.
P/HF. *See* Self-help tips of head and facial areas, page 228, for eye disorders.

Fibromyalgia

Symptoms

The term is often used for any musculoskeletal pain or excessive stiffness; sometimes there is also unexplained chronic aching in the joints that is not connected to any other disorder. There is often a link between fibromyalgia and chronic fatigue syndrome, or ME as it is more commonly known, as both disorders are somewhat similar in as much as they both include impaired muscle function and chronic periods of fatigue after any undue exertion. The aim is to restore a relaxed state; this ensures there is less stress in the body, which may be a cause of the homeostatic imbalance of the whole system.

Areas to work

M/R. Main area of problem. Also work the adrenals for the naturally occurring corticosteroids, which do not cause undue side-effects; these quickly help to relieve pain and inflammation in most parts of the body. Reflexology relaxes all the muscles and tendons, allowing greater freedom of movement, and less pain generally.

A/A. Work the liver and kidney areas to ensure that there is no undue build-up of toxins; these are often released when any chronic inflammatory process is present, and they can cause further tissue damage if not eliminated properly.

P/Hs. TB-5 and HE-4 will help upper limb problems. SI-5 and 6 will help lower limb problems.

P/LL. LIV-8 will aid all four limbs, because it communicates with the gall bladder, the lungs, the stomach and the brain; it has a widespread effect on those organs that are involved in the regulation of the metabolic processes. Also GB-39 helps with any weakness of limbs.

P/AS. Work area of problem.

P/AA. Apex of ear, and apex of antitragus, for inflammation and an analgesic effect. Continue pressures daily on this area.

P/OM. Subcortex will act as a strong analgesic, as this is a functional disturbance of the whole autonomic nervous system.

P/TCM. Shenmen for pain relief.

Frozen shoulder

Symptoms

Chronic pain or inability to move the shoulder joint.

Three bones meet at the shoulder: the scapula (shoulder blade), the clavicle (collar bone) and the humerus (upper arm bone). The shoulders are a diarthrosis or a synovial, freely movable, ball and socket joint. Shoulder problems are very common and often affect the neck, arm and hand. Shoulder mobility normally includes: elevation, external and internal rotation, horizontal flexion and extension, the most mobile point being between the humerus and scapula. Tendinitis, capsulitis and bursitis are all problems that often occur with a frozen shoulder, and occasionally a tendon may rupture. This total loss of mobility does not occur in any other part of the body. Most shoulder problems recover in time but they can last up to a year, going from the limited stage to frozen stage and then gradual mobility, but even up to 3 years later certain restrictions can still occur. Reflexology encourages nature's healing programme. A frozen shoulder seems to occur more in women in the menopausal years, even though I have treated many men; it can also occur in the less used limb. When in the early stages, the medical profession usually respond by suggesting locally acting corticosteroids. These can cause loss of pigmentation in the skin and in certain cases the problem may be exacerbated. Other forms of treatment such as anti-inflammatory pain-relieving medication, in tablet form and in creams, heat, ultrasound and physiotherapy are all tried, but often patients may respond slowly to these. This leaves them confused and depressed because the harder they try the worse the shoulder gets.

When patients first come for reflexology treatment they are so relieved that someone is listening to them. Reflexology treatment enables a patient to relax completely, which helps to relieve the pain and the shoulder gradually improves. Once this occurs we encourage patients to take responsibility for gradual exercise because they realize the healing process has begun. They can now accept this but are often amazed at the results especially if the medical profession were unable to help.

While shoulder problems persist, as described, the arm should get as much rest as possible, with no heavy lifting or straining, just normal movement as much as possible, and within 8 weeks nine out of ten patients will be almost completely recovered. Even though the shoulder is often more painful in the early stages, once it becomes frozen it may be limited in its use, but it is often more comfortable when sleeping. It is of the utmost importance that sleeping patterns are looked at for this condition (*see* Behaviour patterns, chapter 3, page 89). When the arm begins to be more mobile then the patient is encouraged to do gentle exercises. Measure the amount of increased movement each session, by getting the patient to lift to a certain point on the wall. It is amazing how each session brings about more mobility.

Areas to work

M/R. The main shoulder and axillary area, and the shoulder muscle and chronic neck point for the sternocleidomastoid muscle, as movement of the neck affects the shoulder and the pectoralis muscles.
A/A. Cervical spine as the brachial plexus serves the whole region. Also the adrenal glands for the naturally occurring corticosteroids that do not cause undue side-effects, but quickly help to relieve pain and inflammation. This affects all the muscles in the shoulder region as they work in combination with one another; if they are stiff or inflamed, reflexology relaxes them allowing greater freedom of movement.
P/Hs. SI-4, 5 and 6 for all arm and shoulder problems. LI-4 is essential for any painful shoulder impediment.

Warning! LI-4 can only be used providing the person is not pregnant, as it is an empirical point to promote delivery during labour.

P/LL. ST-38 is marvellous for relieving a stiff shoulder; apply pressure to the point and get the patient to move the shoulder at the same time as this firm pressure is maintained; the pain and stiffness are gradually relieved. Also GB-43 helps shoulder and axillary areas.

P/AS. Firm pressures on shoulder and cervical point.

P/AA. Apex of ear, and apex of antitragus, for inflammation and an analgesic effect; continue pressures daily.

Self-help tip: use a cotton wool bud or the bottom end of a matchstick with a little cotton wool around it to apply firm pressure on the points; if you are unable to do this get your partner or friend to apply these pressures.

P/OM. Adrenal glands; this point has strong analgesic properties.

P/TCM. Shenmen for pain relief.

(*See* figure 5.9a for upper limbs.)

Gall stones

Symptoms

Pain and discomfort often appear in the shoulder region between the shoulder blades or high in the upper abdomen. Certain foods can bring on an attack, and the person may be sick. Gall stones are hard masses of pigment made up of cholesterol and calcium salts. These may be present over many years without causing any undue discomfort or pain, unless they block a bile duct. It is imperative that diet is addressed, so that the patient is aware of cholesterol-forming foods, as these must be eliminated from the diet. Patients should be encouraged to increase their fibre intake and the amount of water they drink.

Areas to work

M/R. The liver/gall bladder to regulate any excesses of cholesterol levels; this also calms down the biliary tract by normalizing the body's own production of bile acids, which then in turn act on the stones to break them down.

A/A. The thyroid/parathyroid to balance the levels of thyrocalcitonin; also ribcage relaxation.

P/Hs. PE-6 and TB-3 are both involved in normalizing the liver.

LI-4 can be used as a calming point as it has an antispasmodic action.

Warning! LI-4 can be used only providing the person is not pregnant, as it is an empirical point to promote delivery during labour.

P/LL. GB-40 helps all the upper hypochondrium.

P/AS. Liver/gall bladder points.

P/AA. Centre of superior concha for abdominal pain.

P/OM. Sympathetic nervous system (antihelix), for all biliary colic.

P/TCM. Shenmen for pain relief.

Gastritis

Symptoms

Pain and discomfort are often similar to the pain of an ulcer; severe discomfort is felt in the upper abdominal area. This may occur immediately after eating, or within a short period of about 3 hours. This problem arises because of some irritation to the stomach lining, which becomes inflamed. This can be caused by many things such as: alcohol, smoking, or too much stress in everyday life. Occasionally it can be due to an autoimmune disorder, whereby the body's own antibodies destroy the tissue and inflammation manifests in the stomach lining, creating a problem.

Areas to work

M/R. The stomach area to neutralize the acid and any inflammation, allowing natural healing to take place. Treatment should always be aimed at approximately 2–3 hours after the main meal of the day, as this will help to balance the acid surge that occurs at this time, which is often the culprit of the annoying problem.

A/A. The great toe for the vagus nerve as its nerve fibres serve the stomach and whole digestive tract; it also regulates the acid and pepsin release.

P/Hs. PE-6 and TB-4 are potent points to aid the stomach.

P/LL. ST-35, 36 and 39 will regulate the stomach's activity.

Warning! ST-36 must not be used on young children.

P/AS. All abdominal areas.

P/AA. Apex of antitragus for inflammatory problems.

P/OM. Subcortex and sympathetic nervous system, as both are involved in regulating the autonomic nervous system. Work the vagus nerve directly on the dorsal surface.

P/TCM. Shenmen for pain relief.

Gynaecological disorders

This is dealt with under Menstrual problems (page 305). However, the whole reproductive tract can be treated as disorders often occur because of a homeostatic imbalance within a given area. With treatment hormonal imbalances are normalized very quickly, and these abnormalities once corrected allow normal functioning and healing within.

Haemorrhoids

Symptoms

These are often referred to as piles. Haemorrhoidal veins form the lowest section of the portal system; as they have no valves at this point it is quite common for them to become distended. Any venal distension in the anal area can be painful; as the veins of the rectum become distended and the anus becomes aggravated many factors can irritate them. This can be due to constipation, in which case the diet must be altered to include fresh vegetables and fruit. Daily exercise or regular walking will improve the circulation in general, especially the portal circulation. Other known causes are pregnancy and the repeated use of laxatives; even sitting on cold surfaces can irritate. People who lead a sedentary lifestyle with little exercise are often prone to this problem. This is why behaviour factors are studied as occupation can also aggravate or cause the problem. People who may be vulnerable are lorry drivers or sales people who spend long hours driving, and office staff who sit for long periods on synthetic seats with little movement; these occupations can exacerbate an already existing problem causing a sluggish bowel action and pelvic congestion.

Fluid is absorbed throughout the large intestine, therefore the longer the waste matter is retained, the more it becomes dehydrated and the more difficult to pass.

Areas to work

M/R. Work the solar plexus and diaphragm reflexes to reduce stress and normalize functions of the abdominal organs. Liver and gall bladder reflexes aid digestion and release bile to act as a mild laxative; this makes it easier for stools to be passed. Also work the spinal area as the pudendal nerve serves the anal sphincter.
A/A. Pancreatic reflexes to secrete digestive juices, changing acidic contents leaving the stomach to alkaline. Stomach and intestine

reflexes to perform their digestive secretions and absorption, and to encourage peristalsis to move the contents onwards. Adrenal reflexes to increase metabolism and aid in any inflammation that may arise.

Always finish treatments with relaxing techniques, friction, moulding, spinal twist and solar plexus relaxation, with crossed hands to balance energy. Do solar plexus deep breathing so that client enjoys the treatment and has a positive attitude to good health and vitality. Often people who are constipated have a reserved nature, and tend to withhold.

If it is a client's first treatment I would give a complete but gentle treatment to both feet, so as to chart the sensitive reflexes. The signs of imbalance of areas of the digestive system should show up in sensitive areas, in the appearance of creases, calluses, or the condition of the nails. Reflexology treats the body as a whole, to normalize all bodily functions. Ask the client to note changes and responses to treatment. After a couple of days, depending upon the results, a further treatment paying special attention to specific complaints in specific areas of reflexes may be required.

P/Hs. LI-2 and 4 for all intestinal disorders. Also TB-4 to aid in elimination.

Warning! LI-4 can be used only providing the person is not pregnant as it is an empirical point to promote delivery during labour.

P/LL. SP-5 aids any constipation and haemorrhoids.

P/AS. Rectum and anus point.

P/AA. Apex of antitragus for inflammatory problems.

P/OM. Subcortex and sympathetic nervous system, as both are involved in regulating the autonomic nervous system.

P/TCM. Shenmen for pain relief.

P/HF. Chengjiang (CV-24) point on the lower lip helps all constipation.

Self-help tips: spray cold water to the area, ensure the diet contains sufficient fibre, and drink at least six glasses of water daily.

Hayfever

Symptoms

Some people are hypersensitive to pollen or spores that are all around us in the air we breathe. If the person inhales this allergen then a substance known as histamine found in all tissues of the body is released; this is often known as the defence mechanism, but its release may cause dilation of the blood vessels as a response and this may cause inflammation of the mucous membranes. The excess fluid production takes place in the delicate lining of the nose, sinuses and the eyes, causing unpleasant irritation of all surfaces. Treatment is similar to eczema, which is also often an allergic reaction. Reflexology treatment should commence prior to the hayfever season starting. The client should try to avoid situations that make the problem worse; eg when driving keep the windows closed and use the air conditioner if possible.

Areas to work

M/R. Reflexology is a marvellous way to detoxify the body, working on the liver reflex will help to eliminate any excess toxins from the body. The skin is related to the lungs according to the Chinese theory; it is amazing how many asthma sufferers have eczema and/or suffer from hayfever.

A/A. Stimulation to the adrenal glands, with its powerful anti-inflammatory properties, will calm and relieve any tendency to wheeziness, breaking up any stubborn congestion, and facilitating the whole breathing process.

P/Hs. LI-4 is a good point for hayfever.

Warning! LI-4 can be used only providing the person is not pregnant, as it is an empirical point to promote delivery during labour.

P/LL. SP-1 and GB-44 help all nose and lung problems.

P/AS. Adrenal glands point, as the corticosteroids aid in calming even the most inflamed area.

P/AA. Apex of ear helps in all inflammatory disorders.

P/OM. Adrenal glands (tragus) for its marvellous anti-inflammatory and antiallergic properties.

P/TCM. Shenmen for pain relief and as a calming point. Wind Stream, an allergy point.

P/HF. There are many eye and nose points (*see* chapter 7, page 212).

Hazardous lifestyle

Tobacco

Smoking can cause the bronchiole to constrict, producing mucopus. Smoking can paralyse the cilia, the little hairs that line the upper respiratory tract, for hours and irritate the sensitive lining of the airways producing even more inflammation. Smokers often develop an irritating cough to remove this congestion; persistent coughing drains and damages the lungs and reduces their efficiency. Tar droplets remain in the lungs, and chemicals from tar can cause growths which can develop into cancer of the bronchial tubes. Carbon monoxide is a poisonous gas inhaled while smoking; it can reduce the ability of the blood and interfere with its oxygen-carrying capacity.

Nicotine is another poisonous substance in tobacco; it is also strongly addictive and can increase the pulse rate and blood pressure. Nicotine disturbs the balance of fatty substances in the bloodstream. Poisoning can occur owing to excessive amounts of nicotine. In the first instance there is overstimulation of the central nervous system and the autonomic nervous system; this is closely followed by depression of these systems. Prolonged inhalation or ingestion of this toxic substance leads to a decrease in the diameter of the blood vessels (vasoconstriction) of the hands and feet, and peripheral vascular disorders may develop. Patients may complain of pains in their hands, arms, feet or legs. The tips of the toes may have a loss of sensation on the plantar aspect of the feet; the lung reflex appears yellow, and the liver reflex is very tender owing to this toxic substance.

Smoking is one of the main causes of lung cancers; just a small percentage of these cancers are caused by atmospheric pollutants such as sulphur dioxide and nitrogen oxides. Smokers are also more at risk of a heart attack than are non-smokers. Because of the carbon monoxide reducing the amount of oxygen in the blood, the heart has to work much harder but gets less oxygen. A quarter of all deaths from heart attacks are thought to be caused by smoking. The nicotine and carbon monoxide make the blood more prone to clotting, accelerating the furring up of the coronary arteries so blocking them.

Nature's way of dealing with this problem is to try to get rid of all excess bacteria produced by mucus congestion by coughing and sneezing. It is only when the airways become blocked up and congested that you need to resort to other methods. Reflexology applied in the right way will ease this congested state.

There are several stages to stopping smoking and several attempts may have to be made before succeeding, the main point is to want to stop. Making a simple list of the incentives to stopping is helpful. The most important factor is to be aware of vulnerable times. At these times the main objective is to keep busy but try to relax. Reflexology helps put the person in a more relaxed state, prior to starting any withdrawal or eliminating programme. It makes them more determined, easing the withdrawal stage, and helps to eliminate any mucus or congestion, so breathing improves.

(*See* plate 9 of a smoker with irritable bowel syndrome and wheat intolerance.)

Areas to work

This is a total functional disorder, so a complete treatment over many weeks, together with a change in lifestyle, can only be beneficial. (Refer to The zones of the respiratory system, chapter 5, page 136, for lung imbalance.)

M/R. When there is a problem with the respiratory system in whatever form it is most important to work the intestinal areas thoroughly as this is an area that will assist in the removal of any excess mucus. This includes upper respiratory problems such as a sinus infection; this infection spreads from the pharynx and the congested mucosa can become even more infected by bacteria and become a chronic problem. Pharyngitis, laryngitis and tonsillitis are all related to the same viral and bacterial infection with a great deal of excess mucus (*see* Colds, page 271).

A/A. As well as covering all respiratory areas, work intestinal points to eliminate any excess mucus; the lungs and intestines have an intimate contact according to TCM.

P/AA. Apex of ear as a soothing analgesic effect.

P/TCM. Ear Shenmen point will help any withdrawal syndrome; it also helps any associated anxiety by tranquillizing the mind.

Alcohol

Alcohol is a chemical substance that alters the functioning of the body. Heavy drinking over a period of many years may cause long-term ill-effects on the body. These can take place from the brain downwards, damaging body tissue, the main two problems being cirrhosis of the liver because this organ is responsible for metabolizing alcohol from the blood, and cardiomyopathy, which can lead to a reduction in the force of heart contractions, and in turn to a decrease in the efficiency of blood circulation. In certain cases peripheral neuritis is evident with numbness or tingling felt on the extremities.

Areas to work

As for the previous disorder, also the kidneys to assist filtration and absorption. Stimulation should be firm but not too heavy. The result is the kidneys respond according to the body's needs.

Excess stress

Most people experience stress at some time in their lives; this stress can take place at home or in the workplace, or certain life events can produce extreme stress, eg birth of a baby, death of a loved one, divorce, physical violence, family conflict, moving house, loss of a job, unpleasant thoughts, unpleasant sights, accidents, too much heat, cold or noise; these are only a few of the many aspects of life that may cause an overload of stress. Any stressful stimuli can immediately change the internal environment of the body.

Reflexology is a must for any stressful situation, it is a complete stress buster often within one treatment. (*See* Stress disorders, page 343, and chapter 10 for a detailed discussion.)

Diet

Diet can be a key factor in many disorders. The right choice of food is most essential to help maintain a healthy heart. Basically eat less fat, salt and sugar and more starch and fibre, especially more fruit and vegetables. A high intake of natural vitamin C from fresh vegetables and citrus fruits is a health booster. Also increase water intake, drinking at least six glasses of water daily, and cut back on stimulants such as tea and coffee. (*See* chapter 11 for a detailed discussion.)

Physical activity

It is advisable to become more active gradually; there are many things that can be done to improve fitness levels. People of all ages can enjoy a brisk walk; walking can be encouraged instead of always using a car or taking a bus. Little adjustments to daily activities, like walking up stairs instead of using a lift or escalator, are beneficial. As strength and stamina improve through gentle exercise then everyday activities will become easier. Walking will also strengthen the heart muscle.

The most important point is to enjoy the exercise, and aim to increase any exercise routine slowly. If in doubt about health always check with a medical practitioner first.

Areas to work

A general treatment working all heart reflexes on hands and feet, cervical and thoracic spinal areas; this helps all areas of the thoracic cavity down to the diaphragm as these nerves arise from three levels of the cervical trunk, then descend through the thoracic inlet and end in the cardiac plexus. Their fibres reach the lungs and all associated viscera as well as the heart. The vagus nerve arises from the brain and emerges at the medulla oblongata around the ear and continues through the neck to the thorax and then on into the abdomen. A reflexologist will work all these areas in a full treatment.

Self-help tips: many points help to calm a person down and normalize the heart function. First pressure points on the hands are PE-4, one hand's-width above the crease of the wrist, which will help the heart. The heart meridian from HE-9 down to HE-5 will help irregular heartbeat and palpitations; these are calming points and will strengthen the heartbeat. Stroking the ear on the sympathetic point at the top of the ear between the helix and the antihelix helps the circulation as there is stimulation to the autonomic nervous system at this point. The subcortex on the medial side of the antitragus regulates the circulation and the whole cardiovascular function. The vagus nerve can be contacted by stroking behind the ear. KI-1 on the plantar aspect of the foot for all acute problems. Duyin on the middle of the second toe is for cardiac pain, and the Qiduan reflex points on the tips of the toes are for helping the nervous system. Shixuan points are for all acute problems; these are on the fingertips. Press in with opposite hand as near to the nail as possible, and do both hands; this has a good calming action.

Headaches

Symptoms

Patients often complain that they are prone to headaches and worry that it could be some underlying disease. The pain is not from the brain itself, however, which has no sensory nerves; it is from the meninges and the blood vessels surrounding the brain and also the muscles of the scalp. The pain may be in a specific area, a general to deep throbbing or even stabbing pain, which can sometimes lead to vomiting and visual disturbances. Many headaches have common causes such as: hangovers, poor ventilation in home or office, excitement and even excessive sleep. Certain foods can act as a trigger to bring one on; the known irritants are: chocolate, red wine, cheese, and food additives (which are in most packaged foods). Sinus problems and migraine itself can be severely debilitating problems; neck strain, constipation, high blood pressure, eye strain and indigestion all play a part in causing this distressing disorder.

Areas to work

M/R. Work the liver to detoxify and cleanse the system. Often the simple explanation is that high toxic levels in the system have reached the brain barrier or the cranial arteries are dilated, causing pressure. Often, stimulation of the vagus nerve can cause a normalization of such dilation. Reflexology relaxes and acts as a sedative; it has antispasmodic action on the muscles of the neck and scalp, and it stimulates the cerebral circulation and tones up the central nervous system. However, persistent headaches should be checked with a GP for any abnormalities.

A/A. The fifth cranial nerve (the trigeminal nerve, a paired nerve) arises one each side from the pons varolii, part of the brainstem. The skull is innervated by the trigeminal nerve, which splits into three main branches: the ophthalmic nerve, which serves most of the scalp and upper eyelids, tear glands and cornea; the maxillary nerve, which supplies the upper jaw, sinuses and teeth; and the mandibular nerve, which supplies the lower jaw and the muscles involved in chewing and the production of saliva. This nerve can be reached on the lateral edge of the great toe, and it relaxes the jaw area, which is often held tight with the teeth firmly clenched, creating further problems.

P/Hs. SI-1 for headaches and LI-4. This can be used as it is a calming point and has an antispasmodic action on any facial neuralgia.

Warning! LI-4 can be used only providing the person is not pregnant, as it is an empirical point to promote delivery during labour.

P/LL. BL-67, GB-44 and LIV-2 for headaches.

P/AS. Brain area.

P/AA. Midpoint of rim – aids the cerebral cortex.

P/OM. Subcortex for its analgesic properties.

P/TCM. Shenmen for pain relief, and Liver Yang (helix).
P/HF. There are many points for headaches (*see* chapter 7, page 224).

Heart disorders

We would all like to discover what causes heart problems. For years scientists have studied many different factors, but there seems no one isolated cause that will increase the risk of a heart disorder, and in fact there are many contributing factors. Statistics are supposed to show that men are predominantly more at risk than women. It is quite natural as part of the ageing process for our arteries to narrow, but many factors can exacerbate this natural ageing process of hardening or loss of elasticity and furring up of the linings of the blood vessels, which may lead to angina or a heart attack. The vulnerable years used to be from 50 years old onwards in women, possibly due to a reduction in hormones that had given some protection in earlier life. In men the danger time seemed to be from the mid 40s onwards. However, there seems to be an increased risk in all age groups.

Inherited abnormal genes or genetic variations cannot be controlled by the individual. However, many things can be done to help maintain a healthy heart. A hazardous lifestyle may be increasing the risk, and this is one of the three major factors that needs to be embraced; the other two are diet and exercise.

(*See* plate 10, of a patient with heart disease, *also* the circulatory system and foot analysis, chapter 5, pages 150–7. *See also* Circulatory disorders, page 270 and Hazardous lifestyles, pages 291–5.)

Areas to work

M/R. Work heart reflex, but remember many other factors are involved. Working the liver area helps to detoxify the system.
A/A. Stimulation of the whole system will balance any irregularities.
P/Hs. HE-5, 7 and 9, and PE-4 will regulate and strengthen the heartbeat.
P/LL. SP-4 is specifically for cardiac inflammation.
P/AS. Heart and cardia.
P/AA. Centre of ear; as this point contacts the vagus nerve directly, it will have a calming influence and slow down the heart.
P/OM. Subcortex; because this point contacts the functional areas,

it controls and regulates many of the visceral activities, such as the heart rate.

P/TCM. Shenmen for pain relief, and as a calming point.

Self-help tips: if tense or agitated you can stimulate your parasympathetic nervous system just by stroking or palpating the ears to the back of the auricle; this calms you down immediately. It supplies sensory fibres to the ear. The point is almost at the hinge of the jaw; it is where the vagus nerve passes through the neck on its way to the abdomen. Also fingertip first aid working on the heart and pericardium pressure points will help. Stroke the wrist area, below the little finger, over the creases. Apply pressure between the tendons a palm's-width up the arm; this point will help angina and any increase of heart rate above normal.

A case history of heart disorder is given in box 8.7.

Box 8.7   CASE HISTORY: Heart disorder

Male, aged 55 years, retired headmaster.

Psychological state.   He is very aware of his position within his small community; he is a regular attender of his local church, and has always helped in compiling the church accounts. A very pedantic man, extremely aware of his appearance; he used to be a keen keep-fit enthusiast. The wife is the deputy head of a local primary school, and they have two children, a daughter and son. The son had caused them many problems since the age of 14 years old; he had dropped out from college and had been a constant source of worry ever since. The daughter had completed her studies, was most supportive of the brother, and had no conflict with the parents.

Clinical problems presented at first treatment.   He could not walk straight and veered to one side, also he had a droop to one side of the face.

Background medical history.   He had suffered a stroke about a year before, and also had high blood pressure. He was awaiting a triple heart bypass operation owing to a blocked coronary artery.

Medication.   Propranolol – Niazinopol.

Observation of the hands, feet and general evaluation.   The feet and hands were very moist, and the feet and parts of the legs and arms had many eruptions. There were excessive amounts of perspiration of hands and feet (hyperhidrosis). The feet were extremely yellow in the colon area; there was also a raised area on the bladder point, and a rash present on both feet up to the ankle area. He was very breathless on arrival.

Over the first few treatments I worked very gently, because of his problems; because of open areas I wore surgical gloves. The area to the kidney reflex was extremely tender. The rash persisted even though there was general improvement in his walking. His face had lost the drooping look on the right side and he no longer dribbled. He decided to go to his GP because the rash was not clearing as he wished and he was prescribed steroids.

Current health status. Over several weeks he received treatments that resulted in a great improvement to his general well-being, but his breathlessness had increased, even with the slightest exertion. He underwent his triple heart bypass operation and returned 10 days after leaving hospital because he was in severe pain in the sternum and clavicle areas owing to his surgery. The first thing I noticed was the complete absence of any rash on his feet and ankles. We went through all the things that he had not eaten whilst in hospital and the missing ingredient was his fish oil capsules! After his treatment he no longer had pain in the sternum area. He now attends on a regular 6-weekly basis to continue maintaining his good health. This case history proved successful in the case of the skin problem because of the holistic approach to the patient, embracing all factors. This gentleman attends on a 1-monthly basis as a preventative measure.

Heartburn

Symptoms

A burning sensation may be felt in the throat or the oesophagus, a feeling of discomfort may occur after eating.

Areas to work

M/R. The great toe for the vagus nerve to normalize acid and pepsin release. Work the solar plexus, diaphragm reflexes and stomach reflexes to regulate the functions of the abdominal organs. Work on the adrenals in case the oesophagus is inflamed.
A/A. The spinal reflex will aid and control the general speed of the passage of food and the rate that digestion takes place; digestion is

greater and takes only a short time if you quietly rest after taking any food.

P/Hs. LI-3 for any flatulence.

P/LL. SP-2 and 3 aid digestion in general.

P/AS. All digestive organs.

P/AA. Subcortex for all functional disturbances.

P/TCM. Sanjiao as it contacts the vagus nerve, and increases the digestive process.

Indigestion

Symptoms

Indigestion is a general term for abdominal discomfort, usually this occurs just after eating. It has many causes, and investigation is necessary in order to improve or cure the condition. This is where the initial consultation is very useful; however, some clients may not feel totally at ease on the first visit. The client will develop confidence in your treatment and you, and problems can be discussed in more depth on subsequent visits. Starting with the mouth, bad teeth or ill-fitting dentures or even teeth that are missing owing to extraction will certainly affect the mastication of food. Other causes may be missing breakfast or lunch and then having a large meal at night to make up for it, or eating the wrong foods – those that are high in fat or too spicy – eating when not hungry, or eating when stressed. How long after a meal the pain occurs can help identify the problem. Disorders like stomach ulcers and duodenal ulcers, and gastric ulcers or, higher up in the tract, heartburn, are often caused by the presence of acid, pepsin and bile breaching the mucosal lining of the organ or tract. Eating too quickly or an excessively large meal can cause heartburn and indigestion.

Constipation, flatulence, haemorrhoids, nausea, stress, depression, and insufficient secretion of bile or pancreatic juices to neutralize the acid, all affect the digestive system; they can, if allowed to continue, cause chronic problems. Prevention of a large number of digestive disorders can be achieved by more careful attention to everyday things, like washing fruit and vegetables (as these are often sprayed with pesticides), storing frozen foods at correct temperatures and thawing them out properly before thoroughly cooking, thus preventing multiplication of bacteria like salmonella and listeria, which cause food poisoning. Observance of proper hygiene when handling food should always be adhered to.

Flatulence is often present in tense or stressed people. These people often swallow air as they eat and gas is produced from the bacterial fermentation of the intestinal contents. If there is a bloated, uncomfortable distended feeling this is often due to excess gas in the stomach and intestines. Anyone prone to this problem should be aware that certain foods, such as beans, may cause it.

Constipation or irregular bowel movement may be due to ignoring the signal to evacuate the bowel; further dehydration of contents takes place and stools become even more solid, while gas is produced.

Areas to work

A general treatment will aid indigestion or dyspepsia. Work the solar plexus, diaphragm and stomach areas; also the pancreas reflexes to release digestive juices and the enzymes necessary for digestion. Stimulating the liver reflexes removes waste and toxins; the gall bladder is worked to stimulate bile release; this acts as a mild laxative and the alkaline effect also helps stimulate peristalsis in the duodenum. Working the stomach and intestinal reflexes regulates digestive, absorptive and excretory functions.

(*See* Digestive disorders, page 279 and Gastritis, page 288.)

Insomnia

Symptoms

The client is unable to sleep; this may cause further problems such as a debilitating tiredness. Many factors may be involved, from simple anxiety about a task that has to be undertaken, to a medical reason, or great grief. Relaxation is the key word; most people who have reflexology state how their sleep patterns improve and problems become negligible.

Areas to work

M/R. A full treatment will help to regulate sleep patterns at all ages, including children and older people who need less sleep, or who often rise early. A good bedtime routine is essential, with no stimulating drinks such as coffee, tea, or an alcoholic drink. The latter may make you drowsy but it often disturbs your sleep patterns over a period of time. Work the hands every evening.

A/A. Work the whole digestive system, to ensure that trouble-some disorders like indigestion or constipation are not the cause.
P/Hs. Specifically HE-6, a good point for insomnia.
P/LL. On the base of the heel, the Shimian point.
P/AS. A gentle ear treatment as many points will aid in this problem; treatment creates a relaxed state owing to the analgesic effect.
P/AA. Centre of ear, as this point contacts the vagus nerve, slowing the heart rate.
P/TCM. Ear Shenmen for insomnia.

Jaundice

Symptoms

Gilbert's syndrome is a mild form of jaundice that over 2 per cent of the population suffer from. There is a homeostatic imbalance of the bilirubin; this is often a sign that the liver is slightly impaired in its normal functioning. Usually the patient has yellowing of the feet, hands or eyes; the inference is that the system is toxic; this can be caused by micro-organisms and many aspects have to be considered. Other causes could be gall stones, or a dysfunction of the liver cells. (*See* plate 11 of person with Gilbert's syndrome.)

Areas to work

M/R. Commence on the hands as the liver point may be extra tender; because of the highly toxic state it is necessary to treat gently, so that the body can adjust to the healing process. The hands and ears release fewer toxins.
A/A. Work the whole digestive system.
P/Hs. Specifically PE-6.
P/LL. KI-1 for all acute problems.
P/AS. Liver/gall bladder point, and spleen and pancreas areas to calm the liver.
P/AA. Centre of ear, as this point contacts the vagus nerve.
P/TCM. Sanjiao for the vagus nerve.

Kidney stones

See Gall stones for any calculus.

Knee problems

Symptoms

Any pain or discomfort when carrying out everyday procedures. This complex joint is vulnerable to injury and strain. Often there can be a simple cause of strain of the ligaments or tendons; these strong fibrous bands are at each side and they limit any sideways movement. As the knee is situated between the femur (thigh) and the tibia (shin), with the patella lying across the front, it is partly a hinge and partly a gliding joint, lined with synovial fluid membrane, and two crescent-shaped structures of fibrocartilage (meniscus) divide the cavity. The knee has a range of movements such as flexion, extension, and slight rotation when being flexed. The two discs of cartilage protect and cover the surfaces of the femur and the tibia; this reduces any friction and also increases stability. The quadriceps muscle is important because its tendon forms a considerable part of the capsule of the knee, and it is involved in extension and straightening the joint; if there is any damage this muscle can atrophy very quickly, often within a few days if the knee is not being used properly. The hamstring muscles behind the knee flex the knee. Problems often arise when the muscles are not being used, as this can lead to stiffness and limited movement; often the knee gives way when weight is put on it.

Areas to work

M/R. Knee reflex and hip- and leg-related areas, also spinal areas.
A/A. Stimulation to the adrenal glands will help to activate their powerful anti-inflammatory properties, and this will calm the whole area down.
P/Hs. SI-5 for knee disorders.
P/LL. GB-34, 35, 36 and 37 for all knee and leg problems, and LIV-7 for any knee disorder.
P/AS. Knee point.
P/AA. Apex of ear for any inflammatory disorder.
P/OM. Adrenal glands for any inflammatory disorder.
P/TCM. Shenmen for pain relief.

Leg and foot problems

There appears to be insufficient literature available in the field of reflexology regarding leg and foot problems. We know that sudden onset of back pain can be helped quite quickly with reflexology. Chronic back pain is usually the result of the problem being ignored in its early stages and this often develops as a pain in muscles (tendon and ligament) going down to the lower limbs. I deal with many sports injuries, particularly in athletes, and this has led me to take a deeper interest in the lumbar and sacral spinal nerves and the distribution to some of the voluntary muscles, to help leg and foot pain. As well as an ability to acquire injuries, we also have a remarkable ability to repair and recover, and reflexology facilitates this healing process. Bone is a living structure; its cells are constantly renewing and repairing themselves when necessary. The ligaments joining bone to bone are composed of strong fibrous tissue; they are also flexible and can adapt to change. If a ligament is under tension it will extend, whilst if it is allowed to become slack it will shorten. This is also true of tendons. One difficulty with tendons and ligaments is that they do not have a rich blood supply, so often their rate of healing is a little slower compared with the other tissues. Strain of a muscle is caused by excessive stretching or working of a muscle; this can result in severe pain and swelling of the muscle. Damage to the tissues then gives rise to an inflammatory process.

Reflexology to the points stated stimulates the nerve and blood supply to the involved region; also working the adrenal glands stimulates the naturally occurring glucocorticoids, which have a very powerful anti-inflammatory effect when treating conditions involving inflammation. The leg muscles have great vascularity; the muscles at the back of the calf are very important for the pumping action that helps the blood in the veins return to the heart. If muscles are overused or deprived of oxygen they become painful. This is a common problem in some athletes, and the thigh, leg or foot can become swollen and stiff.

Reflexology can help the healing of bones, relieving tension in locked muscles, ligaments and tendons. As holistic practitioners we stimulate the body's healing mechanism to accelerate the healing process. (See chapter 5 for biomechanics of the foot and foot exercises pp. 121–6, 159–88.)

Areas to work

M/R. Main area of problem: leg, knee or foot.
A/A. All spinal areas.
C/R. Work hand area, or wrists for ankles, forearm for foreleg.
P/Hs. SI-3 for spinal area.
P/LL. GB-34, 35, 36 and 37 for all knee and leg problems, LIV-8 for any disorders of all limbs, B-58 for lower leg problems.

P/AS. Area of problem, such as leg point if lactic acid has built up in the muscle tissue; if there is muscle fatigue, apply firm pressure to this point.

P/AA. Apex of ear for any inflammatory disorder.

P/OM. Adrenal glands for any inflammatory disorder.

P/TCM. Shenmen for pain relief.

(*See* Sports injuries and Knee problems, pages 339 and 303. Also figure 5.9b for lower limbs and the nerve pathways.)

Menstrual problems

The menstrual cycle brings great hormonal and internal changes, many different and sometimes often quite distressing complaints, but quite common to lots of women. Symptoms can vary in duration and severity.

Amenorrhoea. This is scanty menses or cessation at a time when it is not normal. It is usually due to a hormonal imbalance, or it could be a disorder of the hypothalamus; in some cases an ovarian or thyroid deficiency, even stress and anxiety, can cause this problem. Sudden shock, as in the case of death of a loved one, can cause complete cessation of the menstrual cycle and early menopause. Even a little stress, or changes in body-weight, from excess gain to great loss of weight, can cause it. If this is not the cause of the problem it is important that the person concerned visits their GP to have their hormone levels checked.

Dysmenorrhoea. This can be painful and heavy periods, with lots of abdominal pain. Any difficult menstruation may be due to inflammation of the membranes and lining of the womb, the endometrium; the womb reacts to bacterial substances upon this delicate mucous membrane lining, and if left this could lead to a disorder known as endometriotis. Often there is excessive menstrual bleeding and pain and discomfort in the lower back and legs, abdominal pain and cramps. At worst, ulcers could be forming in the membrane lining or even tumours in the myometrium, the muscular tissue of the uterus (womb) that surrounds the endometrium. So a check-up is always wise to ensure that there is no medical cause for the problem.

Menopause (climacteric). Menstruation ceases at the menopause. This is not an illness but a natural stage in life, but it does bring certain biological changes. Sometimes there is a gradual decrease of periods or complete stoppage of the monthly cycle; this, together with the change in the balance of hormones, can prove uncomfortable for some. Problems include hot flushes, dizzy spells, vaginal dryness, nervousness, tiredness and mood changes; these are quite natural and often due to the ovaries not producing the hormone oestrogen. The hot flushes can be mild or so severe they disturb your sleep. These can last for 1, 5 or even 10 years and eventually stop as the body becomes used to lower levels of hormones. Again reflexology at this stage helps enormously.

Regular and sensible exercise – cycling, brisk walking, jogging and keep-fit, tennis, badminton, swimming – or activity of any sort is better than none at all. A recommended routine would be 30 minutes to 1 hour three times a week. You can start off lightly and then gradually build up as you become fitter. This helps to build bone mass. Many women worry about the menopause and the effects of hot flushes; they are often so intense they feel red all over. However, this is often unnoticeable to other people. It is wise to dress in layers, so that you can remove clothing gradually. If shopping, and in and out of shops, it is better to have a lightweight coat with a thicker and heavier scarf, which can be removed easily. One of the pluses is that the increased perspiration often keeps the skin more supple and less prone to lines of ageing. Another benefit is the end to most women's problems, such as 2 weeks out of 4 suffering tiresome symptoms, possibly with premenstrual tension (PMT) followed by painful menstruation.

Vaginal dryness may be a problem; it is caused by lack of lubrication, or sometimes a thinning of the vaginal walls. The vagina shrinks in a woman who chooses not to have intercourse, and then subsequent lovemaking can be slightly painful because of the loss of elasticity. Use of a lubricant during intercourse will help prevent increasing rigidity and shrinkage of the vaginal tissues, keeping the vagina healthy. In addition there are no worries about contraception, so this can be a wonderful change for the better. Women should be encouraged to think positively about this change, and not just expect problems. It is often stated that over two-thirds of women experience no change apart from cessation of menses. Because of the publicity in magazines about hormone replacement therapy (HRT), many women expect problems. Also doctors disagree about the possible side-effects of prolonged taking of HRT. Some people look on HRT as a magic potion. It does not stop you getting old, but can help prevent osteoporosis, which is one of the serious side-effects of the menopause (*see below*).

Osteoporosis.   The term is from the Greek and literally means 'porous bone'. Bone tissue becomes softer, weaker and thinner with this condition. It often develops slowly after menopause; declining oestrogen levels are often responsible for the body's inability to absorb calcium from food. Women should not wait for this problem to occur. Calcium is an essential nutrient to the bone-building process, and extra calcium can be taken before the meno-pause to increase bone density. Cheese, milk (either skimmed or whole), and green vegetables such as broccoli, spinach and green beans, all contain calcium; the latter are less fat forming than whole dairy products. Inactivity can cause demineralization of bone; this is often seen in elderly men and women.

Only a GP may prescribe calcium supplements, but many people take these, whether there is a need to or not.

Pelvic inflammatory disease.   This includes salpingitis (inflamma-tion of the Fallopian tubes) and endometriosis. If left untreated, scar tissue can form; this can also spread to the ovaries and possibly the patient could have trouble conceiving at a later date. The membranous lining of the womb breaks away and fragments are found in other sites within the pelvic cavity. There are many different stages, from primary endometriosis to severe. The symptoms often do not appear during pregnancy or after the menopause, but these can be very painful and distressing problems over a period of many years.

Many women put up with undue pain and congestion, thinking that it is normal to suffer at the time of menstruation. Vasodilation of the pelvic organs is often the cause. Reflexology gives deep muscle relaxation and, using stimulation to the main acupoints, pain relief is very quick.

Premenstrual tension (PMT/PMS).   This can be a complex list of symptoms, from just general nervousness and irritability to outbursts of emotional disturbance, headaches, often depression for no reason, and fluid retention or bloating, which is often associated with excess salt and water in the tissues. It can affect women in varying degrees. A good diet is essential, as is regular exercise and plenty of relaxation. Sometimes supplements of vitamin B6 (pyridoxine) help, or evening primrose oil, which is rich in gamma-linoleic acid (GLA); the latter is associated with the production of tissue hormones (prostaglandins) that help normal-ize menstruation. Fennel tea and water are nature's diuretics; these are excellent for fluid retention, and fennel is known as a hormone precursor. Together with reflexology they encourage normal regulation where there is a hormonal imbalance; also reflexology acts to stimulate or inhibit nerve impulses to the brain, where many hormonal signals are received. There is a link between the endocrine and neural activity.

Areas to work

Refer to reflex zones to work to help the following:
Menstrual problems could be due to an imbalance in the hypothalamus/pituitary function. This tiny structure attached to the underside of the hypothalamus synthesizes and releases vital hormones that act on the ovaries and testes (gonads) to promote the production of the sex hormones, sperm and ova. Two important secretions are follicle-stimulating hormones, helping the ripening of the follicles in the ovary and formation of sperm in testes, and the midcycle surge of luteinizing hormone that results in ovulation. This latter hormone stimulates ovulation, corpus luteum formation and synthesis of progesterone by the ovary. If any of these hormones are out of synchronization it shows that there is a homeostatic imbalance in the endocrine system.

Reflexology often helps unexplained infertility problems, such as lack of ovulation, decreased sperm production, even amenorrhoea. Stimulation to other endocrine glands such as the thyroid is very necessary. In the thyroid, iodine is essential to formulation of the hormones thyroxine (T_4) and tri-iodothyronine (T_3), so a good healthy wholefood diet is necessary as we ingest this from food. Extra stimulation of the adrenal cortex, which lies on the medial edge of the plantar area of the foot, helps many problems, especially during menopause. The adrenal cortex is vital for many functions of the body, as it produces three kinds of corticosteroid hormones. Its secretion is stimulated by ACTH, a hormone from the anterior pituitary lobe; it affects carbohydrate metabolism (through glucocorticoids, which have a widespread effect), and electrolyte metabolism (through mineralocorticoids, mainly aldosterone). The gonad corticoid is allied to the oestrogens produced in the ovaries and the male hormones the androgens; this latter hormone is synthesized in small amounts. The female androgens are important as they aid the libido and are necessary as they can be converted into oestrogens as the normal ovarian function decreases.

The parasympathetic nervous system (second, third and fourth sacral nerves, *see* figure 2.5, page 40) helps increase the diameter of blood vessels (vasodilation) especially in the arteries. In this system there are many long preganglionic fibres; in the head and neck these synapse in ganglia close to the base of the skull, but in the rest of the body they synapse with a second neurone in the walls of the pelvic organ. Stimulation of the great toe or thumb and the sacral reflex on both limbs will help most menstrual abnormalities. Stimulation to the area of the sacral vertebrae helps the five points of spinal nerves that emerge at that point. These nerves carry sensory and motor fibres to and from the anal area and the genital regions. The fibres of the sacral nerves leave the spinal cord and synapse with nerve cells in the walls of the pelvic organs; the effects of stimulation are variable according to the stage of the menstrual cycle. The lumbar area is also worked to contact the lumbar plexus. Nerves that may be stimulated include the iliohypogastric nerve, ilioinguinalis nerve and genitofemoral nerve, which all arise between L1 and L2. The femoral nerve arises from L2, L3 and L4. These nerves supply muscles and skin in all areas of the lower abdomen. So you can see how working the spinal reflexes will help many disorders.

The sacral outflow of parasympathetic nerve fibres, together with the lumbar outflow of sympathetic nerve fibres, gives a double stimulation of nerve supply to the reproductive organs. Stimulation of the spinal area, hand or foot, will help balance the nerve supply to this region and is of much benefit to people who have a problem in this area.

Stimulation of all endocrine glands and the reproductive organs helps balance the hormones. There is a theory that we may block certain types of prostaglandin that are released from the tissues of the body, which in excess cause dilation of many of the peripheral blood vessels, leading to headaches during the menstrual cycle and painful spasms in the uterus. Does reflexology block these prostaglandins? This is a question I have often given great thought to. It can inhibit excess nerve transmission so it must be able to normalize this secretion. Many people attest to reflexology actually helping them, with often the hot flushes disappearing completely or, if one does arise, it does not seem to the same intensity as before. With reflexology, menstruation problems become a mere minor interruption to everyday life – bloating and menstrual cramps become a thing of the past, and backaches that often occur at this time are less troublesome.

Areas to work

For painful menstruation:
M/R. For painful menstruation work all reproductive areas and

the endocrine system. Also the adrenal glands as this will help if there is any inflammation.

A/A. Sacral nerves supplying the region.

P/Hs. LI-4 has an antispasmodic effect on the uterus so is a good point to work on the hands.

P/LL. SP-1, 6 and 9, LIV-8, BL-60, KI-1, 2, 3, 4, 8 and 10 and GB-41 can be stimulated quite firmly. For amenorrhoea these above points are marvellous, in normalizing menstruation.

Warning! LI-4, SP-6 and BL-60 can be used only providing the person is not pregnant, as they are empirical points to promote delivery during labour.

P/AS. Work all reproductive organs and the endocrine point.

P/TCM. Ear Shenmen, for pain relief, if necessary.

Area to work for mastitis due to a hormonal imbalance:

P/LL. GB-42.

P/AS. Chest/breast area.

P/AA. Apex of ear as it has a soothing and calming effect on all the above disorders.

Multiple sclerosis

Symptoms

This is another degenerative disorder of unknown cause, in which there is a progressive destruction of the myelin sheath around the nerves of the brain and spinal cord, disrupting their function. Symptoms may vary from muscular weakness, causing an unsteady gait, tremors in the limbs, and tingling or burning in the extremities. The vision becomes disturbed, with involuntary eye movements, double vision, and blurring; the symptoms can be endless depending on the severity. There are often periods of remission, and attacks may also vary greatly. A general treatment will alleviate many of the everyday problems such as constipation or indigestion.

Areas to work

M/R. In case this is an autoimmune problem, lots of work on the thymus area; this helps the whole autoimmune system. Also the adrenal glands are worked for the corticosteroids and their powerful anti-inflammatory properties. Brain and spinal areas can be worked daily.

P/AA. Apex of ear as it has a soothing and calming and analgesic effect. Spinal cord on dorsal surface.

(*See also* Nervous disorders, page 312.)

Nasal problems

Symptoms

Inflammation of the mucous membranes causes a heavy head and tenderness in the facial area. This problem may be caused by an allergy or infection, which can lead to many other distressing complications. As the person eats they often have to take in air through the mouth as they try to chew; this can lead to flatulence and abdominal discomfort. If mucus passes down the back of the throat it can cause catarrh of the stomach. Often there is a loss of the smell reflex; this can impair the taste of food. Many nasal problems are greatly helped with reflexology, especially sinusitis. Most clients have suffered over many years with intermittent periods of relief; they are often amazed at how reflexology embraces lifestyle and eating patterns in this disorder, but it is important to reduce all mucus-building foods as these add to the problem.

Areas to work

M/R. Nose and facial areas.
A/A. Intestinal areas will help all upper respiratory tract infections. Also the liver to remove any excess toxins from the system.

(For more information *see* Asthma, page 249, and Sinusitis, page 336.)

Neck problems

Symptoms

These include pain or stiffness when turning the neck. The cervical region of the vertebrae is made up of seven small bones; it acts as a channel for the spinal cord. The area is richly supplied with nerves entering and leaving the brain, and is endowed with eight cervical nerves, which are divided into two plexuses, the cervical plexus C1–C4, and the brachial plexus C4–C8, and the first thoracic nerve. These nerves serve the areas from the head to the diaphragm, so are important to stimulate for any disorder occurring within that area; many arm problems are due to some disorder of these nerves. The muscles of the neck that flex or rotate and turn the neck are innervated by these nerves, and spasms in their muscles can be very debilitating. The innervation of these muscles comes from certain spinal segments of the peripheral nervous system. Injury or disease of peripheral nerves can cause many problems, as peripheral nerve innervation to the skeleton closely follows muscle innervation, the bones being motivated by the same nerves that supply the muscles attached to that bone.

Most neck problems can be avoided (*see* behaviour patterns, chapter 3, page 89). Incorrect postures are nearly always the cause.

Areas to work

M/R. Cervical region, and chronic neck points.
A/A. Adrenal glands for their powerful anti-inflammatory properties. Also the axillary area.
P/Hs. LI-1, SI-1, 2 and 3.
P/LL. BL-60 and 65.

Warning! BL-60 can be used only providing the person is not pregnant, as it is an empirical point to promote delivery during labour.

P/AS. Neck and cervical vertebrae.
P/AA. Apex of ear for an analgesic effect.
P/OM. Adrenal glands for their anti-inflammatory properties, if there is any rheumatic tendency.
P/TCM. Shenmen for pain relief; it is also a strong analgesic point.

(*See also* Frozen shoulder, Torticollis or wry neck and Whiplash injury, pages 285, 348 and 353.)

Nervous disorders

There is a common link between certain disorders of the nervous system that also are autoimmune disorders. Sometimes these disorders are of unknown cause, such as myalgic encephalomyelitis (ME) or chronic fatigue syndrome (CFS) as it is now known, myasthenia gravis, and multiple sclerosis, Ménière's syndrome and Parkinson's disease. These are all due to a homeostatic imbalance within the nervous system, or within the neurotransmitters.

Sometimes these disorders are of gradual onset; sometimes there is an acute onset becoming slowly progressive. Symptoms seem to vary considerably. Many of these systemic disorders have peripheral neuropathy; the receptors in the muscles are gradually destroyed or for some reason the nerve transmission is not passed on.

Many people suffer from general myalgia and general muscle weakness affecting many parts of the body. Optic nerves may be involved because of weak nerve transmission to the muscles of the eyes; this may cause drooping eyelids or general problems in the facial area. There may be a general weakness in the throat and larynx (voicebox), and speech can be affected, swallowing can be difficult, there is numbness and tingling in the skin, and general lack of co-ordination. The list is endless, with depression and tension often setting in and exacerbating the problem. We know a good diet can help enormously, together with the simple but powerful stimuli of reflexology.

A certain amount of stress is a necessary part of our daily living. This can be a beneficial stimulus to get us activated. However, too much stress leads to anxiety and apprehension. When symptoms such as anxiety arise this shows the balance of certain chemicals in the brain has been disturbed, and an anxious state will increase the activity of the brain even more, often stimulating the sympathetic nervous system into overdrive and the result being a further increase of physical symptoms, such as palpitations, breathlessness, tremors and shaking, even digestive disorders and headaches, backache, pains in the neck and general fatigue and tiredness. All these physical symptoms are produced by an increase in noradrenaline, creating this fight or flight response. This excess stress creates brain dysfunction. Any homeostatic imbalance between the excitatory and inhibitory neurotransmitters (*see* chapter 2, page 45) may cause nervous disorders, such as anxiety, depression, insomnia, Parkinson's disease, myasthenia gravis, multiple sclerosis, etc.

Noradrenaline is also responsible for neural stimulation to the pineal gland; the hormonal output from the gland is melatonin, which is thought to synchronize the circadian rhythms. The exact function is still not quite understood, but it is thought to be responsible for inducing sleep, helping to modify mood, emotional performance and fatigue, and alleviating depression. There is a very fine dividing line between the amounts of noradrenaline released as a neurotransmitter, and as a hormone, and then the subsequent stimulus to the pineal gland and the release of melatonin. Melatonin is produced and released in larger quantities in the dark. Its synthesis is discontinued when any bright light enters the eye, which is the reason why jet lag is never quite so bad when you are away on holiday as the bright light inhibits the release of melatonin. If this regular apportionment of light and dark is disrupted by air travel, the internal body clock is unbalanced; too little or too much of the hormone can cause a problem in the body. The natural substance melatonin is formed from different constituents, one being serotonin, a hormone that has certain properties including the ability to induce sleep; low levels cause insomnia. Balance of these substances is of the utmost importance. Serotonin is also thought to play a part in our sensory perception and the overall control of our moods. This is the reason that melatonin is referred to as the mood enhancer and known as an antistress, antipanic and antiageing hormone. It is also thought to be helpful in immunity, and to play a part in decreasing pain sensitivity. In many countries it is taken to alleviate jet lag.

Seasonal Affective Disorder syndrome (SAD).   This is a form of depression, often exacerbated at the onset of winter or by too long a time spent indoors. Again this is linked to disturbance of the light–dark cycle, and seems to be associated with abnormal levels in the production of melatonin. This is thought to be responsible for the many stress-related problems. (*See* SAD, page 334.)

A hypothesis is that by administering melatonin the symptoms are subsequently relieved. The medical profession prescribe melatonin, which sometimes can lead to the exacerbation of symptoms, making the patient even more depressed. It is freely on sale in some countries, but we are not sure of the long-term side-effects. Working on the great toe and brain areas of the foot helps all these disorders without the use of drugs.

Myasthenia gravis.   This disorder affects the muscles of the body, because there is a fault in the transmission of neural impulses to them. Acetylcholine is a most important neurotransmitter and is released by neurones connected to skeletal muscles, often causing them to contract. It also transmits messages between the brain and spinal cord. Interruption and interference with this action of acetylcholine on skeletal muscle is the cause of myasthenia gravis. It is also thought to be one of those autoimmune disorders whereby the immune system has a homeostatic imbalance and produces certain antibodies that confuse the signals being transmitted. Abnormal antibody activity destroys many receptors, reducing the stimulation of muscle cells. The consequence of this is that there is intensifying muscular weakness. The thymus is thought to be the culprit; however, removal of this organ does not guarantee an alleviation of the disorder. Also many of the strong drugs used are only palliative; they do not cure the disorder, and most of them have very debilitating adverse effects. We know reflexology helps many nervous disorders and patients have found great benefit, though not complete cessation of problems.

Alzheimer's disease.   It is also thought that Alzheimer's disease may be caused by a depletion of nerve cells that release acetylcholine in the brain. It is a very debilitating disorder. Reflexology can only help the whole nervous system to achieve balance, which allows the stabilization of the homeostatic function of this vast and complicated arrangement of interconnected neurones.

Parkinson's disease.   This is caused by deficiency of dopamine, another neurotransmitter (see Parkinsonism, page 319).

Dopamine is also known as one of the group of catecholamines; these substances have various roles. For instance, there is a hypothesis that schizophrenia is caused in part by abnormalities in the metabolism of this neurotransmitter.

A case history of myasthenia gravis is given in box 8.8. (*See also* plate 15.)

Box 8.8   CASE HISTORY: Myasthenia gravis

Female, aged 28 years.

Clinical problems presented at first treatment.   Myasthenia gravis. Both her eyes were drooping, she could not swallow liquids, but could only sip slowly, suffered extreme tiredness and fatigue, with problems in her arm muscles, and was unable to do her hair. Her arms constantly ached and she could walk only short distances, her speech was very slurred and she had a drooping mouth on the right side. This young lady had a general malaise especially after even slight activity; this affected her appetite later in the day. Her vision was blurred and when she was very tired she complained of double vision.

Background medical history.   This young lady had suffered over a period of 5 years with the above disorder, but it was only diagnosed in 1994. She has taken several courses of antibiotics over a period of time but these only gave temporary relief. Drugs were also given to improve muscle function, as were corticosteroids. She experienced quite a lot of side-effects with these medications and when she went to see her medical practitioner, because she did not want to continue, he suggested removal of the thymus gland. In the latter part of 1993 she stopped all orthodox treatment and then commenced treatment with a homeopathic doctor. Her diet was changed and different preparations were taken and a mild improvement was felt but problems at work (which was now only part-time, mornings, as she was too fatigued by the afternoon) seemed to set her back as before and she lost confidence in her treatment, as she felt that her muscles were getting weaker. She presented herself to me in early 1994.

Observation of the hands, feet and general evaluation. The feet were very yellow and moist, with poor muscle tone and flaccid; the nails were normal but the second toe of both feet was quite rigid. The hands were also hot and clammy, and very red. She had a simian line on her hand and this appeared very red (*see* hand analysis, chapter 6, page 194).

After the first treatment, which was given on parts of the hands and feet over a period of a few days, she felt relaxed and the first great improvement was that she could swallow with more ease. Over a period of treatments, first her eyes improved, with the double vision and drooping eye on the right side diminishing, then her boyfriend commented that her speech was not so slurred. Over a period she noticed she did not want to go to bed in the afternoons; it was also easier to do her hair. I would work many combination points on her hands, ears, feet and legs; invariably she would have a bean in her ear at strategic points.

General improvement was felt over the next 3 months. I taught this young lady to work on her own hands and she was delighted when she felt a response; if she had a bad day she could work on her own hands and this stimulated her and she could cope better. To date we have not had any great relapse; successful treatment is still continuing. Each full treatment consisted of extra work on the thymus, adrenals, all the toes and fingers (brain area) in the web of the thumb and index finger and spinal area on feet and hands, reflexes being worked firmly and with lots of relaxation techniques. As the reflexes of the hands and feet improved, pressure was increased. Each treatment I utilized the ear points and applied a bean if necessary. The colour of her hands and feet improved on each visit, as did the temperature. Her general muscle tone has improved generally.

Foot observations at end of treatment. Her feet became a better colour, not so yellow and moist, muscle tone had improved and the second toes on both feet were now normal; her hands were also a better colour and the simian line on her hand was very feint. This young lady now attends once a month.

PATIENT'S COMMENTS. I was diagnosed as having myasthenia gravis (MG) in January 1994, which basically means that the involuntary muscles can weaken quickly after normal/ repetitive use. I had originally gone to the doctor's in 1993, as my boyfriend had noticed my right eyelid drooping. The doctor could not find any problem or reason for this and recommended a trip to the optician. They too could not find any abnormalities. The return visit to the doctor's ended in an appointment at Harlow Hospital with the neurological consultant.

At the hospital I had a medical examination, as well as being questioned on fine details of my physical well-being and performance. They had their suspicions on the cause of my weakness, but needed to check this by doing a blood test. This proved positive; I did have this disorder. I was very shocked, which was only to be expected. I had led a fairly active healthy life, but I had noticed that for the last few years I had been feeling generally weaker. I had put this down to being overworked or something!

The treatment the hospital had to offer was that of drugs, Pyridostigmine Bromide initially, then removal of the thymus gland, and then maybe steroids. I was horrified. I read as much as I could on the subject of MG, the treatment, as well as meeting with other sufferers. I decided I was going to try complementary therapies. I started to see a homeopath for a while, which helped me to sort out a healthy diet, but I felt healthier in other ways. But my MG symptoms were getting really quite bad. I'd heard of Beryl Crane and reflexology, so I thought I would try it out. At this point I was tiring fairly easy, I felt very heavy limbed. I had double vision and could only sip at drinks of water because if I tried to drink any faster it would come out of my nose.

I remember my first visit. Beryl asked me about the condition and the effect it had on me, as well as other health questions. She came across as a very friendly and positive person, which is really what I needed. The reflexology on my feet was lovely. She could pinpoint problems/imbalances, as she worked different areas. I remember at the end of the treatment she said, 'Now go home and drink plenty of water' (I'd told her this was not possible, I could only sip). She confidently said, 'You'll be able to now!' I went home and I could; it was so good.

After following treatments, I felt stronger and more in control of my health than I had done for a long time. I was also sticking to a fairly strict diet at this time. I remember coming home after one treatment and cleaning all the windows – absolutely impossible before. I had so much energy, I began cycling again to work and feeling much happier and not feeling so tired all the time. Simple things such as hanging up my washing became so enjoyable; this would have previously made my arms ache but now this was not a problem.

At times I would overdo it. After not being able to do hardly anything, I wanted to do everything! I have had some pretty bad periods too, but this I think was mostly due to stress. It is also a case of realizing your capabilities, and this is what Beryl often told me.

I was visiting her once a week but now it's about once a month. Each visit she deals with each problem I have; these can be new or old recurring ones. Not long after my first visit, she showed me how to work on my hands, which I do every morning, which gives me a sense of control and independence with the MG. My double vision has not occurred for over a year. Each visit is so good, it really works for me. The tender parts she works and works. Sometimes it is a little tender, then Beryl lessens her pressure; it is never so uncomfortable that I do not enjoy it, and I know it is doing me good. I recommend it to everybody and am glad I chose to have reflexology, as opposed to other treatments. I feel lucky that Beryl is a knowledgeable, friendly and positive reflexologist. I have tried to get treatment on the NHS as I think it should be available to all people who have a debilitating disorder like this.

In the last 2 years I have taken trips abroad to Turkey and Sri Lanka back-packing, mountain walking, and snorkelling, which I am sure would be an impossibility without the reflexology and/or if I'd gone with the original drug option. Thank you, Beryl.

Oedema

Symptoms

Swollen legs or ankles, ie subcutaneous oedema, may be noticeable prior to menstruation; bloating and weight gain are quite common at this time. Any other accumulation of fluids should be investigated by a medical practitioner. General oedema in the area of an injury is normal. Simple self-help tips are to increase the water intake as this is nature's diuretic, elevate the legs and rest them for a period. Regular treatment helps to alleviate this problem.

Areas to work

M/R. Kidneys, to get rid of any excess fluid.
A/A. Heart and liver to stimulate the circulatory system, and help to remove any excess toxins from the system.
P/Hs. TB-4 stimulates elimination.
P/LL. SP-5 and ST-41; the former is good for oedema of the abdomen while the latter is for the ankles.

Oesophagitis

Symptoms

In oesophagitis there is a bitter-tasting regurgitation; eating may be difficult as it can feel as though there is something in the passageway. Even swallowing may be difficult and food seems to remain in the gullet.

Areas to work

Note. One patient who had suffered for many years had lost weight and could not lie down because of the acid reflux. For five sessions I only worked his toes, owing to his work commitments. He had such a marvellous response that he made time for subsequent sessions. He now attends periodically if he gets any trouble. His main problem is that he does not give himself any thought until a disorder manifests.

M/R. Lots of work on the great toe. The cranial nerves help this whole region. Acid and pepsin release is regulated by the vagus nerve.

A/A. Pancreas and liver; both of these areas help in calming, while the alkaline properties of the pancreas help to buffer the acidic gastric juice.

P/Hs. PE-6 and TB-3 both help all digestive disorders.

P/LL. ST-35 helps any gastritis. SP-2 helps the digestion.

P/AS. Area of problem.

P/OM. Sympathetic nervous system.

P/TCM. Sanjiao helps all abdominal problems and the oesophagus, as the vagus nerve and all its tributaries pass through at that point.

Parkinsonism

Symptoms

This is a progressive disorder that may occur from midlife onwards. The condition has an unknown cause. There is a homeostatic imbalance in the neurotransmitter dopamine, often due to degeneration of the basal ganglia. Dopamine is a neurotransmitter released at nerve endings, in the brain and around some blood vessels. It blocks activity in specific nerves and is important in the control of body movements. A deficiency of this transmitter within the basal ganglia causes Parkinson's disease; symptoms are tremors in the head and limbs, muscular stiffness and the inability to control or initiate movement. A finely tuned balance between acetylcholine and dopamine is necessary to bring about co-ordination of movement. When there is a degeneration of dopamine-producing cells, Parkinson's disease is the result, while overactivity of acetylcholine causes a state similar to anxiety. Certain drugs can boost the effects of dopamine but, because many drugs are poorly absorbed or cannot pass directly from the bloodstream to the brain, other chemicals are used and many counteracting drugs also have to be used.

Rigidity of the muscles can affect the face, and voice. Tremor of the limbs starts in the hands and then spreads to the other limbs. Stimulation to the brain and spinal cord helps normalize some of the tremors.

Area to work

A full treatment session is recommended. (*See* Nervous disorders, pages 312–18).

Pregnancy and prenatal care

Reflexology can be used as a preventative treatment to boost the immune system, either prior to pregnancy or during the first trimester if the person is used to reflexology. It is wonderful for balancing the body to help protect against any irregularities that may occur. Not only does treatment help on physical levels but it also helps on the spiritual level, which is all part of the healing process. At all times the patient should be encouraged to discuss the reflexology treatment they are receiving with the doctor and antenatal clinic. Treatment can continue throughout the pregnancy period. It helps many of the irritating problems that mothers-to-be often face.

Antenatal reflexology

In morning sickness, reflexology helps to settle acid reflux and calm the muscles as well as the nerves of the abdominal wall and the muscles of the diaphragm. The vomit centre is in the brain; often there is an irritation of this centre. Work on the great toe right down to the base and around the ball of the foot to help calm the oesophagus; also work the pituitary to balance the hormones, as high levels at this time are often the cause of the problem. Psychological stress or great emotional disturbance can cause vomiting; it is imperative that the mother-to-be remains calm. Ample rest must be taken and reflexology will soothe the whole nervous system. For unexplained continuous nausea or vomiting, or in the case of hyperemesis gravidarum (pernicious vomiting of pregnancy), medical aid should always be sought in case it may be some other disorder. Useful tips for nausea are sipping dry ginger ale, or eating a dry biscuit. Fitzgerald always spoke of eating popcorn for morning sickness. Cantaloupe melons are high in B_6 (but pregnant women should never take vitamin supplements without consulting their doctors).

During this period some women experience extreme tiredness and fatigue, and change of mood; sometimes they are irritable owing to the hormonal changes. Again, minor discomforts such as constipation, frequent urination and troublesome discharge can all be helped with reflexology. Lower back pain is a common problem as pregnancy progresses; it is often due to the increased weight, or it may be faulty posture. Back pain is relieved with gentle treatment; also useful self-help tips can be used.

In the second and third trimester oedema may occur; with an accumulation of fluid in the tissues, the swollen legs and ankles can be quite troublesome. Reflexology helps normalize the water balance of the body, especially the lymphatic system, balancing the electrolytes and proteins, etc. As the expectant mother tends to slow down, this stimulation to the kidneys and lymph areas is most beneficial as it helps the body to excrete excess fluid, increasing the output of urine from the kidneys without resorting to drugs or diuretics. Water is nature's diuretic, and drinking six to eight glasses daily helps to reduce retention of excess fluids.

Hypertension is quite common in pregnancy. Mothers-to-be should be encouraged in self-help: weight gain should not be in excess, smoking should be discouraged, and gentle exercise is a must at this time. It is of paramount importance that during pregnancy the person remain stress free as much as possible, as all these factors can elevate blood pressure levels. Reflexology helps by keeping the mother totally relaxed throughout this period and usually the blood pressure normalizes. Reflexologists work on the endocrine system to balance hormones. Homeostatic imbalances in the following hormones and the organs that synthesize them are often the underlying cause. The kidneys may release excess renin in response to stress, which in turn may activate a protein in the blood called angiotensin II; this is a known elevator of blood pressure and causes the adrenal cortex to overproduce aldosterone, which can create imbalances in the amount of potassium, sodium and water in the blood, one of the many causes of hypertension. Work the liver and cortex of adrenals for aldosterone and angiotensin.

The aim of the reflexologist is to maintain balance within the internal environment. If the sympathetic nervous system goes into overdrive for too long and there is too much stress, the whole autonomic nervous system is affected. Stress responses send messages to the adrenal glands directly to create alarm reactions in the adrenal glands. This is the first stage of the fight or flight syndrome, which is our normal response to stress and very necessary in times of any emergency. These responses are instantaneous reactions to activate the body's reserves for the required extra physical activity. However, prolonged stimulus causes more long-term problems to manifest. There are many organs that may be affected, such as the liver, and thyroid and the adrenal glands; these organs become overworked and enervated. This can cause inhibition of the whole digestive processes, and create many stress-related disorders (*see* chapter 10). An increase in blood pressure may cause headaches, shortness of breath and even giddiness. Reflexology induces relaxation, calming the nerves and restoring balance and homeostasis.

It is better to use reflexology only after the first trimester. This is only if the person has never received reflexology before, or if there is a history of miscarriages. We do not know how a new patient may react to treatment, so it is better to wait until the fetus is almost fully formed. Stimulation is then less likely to cause any problem to the developing child. With the GP's consent we can then begin reflexology sessions. This is because there are great changes in hormone production during pregnancy, much greater than in the menstrual cycle. There is a steady increase of both progesterone and oestrogens throughout the 40 weeks of pregnancy. Often it is these changes that may cause imbalances internally. Too much stimulation to the endocrine or reproductive area may normalize a function in a direction that we cannot foresee. So it is better to delay reflexology until the third month when the pregnancy is more settled.

Areas to work

A full but gentle reflexology treatment will aid and help relieve most problems throughout pregnancy, or used with combination points of the hands, lower limbs, and auricular points for a more energetic response.

Note. Do not affix beans to the ears. Do not apply any extra pressures on the pituitary reflex point and chronic uterus reflex point during reflexology treatment.

For specific problems, work areas as listed below.

M/R. Spinal areas for low back pain or soreness. Also musculature of the hip and pelvis.

Warning! Do not work on the lateral malleolus as the acupoint BL-60 is a known elimination point; save this for during labour.

P/Hs. LU-8 helps to calm the oesophagus in extreme vomiting or morning sickness in the first 3 months. PE-6 is a very safe area to work for any nausea, also scratching the dorsal surface of the hand aids nausea. SI-5 is for lower back and knee problems. H-9 and SI-1 are for headaches.

P/LL. ST-36 and LIV-3 are for any general malaise or abdominal discomforts, and headaches. GB-41 is a safe point for lumbar problems or any pain in the body. For headaches B-67.

Warning! Do not use B-67 in the last 2 months of pregnancy as it is a point for malposition of the fetus. GB-44 is a safer point to use for headaches. SP-6 and LI-4 are not to be used during pregnancy.

P/AA. Lumbar on dorsal surface. For hypertension the lower ear root and groove of dorsal surface. Superior triangular fossa pressure will lower blood pressure.

Exercises for pregnancy

- To reduce any swelling, step into a bowl of tepid water. Lift one foot up at a time as if marching in the water. *Note.* Take extra care that you do not slip; put a chair in front of you to hold on to.
- Sit down and put a towel under your foot and, holding either end, lift the leg up; repeat on the other foot.
- Walking barefoot on the spot will help strengthen the spine or reduce any swelling of the ankles.
- Elevate your feet each day for at least 15 minutes. The feet should be higher than your hips. This will reduce any further swelling and helps to relax the feet.
- Last of all, get some kind person to massage a moisturising cream into the feet. Bliss is achieved in approximately 20 minutes. This short exercise repeated daily will bring about harmony and relaxation to the body.

Reflexology in labour

This is a sequence of events that leads to the process by which the fetus is expelled, followed by the afterbirth. This is divided into three stages.

First stage.   Dilation and spontaneous rupture of the amniotic sac take place. At the onset of labour, intensive contractions begin; with each one the cervix dilates until it is fully dilated at 10cm. The duration of this depends on many factors and this period can be painful and tiring. Reflexology seems to relieve the nagging pain without retarding the process; in fact it seems to promote dilation, often quickening this first stage, which often lasts many hours in a first delivery. Reflexology relaxes the mother-to-be and she feels much more in control and confident. Stimulate the pituitary and uterus areas, working all spinal areas together with certain acupoints to help the contractions of the uterine muscular wall; it also helps relax the cervix muscle fibres and the nagging pain, often to the amazement of all concerned. Lots of stroking on the front of the foot helps abdominal wall; also pressure applied to the heels aids in the very powerful intermittent contractions. On full dilation of approximately 10cm the second stage of labour is reached.

Second stage.   This is the expulsion. During this period from full cervical dilation until vaginal delivery the mother-to-be needs to be calm and aware. The second stage is hastened with reflexology; it promotes delivery without undue strain. Work on the pituitary and chronic uterus areas, again with the spinal areas, as this helps the pudendal nerves and seems to give some pain relief, making the mother-to-be less tired and the procedure not so strenuous. The pudendal nerve arises from S2–S4 and serves the skin and muscles of the anal and perineal area, ending in the urogenital region where it serves the perineal area and a dorsal nerve to the clitoris. Working the spinal area also stimulates the genito-femoralis nerve, a mixed nerve arising from the lumbar plexus between L1 and L2, and the sacral autonomies, all helping the pelvic viscera and the reproductive organs.

Stimulation of the pituitary area throughout helps release oxytocin. To expedite the delivery it is advisable to apply pressure as the mother-to-be has the first inclination to bear down. Working together apply pressure on acupoint SP-6 and on the corresponding reflexology areas. Delivery seems to follow quickly without the use of analgesics or narcotics, which can only be beneficial as often these can affect the baby. It is during this period that there is a temptation to use pain-relieving drugs to help. Some may make the baby less responsive or cause breathing problems, or have the more dangerous effect of causing a brief drop in fetal heart rate. GB-21 promotes delivery, aids in placental retention and stimulates lactation. This point can be found on the depression of the shoulders just above the internal edge of the scapular, in line with the ear and the breast.

Third stage.   This is from delivery of the fetus to delivery of the afterbirth (which includes the placenta, umbilical cord and all the ruptured membranes). This stage is usually quite quick, between a few minutes to 30 minutes, but sometimes drugs are used to aid this expulsion. Reflexology is such a powerful stimulant, so surely it is better not to introduce a synthetic oxytocin when stimulation to the pituitary reflex and chronic uterus point will induce the natural progression and expulsion of the placenta and also stimulate milk flow. Lots of stroking on the backs of hands and feet, working the spinal areas, helps the uterine muscles and myometrium to contract; reflexology treatment will also aid the healing of blood vessels and promote lactation. In lactation, the baby's sucking action sends an important message to the pituitary gland to release oxytocin to stimulate milk flow. Stimulation to the pituitary reflex area on the feet and ears promotes activity of prolactin and oxytocin to stimulate afferent nerves to release and let down milk from ducts.

It is every woman's right to choose if she so wishes the type of birth she would like and an increasing number of women are choosing reflexology because it is a totally natural, non-invasive and drug-free therapy that gives pain relief, relaxes and gives energy at this vital time. Reflexology does induce relaxation during labour and anything that can be achieved naturally and non-invasively is wonderful. However, any woman who chooses a complementary therapy must ensure their midwives and obstetrician are happy regarding procedures as always treatment must be compatible with safety. The motto should be best and safe practice at all times.

Many of my patients bring their husbands along in the latter half of their pregnancy for instruction on which reflex point to work on to help with any discomfort. During the prenatal period it helps blood pressure, general well-being, and all neural activity in the spine. In the first stage the backache that is often felt is relieved so bowels and bladder function efficiently and haemorrhoids are eased. Our one thought is always to prevent harm to mother and baby. If a birth needs to be induced we can put pressure on the pituitary to help the labour along. Tests would tell us if more oxytocin was released. During labour sometimes the rhythmic contractions cease. Reflexology helps the labour along; if treatment is given approximately every hour for about 10 minutes, muscular contractions and dilation seem to cause no great problem, and most labours progress quite quickly into the second stage. Reflexology also helps during the third stage. The placenta follows quite quickly in approximately 10–15 minutes especially if the birth is uncomplicated. After labour the mother responds well to reflexology and treatment will benefit the baby too, helping sleeping, colic, and later teething and other minor upsets.

Areas to work

During labour: a full but gentle reflexology treatment will aid and help relieve most pain and discomfort throughout labour. Specific points are SP-6, LI-4 and BL-60. Apply extra pressure on these points throughout labour. For relaxation, tensing and relaxing muscles – start with the feet and move up.

P/Hs. LI-4 has an antispasmodic effect on the uterus.

P/LL. SP-6, BL-60 and KI-4 are stimulated quite firmly.

Afterbirth pains and for general discomforts after delivery:

P/Hs. LI-4 and PE-5 help any uterine congestion or metritis.

P/LL. Use SP-6 and 9, BL-60, LIV-8, and KI-8 and 10 for afterbirth pains.

P/TCM. Ear Shenmen, for any pain and discomfort.

For mastitis:

P/LL. GB-42.

P/AS. Chest/breast area.

P/AA. Apex of ear and apex of antitragus.

Danish reflexology study on childbirth

In 1988, a 4-month-long research project into reflexology treatment and childbirth was carried out at Gentofte County Hospital, Denmark. The purpose of the project was to offer reflexology treatment as an alternative to medical pain relief during childbirth. The project was started by reflexologist Gabrialla Bering Liisberg, who had learnt that reflexology treatment is a standard offer to women in labour at several clinics in Switzerland and Paris. Out of a total of 593 women giving birth at Gentofte County Hospital during the test period, 103 decided to take part in the project. The women were offered reflexology treatment as an alternative in leaflets displayed in the antenatal clinic. During the test period the reflexologist was present in the maternity ward for 39 hours per week.

Sixty-eight women chose to use reflexology treatment instead of medical pain relief. Of these, 61 stated that the treatment had a positive pain-relieving effect, 6 felt no effect and 1 woman experienced increasing pain in spite of the reflexology treatment. Out of the 61 women receiving pain relief through the treatment, 4 needed additional pain-relieving medication. The rest gave birth either completely without forms of pain relief other than the reflexology treatment or with supplementary pain relief such as laughing gas and water therapy.

Forty-nine women chose to try reflexology treatment before medical labour pain relief. Of these, 24 gave birth without medication.

In addition to this, 14 women were to undergo a surgical removal of the placenta in cases where it had not released itself 30 minutes after the birth. These women were given reflexology treatment for 30–60 minutes after the birth, resulting in the release of the placenta in 11 cases. The remaining 3 women had the placenta surgically removed.

Reflexology treatment was also used to attempt to induce labour in 4 women. None of these went into labour following the treatment, but the number of women in this group was judged to be so small by the project managers that no conclusions can be drawn about the effect of reflexology treatment in these cases.

The test results were judged as positive by the reflexologist as well as by the head midwife and the doctor on the ward. It was questioned, however, whether the effect was obtained through reflexology treatment or was more psychologically based. It was also remarked that, because the women made a conscious choice to try out reflexology, the test may be biased, as it possibly selects a particular type of woman who would be open-minded about alternative methods in childbirth.

The research report has not been published but the results have appeared in Danish newspapers: *Berlingske Tidende* (15/6/1988), 'Politiken' (6/4/1989) and *Tidsskrift for Jordemodre*, (Number 3, 1988, a periodical for Danish midwives). The information related above has been confirmed by telephone, by a nurse on the maternity ward at Gentofte County Hospital in November 1989, to Christine Issel, Secretary of the International Council of Reflexologists. These findings are printed with her permission.

Prostate

Symptoms

Pain whilst passing urine, maybe slight fever, abdominal discomfort and discomfort near anus and perineal area. Inflammation of the prostate gland can be caused by bacterial infection.

At birth the prostate gland is basically underdeveloped. By puberty it almost doubles in size as the second sexual characteristics appear. Then continuing glandular development takes place until about the age of 30, when one of two things may happen: either gradual atrophy of the prostate gland takes place, and it shrinks in size, or the opposite may happen – it can increase in size and possibly change shape. At the beginning of the century prostate problems were rare but more recent research shows that they are now increasing rapidly. Diet may play a large part in this. The medical profession often uses surgery as the only answer. As holistic practitioners we believe that prevention is better than cure.

The first sign that there is a problem is usually increased urination, often at night. This is an indication that the prostate is increasing in size. The frequency of urination increases steadily, as does the size of the prostate gland, and then further symptoms often arise; for instance, as the person is urinating the flow slows or trickles out. Sometimes even at the start of urination one may feel the need to pass water but cannot. Often to strain at this point seems to create even more discomfort and pain. Some men experience different symptoms. For example, during sexual intercourse, there may be the discomfort of a full feeling; some experience leakage which can cause embarrassment and further increase problems. The person becomes more stressed and may often panic, being unable to make it to the toilet. By now there may be low abdominal pain, and pain in the groin and the low lumbar areas. Symptoms of course vary from person to person. A nutritional approach is most important; diet, nutrients and reflexology can help problems immensely. Bowel problems nearly always aggravate prostate problems; regular bowel movement is essential to reduce any congestion in the pelvic area. A short fast will always help, but ultimately you must look at diet, exercise and posture. The structure of the body governs the function of the body, and poor posture demonstrates this interrelation: the diaphragm presses down on the abdominal organs and this in turn applies pressure on the pelvic organs (*see also* chapter 3, behaviour patterns, page 89).

The value of a short fast is immense (*see* chapter 11, page 385).

Areas to work

M/R. Prostate reflex; also all other reflexes that may be connected, such as the bladder because it is located beneath, and the rectum, which it lies in front of.

A/A. The adrenals are a powerful aid in any inflammatory problem. Adverse effects from treatment are very rare as it enables the body's natural hormones to function at peak efficiency without disturbing the production of other hormones. Working the groin lymphatics will help relieve any discomfort by fighting any infection if present and stimulating the lymph nodes into maximum filtration, thus effectively removing any micro-organisms or other foreign bodies from entering the bloodstream. Working the spinal nerves of the lumbar and sacral area will help because of the connections and branches that come off this main area. The perinneal nerve that arises from the second to the fourth sacral nerves has scrotal branches. The inferior haemorrhoidal nerve helps to relieve discomfort in the sigmoid (the region between the anus and urethral opening), anus and perineum areas. Work all spinal areas from L4 to S4; this part of the spine reflex will also help all the pelvic visceral nerves.

P/LL. KI-2 to help with any incontinence, BL-66 for all bladder problems and SP-6 and 9 for male pelvic disorders.

P/AA. Angle of superior concha for prostate problems and urinary tract infections.

Quinsy

Symptoms

In this condition there is a difficulty in swallowing. This often is a complication of tonsillitis. An abscess forms near to or on the tonsil and it may need surgical lancing. However, great relief can be gained if the person is unable to attend a medical practitioner (*see* Tonsillitis, page 347).

A case history of quinsy is given in box 8.9.

Box 8.9 **CASE HISTORY: Quinsy**

Female, aged 28 years, supervisor (bank).

Clinical problems presented at first treatment. Repeated sore throat, had a quinsy on tonsil several times. Initially she attended because of loss of voice, and laryngitis.

Diet. Certain foods made problem worse but felt she had a varied diet; drank a lot of coffee.

Background medical history. She had had the problem since her early teens. She had repeated sore throats, and a very husky voice, almost losing it on many occasions. She had just got over influenza and a quinsy on her right tonsil for the umpteenth time. Over the years she had seen many throat specialists; she had also had a laryngoscopy but the results proved inconclusive, and the consultant merely confirmed she had some sort of acute laryngitis. They had tried many things, including inhalations of steam, and antibiotics; these eased the problem for a while but the discomfort and huskiness would return. If she caught a cold it often meant her being in bed for a week at a time; at one time she had been very poorly with laryngotracheobronchitis and she was taken into hospital where she had steam treatment every 2 hours and also a bronchoscopy, where they removed a sample of tissue. Again the results were inconclusive.

History of patient. Her father had died of a heart attack aged 48 years old. Her brother had been diagnosed at the age of 3 with muscular dystrophy and died at the age of 14. The whole family had been affected, especially when it was found to be an inherited disorder; the elder daughter was checked and they felt she could be a carrier. The medical practitioner suggested a series of very complex tests but the elder sister declined and stated she would not have a family. The patient in question was too young at the time, only 15 years old, and 8 years younger than the sister. She was very close to the younger brother and had helped to look after him when the mother was at work part-time. Even though she was very close in age to him she had a wonderful way of being able to calm him and help him. When he was unable to walk it was always she who took him out in his special chair.

Observation of the feet. There was a very cornified area on the base of the great toe, both feet on the medial edge, puffiness on the ball of the foot just below the toes on zone 2 (the right foot more). It was very red in the liver and intestinal areas. Great sensitivity was felt on all toes, plantar and dorsal, and extreme pain in the dorsal aspect of zone 1, and the lateral aspect of the great toe on both feet. Both feet were hot and clammy.

This young lady commenced treatment in August 1994. She had 12 weekly treatments and I worked as much as 20 times on the throat reflex and also used magnetic therapy on reflex points. After week six there was a great improvement; the huskiness of the voice seemed to be lessening and she had a good few weeks without undue discomfort. In mid November she went on holiday to the Balearics; when she returned she went down with a cold and this lasted some 4 weeks. She was unwell and could not attend for treatment.

I started treatment again at the beginning of January and treatments were every 5 days for 3 weeks. The improvement was rapid and the huskiness disappeared almost instantly, as did the sore throat. We extended visits to 3 weeks without any regression and then 4 weeks, again with no return of the sore throat.

She felt well and full of vitality and had been promoted at work; her new job entailed travelling around the country and training other people so she was doing lots of talking, a thing she would not have attempted prior to this. Each time she came I could do a lot of in-depth pressure on C2 just below the nail bed, the cervical spinal reflex, also lots of work on the great toe for the cranial nerves, mainly trying to stimulate the vagus, the Xth cranial nerve, plus the accessory motor (XIth cranial nerve) and the throat reflex. To date we have had no return of the problem, the longest time she has been without pain and discomfort in the throat area.

Observation of the feet at end of treatment. The hard pad of skin has improved, and she had been to a chiropodist at my suggestion. She had made several visits but the hard skin kept returning. I can see an improvement; it does not seem to be thickening up quite so quickly. The puffiness has completely disappeared; her feet are warm to the touch and pink, and feel vibrant and full of energy. This lady now attends on a 2-monthly basis.

Raynaud's syndrome

Symptoms

This disorder arises from an unknown cause. It was first identified by Maurice Raynaud (1834–1881), a French physician. It is a peripheral vascular disorder of the hands and feet; the small arteries become constricted. This is not always due to cold as anxiety has been known to cause this unpleasant problem. Episodes of blanching of any of the phalanges occur causing extremes of numbness and pain. Ischaemia is a restricted flow of blood to that part of the body affected; this can cause cyanosis. As the colour returns it can be very painful, with a burning sensation.

Areas to work

M/R. The aim is to improve the whole circulatory system so that the smaller arteries do not constrict. A full treatment is always recommended.

P/Hs. LU-9 contacts the blood vessels, and TB-2 helps any pain in the fingers.

P/LL. On the plantar surface of the foot, the Shimian and Lineiting points help the toes.

P/AS. The specific area of the problem, eg toes, fingers. Working on the ear seems to promote vasodilation of the affected blood vessels, the relaxation of the musculature of the vessel wall, and seems to promote a quick return of colour with less pain than usual.

P/TCM. Shenmen for pain relief.

Self-help tip: keeping warm, and wearing cotton gloves in the spring, both help. Smokers should try to give up the habit.

Repetitive strain injury (RSI)

RSI does not appear in all medical dictionaries. It means overuse or overstretching of a muscle or ligament, which in turn can lead to injury or damage because of the overtaxing of a muscle or a group of muscles. So we begin to see that many influences or factors causing mental or physical tension or excessive overuse sustained over a period of time can create a lack of functional balance in the whole physiological system, which can create unequal activity in the parasympathetic and sympathetic systems leading to disorders of the autonomic nervous system (*see also* area of problem and behaviour patterns).

Areas to work

M/R. A full treatment session is always needed in case it has been caused by an infection.

A/A. The adrenal glands are powerful in aiding in any inflammatory problem, regardless of whether it is tendinitis or muscular in cause.

P/Hs. SI-4 and 6 are good for all tendon or ligament problems of the wrist, arm or shoulder region. HE-4 is suitable for pains in the wrist and forearm. SI-5 is ideal for knee problems.

P/LL. LIV-8 helps all four limbs.

P/AS. Work areas related to the problem.

P/AA. Apex of ear for any inflammatory disorder.

P/OM. The adrenal glands point can be pressed daily, or a bean can be attached with a hypoallergic plaster to give relief over a period. Adverse effects from treatment are very rare as the body's natural hormones are enabled to function at peak efficiency without disturbing the production of other hormones.

P/TCM. Shenmen for pain relief.

Respiratory problems

Symptoms

This may include any period of severe coughing or difficulty in breathing in or out. Most of the disorders within the respiratory tract are due to homeostatic imbalances. Disorders such as simple cough, asthma, bronchitis, or even emphysema all have one thing in common: that is that there is some irritation or obstruction to the air passageways. Lifestyle must be addressed as smoking is one of the main causes of most lung problems; even passive smoking plays a part in the many related problems. Many of today's respiratory disorders can be linked to environmental pollution, or inhalation of irritants such as pollen or moulds. Even certain foods can cause an allergic reaction. One of the main elements in all lung disorders is the general condition of the person's health. So it is essential that the person is aware of these factors and must protect themselves by improving their health generally so that they do not aggravate their disorder. Reflexology helps to boost the immune system. (People's immunity is always much lower when they are dealing with any illness.) The general circulation also improves, which in turn aids digestion, stimulates the endocrine glands and aids in high or low blood pressure.

Areas to work

M/R. A full treatment is always advised; the aim is to facilitate the breathing process. Extra work should be done on the lungs and the diaphragm area. The cervical region also aids as the phrenic nerve arises at this point between C3 and C5; not only does this aid the diaphragm but it also has offshoots to the pericardium of the heart, and the coeliac plexus. Also work the upper lymphatics.

A/A. The adrenal glands point is worked for anti-inflammatory properties, helping in the reduction of obstruction in the airways, or any narrowing of these passageways; it is amazing how the patient often comments on thick mucus or phlegm that is green or yellowish and how within one or two treatments this muco-purulent substance is broken down and becomes clear and less sticky. The large intestine is always an area of assistance in all respiratory problems; the Lungs and Large Intestine are paired in TCM. Working the large intestine aids in the removal of any excess mucus.

P/Hs. LU-7 through to 11 aids in any respiratory disorder. These points worked daily help any shortness of breath, and in clearing any excess mucus as there is a connection to the large intestine. These points also open up the respiratory passages. Also work points LI-5 and 6 to aid respiratory problems.

P/LL. SP-3 and ST-40 aid asthma, and phlegm breakdown. KI-9 helps to relax and calm the chest area. Also GB-43 aids the lungs.

P/AS. The lung points and trachea help any coughing; initially they may stimulate the cough but keep up the working and there will be a beneficial outcome.

P/AA. Work all the helix area from 1 to 6. This aids all the respiratory tract.

(*See also* Asthma, page 249.)

Rhinitis

Symptoms

This is inflammation of the mucous membranes of the nasal passageways. It can be caused by allergies or repeated colds. Treat as for hayfever (page 290). (*See* plate 8, of a person with rhinitis.)

Seasonal affective disorder (SAD)

Symptoms

During the autumn and winter months some people suffer excess tiredness, lethargy, depression, unexplained craving for carbo-hydrates, lack of libido, unexplained joint pain, and resistance to infection seems to be diminished; this is seasonal affective disorder (SAD). The body is reacting to the changing season, causing many problems ranging from mild to in some cases quite severe. The latter usually is worst in the winter months from the end of September to the end of March when the days are at their shortest, or it may be evident in shift workers if there is a great change in exposure to light. One in 20 people is noticeably affected during this time, and may become anxious, lethargic and depressed, which in turn may upset the hormone balance. As spring arrives symptoms lift dramatically. The theory is that light governs our body clock, and lack of light upsets the balance of our circadian rhythms. The hormonal function of the pineal gland is still not fully understood but it is thought to have a part to play in the light–dark cycle because of the links between the midbrain and the retina as light enters the eye (*see* chapter 5, page 141). At night the pineal gland releases the hormone melatonin in larger quantities, making us drowsy and we sleep and there is reduced metabolic activity, but as dawn breaks the light slowly enters our eyes, gradually awakening us and melatonin production is reduced. In the winter we arise to the sudden sound of an alarm rather than the natural light signal, hence our body clock is totally disorientated; we may feel drowsy, irritable, or may lack concentration (hence the amount of early morning accidents in the winter months). Over a period depression may set in, as melatonin production is still occurring in the day, which may be affecting vital nerve centres in the brain.

Jet lag is another disorder where the 'circadian rhythms' are disrupted and the whole daily pattern is thrown out of synchronization; this is why travellers are encouraged to get into the eating patterns of whichever time zone they enter. The symptoms of jet lag may persist for several days until the internal body clock becomes adjusted once again to the time change.

Areas to work

Reflexology has a part to play in aiding SAD and jet lag. As an international traveller I can confirm its efficacy. Work the brain area to stimulate release of serotonin (known as the mood enhancer) in the pineal gland; also the hypothalamus in the brain reflex, as it is the appetite centre. Do lots of work on the solar plexus and the spinal area; this stimulates all organs and glands to function more efficiently. Use either hand or foot reflexes; also work over all areas of the ears, stroking gently but firmly. This reflex treatment can be done once or twice during the flight and then just before landing. The result is that you will have more energy on arrival and be less bothered by the time change. Reflexology is very beneficial in SAD as it has a direct effect on the excitatory chemicals in the brain, many of which are neurotransmitters (*see* chapter 2, page 45). In depression many of these are not released in the right quantities, and reflexology seems to raise these levels with no dangerous side-effects.

M/R. All the toes and fingers as this stimulates the brain area, calming the mind and the whole nervous system.

A/A. The pituitary gland balances hormone activity.

P/OM. The subcortex helps any functional disturbance of the autonomic nervous system.

P/TCM. Sanjiao helps all levels of the body because the vagus nerve has such far-reaching effects.

Sinusitis

Symptoms

This is an inflammation of the sinuses, the narrow cavities that are hollow to lighten the weight of the head and lend resonance to the voice (*see* figure 5.3, page 137). They are lined with mucous membranes, and if these become infected the fluid accumulation leads to excessive mucus, which blocks the narrow passageway. This often makes the head feel heavy, and there is pain in the facial area. Acute sinusitis should never be ignored as infection could spread higher into the brain area.

Diet is important so that a clogged state does not exacerbate the problem. All dairy and wheat products should be eliminated from the diet, so that the body does not produce even more mucus.

Areas to work

M/R. A full treatment session is always advisable. This helps to normalize the autonomic nervous system, thus ensuring that the nervous system acts as a decongestant and there is constriction of the blood vessels; this allows the swelling to subside. The liver area needs extra stimulation as there are excess toxins in the system.

A/A. The adrenals are worked for their strong anti-inflammatory properties.

P/Hs. LU-10 is a good point for excess mucus.

P/OM. The adrenal glands for inflammation; they also have antiallergic qualities.

Skin

A detailed discussion of the role of reflexology in skin disorders is given in chapter 9.

Areas to work

M/R. The thyroid in general for the skin. The liver if there are any excess toxins in the system.

A/A. The adrenals for the strong anti-inflammatory properties.

P/Hs. TB-6 is an excellent point to use in any skin disorder. PE-4 has a direct contact with the epigastric vein, which in turn connects with the thoracic veins. Stimulation of this point also helps any mucus retention, which is often evident in people with skin disorders.

P/OM. The adrenal glands for inflammation; they also have antiallergic qualities.

P/TCM. Wind Stream is a marvellous point for any allergy or skin irritation.

A case history of skin problems is given in box 8.10.

Box 8.10 CASE HISTORY: Skin problems

Male, aged 72 years, separated from his second wife (first wife had died). Very tall at 6ft 3in (187cm), with a slight stoop.

Psychological state.   He admitted to being a heavy daily drinker. This had ruined his marriage but he assured me he was not an alcoholic and took pains to explain that he found company with others at lunchtimes and evenings at his local public house. This had become a more regular excursion as his relationship with his wife deteriorated. He was a heavy smoker, between 40 and 60 a day, but considered that he had a good diet. He had a little flat and cooked and cleaned for himself. He was extremely polite and kept referring to me as madam. He was scrupulously clean and paid attention to his dress on every visit, almost as if he were going somewhere special; even his hair was slicked down.

Clinical problems presented at first treatment.   A rash over the feet, legs and part of arms and hands. He also complained of shortness of breath and lower back and hip pain in the left side.

Background medical history.   He complained of chest and lower back pains. He was currently attending the doctor for a skin disorder but prior to this he had not attended for many years.

Medication.   Painkillers for low back. Ibuprofen and a lotion for his feet.

Observation of the hands, feet and general evaluation.   I had to wear surgical gloves as the feet were oozing and pustules covered the whole area. I asked what treatment he had sought and he advised me he had been to his doctor, who had prescribed lotions and ointments but none had seemed to help. I could only use my water spray on all areas of the feet. I did this over the next three sessions because of the lesions. I could not apply firm pressure of the jet on any one place for more than a few seconds. By week five there was a little improvement to the skin; it appeared less angry. The one great improvement had been to his back and hips which he felt were much better, he was walking straighter and did not stoop. His breathing was still poor; he often arrived breathless for his treatment. We discussed his cutting down smoking. I suggested hypnotherapy; I often refer patients to another therapist in the next town who has had marvellous results with smokers. The patient assured me he would cut down his smoking. I also suggested an alcohol line, and social services.

On week six there was a good improvement. He had missed a week's treatment due to a heavy cough and cold. I asked him if he had reduced his smoking and he replied that he had not smoked all week until the day of the treatment. There was such an improvement to his foot rash that I believed it was due to the absence of smoking in some way, so I asked him not to return to his 40 to 60 cigarettes a day as the improvement must surely prove to him that his smoking was causing him problems. I then asked him to try and abstain from any alcohol or at least to try and cut down, to see if we could achieve an even better result. He promised he would try not to smoke as much as possible.

The next week I received a telephone call from one of his friends saying he could not attend due to personal reasons and that he would telephone later for another appointment. I heard nothing from him for several weeks and I felt as though I had maybe not handled the situation as well as I should have. Perhaps if I had not pushed him quite so much to seek other help and left him just receiving the reflexology then things might have improved gradually. However, about 3 months after the initial cancellation I was out shopping and came face to face with him. I was extremely shocked by his appearance. I smiled, he touched his forehead and nodded, quickly scurrying away.

Unfortunately, I consider this one of the very few failures; maybe if I had continued treating him without the pressure on him to reduce his smoking I would have had a more successful end result.

Sports injuries

The majority of sports injuries could be prevented if the right precautions were taken. Muscle fatigue is a common cause of many injuries. It is imperative that the participant establishes a gentle warming-up routine before doing any strenuous physical exercise. This increases the blood flow through the tissues, thus increasing the temperature within, which makes all the tissues more elastic. If the tissue is more supple there is less vulnerability to injury.

A fracture is a break in a bone. This can be caused by a sudden powerful force or persistent stress on a bone. Bone is a living structure; its cells are constantly renewing and repairing themselves.

A sprain is a similar injury to a ligament, a fibrous connective tissue composed of strong inelastic but flexible fibres. It often takes much longer than bone to heal, because ligaments do not have such a rich blood supply and their rate of healing is much slower.

A strain of a muscle is caused by excessive stretching or over-working a muscle. If there is a lot of damage to a muscle this can give rise to a widespread inflammatory process.

Tendinitis is inflammation of a tendon. This can occur after excessive overuse and is quite common in the shoulder area in many sports enthusiasts. Tendons, like ligaments, are made of strong bundles of collagen fibres that can adapt to change, but if they are allowed to become slack due to inactivity then they will shorten and a sudden movement when overstretching or lifting may cause an injury.

Typical injuries are:

Achilles tendinitis. This is inflammation of the tendon of the muscles of the calf of the leg, often caused by some irritation to the back of the heel. This can be caused by poor sports footwear; many of today's trainers have a large ridge or tab at the back which can cause friction. The Achilles tendon (tendo calcaneus) is situated at the back of leg; it commences below the calf and attaches distally to the middle of the ankle and to the calcaneus (heel bone). The gastrocnemius and the soleus muscles that flex the toes are often involved, because of their insertion through the tendon. These are the main muscles involved in walking or running. As this is such flexible tissue and can withstand quite a considerable amount of pulling force, injuries are often self-inflicted owing to insufficient care when preparing for sport.

Ankle sprain. This can be due to a tearing of some of the fibres in the ligament that supports the ankle bones. Usually this injury is the result of a sudden wrenching or twisting motion that can even rupture the blood vessels. This happens not only in many sports such as badminton, tennis or squash but also with poor supportive footwear; too-high heels can cause the foot to turn over on to its outer edge. Ankle sprains should never be ignored; care and rehabilitation are a must to ensure that the person is not left with a weak and unstable ankle.

Back pain.   Back pain can strike at any time irrespective of age or gender. If you are a sports enthusiast it is often due to a ligament sprain, a muscle or tendon strain. Severe cases may be caused by displacement of an intervertebral disc. Often problems arise because of excessive twisting, lifting heavy weights incorrectly, or continuous repetitive movements. Typical sports that make you most vulnerable are golf, gymnastics, rowing, or tennis – or anything where you are in a stretched position (*see* Back chat, page 253 and back exercises, plates 22–6).

Hamstring muscles.   The semitendinosus, semimembranosus, and the biceps femoris are the three muscles collectively known as the hamstrings; they flex the knee and extend the hip. The common injury of tearing of some of the fibres within these muscles at the back of the thigh is often due to overstretching as you suddenly sprint off, or you overkick a ball; it is referred to as a pulled hamstring muscle. RSI from sports activities can affect this muscle, which in turn may affect the knee causing painful spasm. The body's protective response is restriction of the knee joint by spasm; however, although this muscle spasm limits further injury the quadriceps muscle will suffer.

Knee problems.   Knee problems affect many people, not only sports enthusiasts. The knee is a complex joint with a similar action to a hinge joint; with the crescent-shaped patella lying across the front of this joint, it can bend and straighten and has slight rotation. It has two discs of cartilage (menisci) that are wedge shaped, being thicker at their outer edge; this helps to protect the knee by reducing the shock of impact or friction and giving stability. It has two strong ligaments on each side to support and limit the sideways movement. On the anterior surface the tendon of the quadriceps femoris muscle supports the patella. There are two fluid-filled sacs (bursae) above and below, together with lumps of fat that act as pads to prevent friction. Synovial fluid is secreted around the joint from the synovial membrane. The quadriceps muscle straightens the knee; it is a very strong muscle and it does not cause too many problems. However, any knee problem that brings about restricted movement or any swelling that limits the full extension of the quadriceps muscle may lead to wasting of this muscle within 48 hours; this in turn can affect the knee even more so that it simply gives way when weight is put on it. So gentle and correct exercise is of paramount importance at an early stage of injury.

Damage to the cartilage can be the result of twisting when the knee is already in a bent position and the weight of the body is forced on to that leg. Tearing of the fibres in any one of the ligaments that support the knee is quite common; the inside ligaments are often vulnerable if the lower leg is forced sideways. Bursitis can be caused by prolonged pressure or friction on the knee if you remain in the kneeling position for long periods; many occupations can cause this repetitive strain injury. A locked knee occurs when there is an inability to extend the knee fully; this may be due to the presence of a loose body in the joint or a tear within the medial meniscus of the knee joint (*see above*).

Shin splints.   This is a vague term that refers to a stress reaction in the lower leg. This problem can remain for a long time and a period of prolonged rest is often advisable. Injury is often caused by tendon or muscle strain owing to incorrect or abnormal foot posture. Pain develops at the front of the leg on any excessive movement. Soft tissue injury can affect different compartments of the leg, and the nerve endings are irritated. The peroneus longus and brevis muscles that evert the foot, rotate it medially and dorsiflex it, become exhausted as they are continuously used in the balancing action, so uneven surfaces create even more strain.

Shoulder problems.   Strain in any part of the shoulder girdle can be very debilitating because of the many areas involved, mainly both scapulas, the clavicles and the humerus as all three bones join at this point. The shoulder is a ball and socket joint; even the radial and ulna bones may be affected, causing pain and discomfort in the forearm and wrist. Excessive use of the shoulder can damage the delicate tissue and tendons surrounding the joint; it is important not to overstrain or overuse any joint. Many people sit in an office all day then go out once or twice a week to play a sport; racquet games are popular and so is golf, and many people do not warm up sufficiently. The usual problem is of muscle fatigue causing an injury.

Tennis elbow. This is inflammation of the outer border of the elbow; it is often caused by overworking the muscles of the forearm. This problem can arise not only in sport but also commonly in repetitive strain injury.

Note.   First-aid measures.

To any soft tissue injury apply the RICE routine: rest, ice, compression and elevation. This will help relieve the immediate discomfort such as pain and tenderness, and also alleviate any swelling.

Areas to work

A practitioner of reflexology comes into contact with many sports injuries. Many patients present themselves with strains and sprains to the back and legs from injuries at work, from working in the garden or from doing odd jobs around the house. Reflexology stimulates the nerve and blood flow to the damaged region, facilitating the healing process, relieving tension in muscles that have gone into spasm and relaxing taut tendons and ligaments. Working on the direct reflex point that is related to the injury and also on the adrenal glands reflex helps stimulate the naturally occurring glucocorticosteroids, which have such a powerful anti-inflammatory effect. It is important to work the reflexes of the spinal area thoroughly as these contact the nerve plexuses, which are very complicated, hence the boundaries may vary from patient to patient. The 31 pairs of nerves either side of the spine (*see* figure 2.5, page 40) can be stimulated or calmed down if there is a shoulder or lumbar injury. (*See also* each individual problem.) Pressure on a nerve can cause decreased sensation, or pain in an area supplied by a nerve. Patients do not always relate leg and foot problems to their backs. A little more intensive work on the spinal reflexes helps leg and foot pain. As holistic practitioners we embrace all aspects, giving advice to prevent problems arising; we also stimulate and accelerate the healing process, helping the patient's injury to repair and recover. If a pain persists despite resting and having reflexology treatment a patient should consult their GP.

M/R. Work reflex of problem.

A/A. Adrenals for any inflammation.

P/Hs. HE-4 and SI-4 for hand, arm or neck problems; SI-5 for any knee disorders.

P/LL. GB-34 to 38 will help all leg or knee problems. GB-38 helps any pain in the whole body. LIV-7 is known as the 'knee gate'.

P/AS. Area of problem.

P/AA. Apex of ear for inflammatory disorders and to have a soothing analgesic effect.

P/OM. Adrenal glands for their powerful anti-inflammatory properties.

P/TCM. Shenmen for pain relief.

(*See* Leg and foot problems, page 303; *see also* Frozen shoulder, page 285.)

Stress disorders

A detailed account of the role of reflexology in stress is given in chapter 10.

Areas to work

M/R. A full treatment session is needed (*see* Nervous disorders, page 312).

P/Hs. Palpation on the heart meridian on the hands is most beneficial, from HE-9 from the inner edge of the nail bed around to the pad and working down to the wrist all on that little finger (the fifth zone) will help anxiety, depression, and stress-related symptoms. (*See* Anger, page 243, for calming the mind.)

P/LL. There is a foot point that is useful for self-help, just below the tuberosity on the outside of the foot (fifth zone). This is BL-64; this reflex calms the mind. KI-1 on the plantar aspect of the foot for all acute problems.

P/AS. Stroking the ears will aid and soothe rebellious liver energy and relieve mental depression.

P/OM. The subcortex aids the nervous system.

P/TCM. Shenmen for pain relief.

A case history of a stress-related hernia is given in box 8.11.

Box 8.11 **CASE HISTORY: Hernia**

Female, aged 41 years, ran own business in domestic cleaning services (quite stressful).

Clinical problems presented at first treatment. Hernia: the patient had suffered pain and discomfort over a period of 2 years. Her GP felt it was unwise to have more surgery. She was told she was overweight, which was adding to the problem. Her main problem was bowel discomfort. She had slight acid reflux, but lots of noises in stomach and bowel area (borborygmus).

Diet.   She felt this was reasonably good. She could not tolerate a high-fat diet and had had her gall bladder removed 15 years previously. She knew she drank too much coffee and tea.

Background medical history.   Over the period of the past 12 years she had had six operations for a hernia and a repair. The hernia was between the midabdomen and breast bone.

Observations of the feet and general evaluation.   There was a striated area on the gall bladder point. It was also very red in the upper arch of the right foot; there was a deep groove near the medial edge of this foot.

This lady was at her wit's end when she came to see me in early July 1994. Specific points that related to the condition were extremely tender. She attended on a weekly basis for 12 weeks, then every 2 weeks, then at 3-weekly intervals. We seemed to stick at this 3-weekly treatment until February this year. Great improvement was felt, with less acid reflux, stomach and bowel noises had normalized and there was no pain in the abdomen area.

In February I also applied magnetic therapy to the corresponding reflex points. This seemed to speed the healing process; the little remaining discomfort disappeared completely. Her comment was: 'It is as if I never had a hernia problem.' She commented that she felt well and full of energy, much more relaxed and positive. She had joined Weight Watchers to see whether she could lose weight.

March 1995.   There is one slight groove still over the gall bladder point. The previously red area is now normal, with a good temperature to the foot. The deep groove on the medial edge of the right foot is barely evident. This lady attends on a 4- or 5-week basis.

Thyroid imbalance

Symptoms

This includes hyperthyroidism and hypothyroidism. In the former the person often feels overstressed, and may have palpitations and interrupted sleep patterns. The skin in general will be hot and sweaty, and the person feels pushed to be overactive; they end up feeling as if they are chasing their own tails, and generally lose weight. In the latter, symptoms are the reverse: everything seems to slow down, there is often a weight increase and the skin becomes more coarse, the hair may also begin to thin. Both of these disorders are easily diagnosed by having a blood test. These disorders often arise because there is a homeostatic imbalance of the thyroid hormones, which are thyroxine and tri-iodothyronine, T_4 and T_3. This can be caused by any major trauma, or emotional upset; the onset often manifests after the death of a loved one. (*See* plate 12.)

Areas to work

The aim of treatment is to regulate the gland, regardless of whether it is underactive or overactive, as a normal reflexology treatment does not make an organ overproduce or underproduce but aids in normalizing function.

M/R. The thyroid area, plantar and dorsal, of the hands or feet; this is aimed at normalizing the general metabolism of the body. It also aids the skin, hair and nails.

A/A. The pituitary gland to stimulate activity of the thyroid gland, and other endocrine glands.

P/Hs. LI-4.

Warning! LI-4 can be used only providing the person is not pregnant, as it is an empirical point to promote delivery during labour.

P/LL. ST-40 helps any lumps especially in the thyroid area.

P/AS. Thyroid point.

P/AA. Apex of antitragus for thyroiditis.

P/OM. Endocrine point.

P/TCM. Shenmen for pain relief; also to aid if sleep patterns are disturbed.

P/HF. For all eye problems ST-1 and 2 and GB-1.

Tinnitus

Symptoms

Tinnitus includes any noises in the ear; this can be ringing or buzzing, or in some cases it sounds like surging water. It can have a simple cause, such as excess hard wax causing pressure. Some medication can also cause this. In Ménière's disorder, there is an accumulation of fluid in the inner ear, causing other distressing side-effects. Often there is no underlying cause; most drugs do not cure, but only help in suppressing the noise and some of the side-effects. Reflexology is a wonderful way of helping to relieve this disorder. Fitzgerald first spoke of helping unilateral tinnitus by raising the nail at the lateral edge of the third finger.

Areas to work

M/R. Ear, eye and facial areas; also the cervical area as in ear disorders.

A/A. All relaxation techniques as tinnitus can create a lot of anxiety in the patient.

P/Hs. TB-2 is a good point for tinnitus, or other ear disorders.

P/LL. GB-43 and 44 aid the head and ear, the former being exceptionally good for tinnitus.

P/AS. Ear and cervical points.

P/AA. Midpoint of rim aids this problem as well as Ménière's syndrome.

P/HF. Self-help tip: the Tinggong point (on the side of the jaw in the depression as you open your mouth) helps all ear problems.

A case history of tinnitus is given in box 8.12.

Box 8.12 CASE HISTORY: Tinnitus

Female, aged 57 years.

Clinical problems presented at first treatment. Ménière's syndrome, recurrent vertigo, tinnitus.

Diet. She had a sensible diet, although she never eats breakfast. She was active and played a lot of tennis.

Background medical history. The patient complained of acute onset, when she would often be debilitated for a period of a few weeks and the tinnitus and vertigo remained with varying levels of discomfort. She had a damaged nail, which had been caused by a falling branch when gardening 2 years previously, and the tinnitus and vertigo had set in only after this. The lady had also undergone radiation therapy and then finally a mastectomy, also 2 years previously.

Observation of the feet and general evaluation. There were great red areas on the third and fourth toes and a corn on the third toe of the left foot. Her left ear was affected, and on the other foot there was a red area on the third toe, which could quite easily be distinguished from paler area on all other toes. The breast that had been removed was in the same zone as her affected ear. She had taken antiemetic drugs over the preliminary stage of reflexology, but she then discontinued all medication and proceeded with reflexology alone. She experienced great tenderness in the brain reflex (toe areas), facial, eye and especially ear reflexes on the third toe of the offending side. The cervical spine area was very tender, as was the liver area. The first treatment commenced on the hands and then the feet, working particularly on TB-1, 2 and 3 of the hands. She actually had relief from the tinnitus during the first treatment, but this returned after the third day. But, as treatments continued, relief was felt in all areas, and her vertigo became less troublesome when changing positions. The slight nystagmus she had in the eye cleared up after several treatments.

Even though we know that the above problem is caused by a change in the levels of fluid in the membranous labyrinth of the inner ear, thus upsetting the balance of the vestibulocochlear nerve (the VIIIth cranial nerve), this in turn may affect the intratympanic muscle, which we contact on the great toe, and the trigeminal nerve on the lateral edge of the dorsum of the great toe. Both help enormously when worked firmly. The client felt she had gained a quick and beneficial effect.

Observation of the feet at end of treatment. The red areas of all toes had disappeared, and the corn on the third toe of the left foot had almost gone, which had never happened before even after repeated visits to the chiropodist. Her damaged nail had come away and there was a new nail showing.

Tonsillitis

For many years it was quite normal for the tonsils to be removed the moment they were a problem. Today the medical profession realize this should not be the first move as there is evidence that the infection would enter further into the body; now they are only removed as a last resort. Tonsils are a mass of lymph tissue and they play a very important part in the protective mechanism of the body. They often react to a faulty diet, and this is often the reason for enlarged tonsils being so prevalent in children today. As the tonsils are part of the lymphatic system they are involved in the filtering and cleansing of impurities, which may manifest due to faulty nutrition. The tonsils are at either side and the back of the mouth, where it joins the throat. They are there to protect against infection and the invasion of bacteria going deeper into the body. When they are removed, if the poor dietary habits continue, the whole system becomes further abused and congested by de-mineralized food, causing complaints to go further into the body. If parents value the health of their children they should limit most confectionery and white sugars, as they have no food value whatsoever. Regular meals lead to internal harmony and a healthy body. This is so essential if the body is to obtain some benefit from food.

Areas to work

M/R. Work the lymphatic system, the tonsils area and the throat. In children work the same areas but with more emphasis on the thymus gland, to aid the immune system.
A/A. Work the bladder, kidneys and adrenals in case the throat infection affects these other organs. The liver helps rid the body of toxins; the adrenals have a powerful anti-inflammatory action, and normalize the system. If there is any temperature then work the hypothalamus and pituitary to help the fever.
P/Hs. LU-8, 10 and 11 for all throat problems.
P/LL. ST-45 relieves tonsillitis.
P/AS. Helix 1–6 is for tonsillitis and any fever; also the apex of anti-tragus is for any 'itis' disorders as it assists in any inflammatory problem.
P/AA. Throat/pharynx/larynx point.
P/OM. Adrenal glands.
P/TCM. Shenmen for pain relief.

Torticollis or wry neck

Symptoms

True torticollis is due to a shortness in the sternocleidomastoid muscle. However, this term is often used for a severe spasm of the neck when there is a restriction to its movement; because the affected muscle is in spasm the neck is often twisted more to one side and there is difficulty in moving the head at all.

Areas to work

M/R. All neck, chronic neck and cervical reflexes.
A/A. The adrenal glands for inflammation; also the brain as the spinal accessory nerve will help. Also work all axillary areas.
P/Hs. SI-1 is a major point for torticollis and neck problems.
P/LL. BL-65 and 66 are good for neck problems, and releasing torticollis. GB-41 is for any pain.
P/AS. All the neck points; also cervical and clavicle points as these aid the whole area, and give instant relief.

P/AA. Apex of ear for the anti-inflammatory properties, and the strong analgesic effect.

P/OM. Adrenal glands for the anti-inflammatory properties, giving swift pain release.

P/TCM. Shenmen for pain relief.

P/HF. Tianzhu (BL-10) on the posterior aspect of the head helps stiff necks.

Trigeminal neuralgia

Symptoms

In this, a sharp, violent pain is often felt on the side of the head and it can affect all regions of the face. Pain of a sudden onset can be caused by any extreme of temperature. It is a painful disorder, which can be greatly helped with reflexology.

Areas to work

M/R. The trigeminal nerve reflex; this aids all parts – the eyes, forehead, the cheek, the mouth, throat and teeth.

A/A. The adrenal glands for any inflammation, all facial areas, and the dorsal aspect of the toes and fingers for teeth.

P/Hs. LI-4.

   Warning! LI-4 can be used only providing the person is not pregnant, as it is an empirical point to promote delivery during labour.

P/LL. GB-44 and ST-44 and 45 are for all facial problems. Also KI-1 for any acute onset.

P/AS. Work area of problem.

P/AA. Apex of ear for the anti-inflammatory properties, and the strong analgesic effect.

P/OM. The adrenal glands for any inflammation.

P/TCM. Sanjiao point is ideal for Bell's palsy, any facial spasm or facial paralysis, and trigeminal neuralgia. Shenmen for pain relief.

P/HF. Yangbai (GB-14) will help trigeminal neuralgia.

Ulcerative colitis

Symptoms

Colon disease is very common and the prognosis is poor; no drugs provide a permanent cure for these problems. There are many types of colon disease or inflammatory bowel disease. In Crohn's disease any part of the digestive tract can be affected; the section between the small and large bowel, the terminal ileum, is the portion most often affected, and this becomes thickened and ulcerated. Dietary habits can exacerbate the problem: sometimes the client is eating too much sugar in their diet; this is a 'dead' carbohydrate and of no nutritional value. In Crohn's disorder there is often malabsorption of nutrients from the diet, and often weight loss.

Ulcerative colitis is a condition in which the lining of the colon (large bowel) and the rectum becomes inflamed. If the inflammation is limited to the rectum the condition is called proctitis, but when more of the colon is involved, the term colitis is used.

For both, symptoms consist of episodes of diarrhoea, which may contain blood and mucus; there may also be a feeling of urgency, of having to rush to the toilet. Weight loss is very unusual, except in severe attacks, and abdominal pain is unusual apart from some feelings of discomfort before a bowel action. Rarely, the skin, eyes and joints can be affected. There is no known cause for ulcerative colitis. It can affect both sexes at any age but is more common in the late teens/early twenties. It is more common in Western Europe and North America than in developing countries. There is doubt as to whether it is hereditary.

Ulcerative colitis is, by nature, an illness that comes and goes throughout life. There may be prolonged periods when the condition will be better. These periods of remission are made longer by maintenance treatment, which should be taken even when the person feels well. At times, when the inflammation flares up, different treatment may be necessary. Over a period ulcerative colitis may even cause eye inflammation, conjunctivitis or iritis, and other disorders like liver problems and jaundice. Arthritis and lower back pain are common problems. Skin disorders and septic spots or rashes may manifest. Ankle swelling, due to oedema, may occur. In the case of loss of blood from the bowel, then the patient may become anaemic.

The majority of people with ulcerative colitis choose to be treated by medication alone. The medications come in tablet, enema and suppository forms and will be prescribed at various doses depending on whether the inflammation is active or not. Steroids may also be prescribed for acute attacks. These can be given as tablets, enemas, suppositories or, in severe attacks, intravenously. The preparation chosen by the doctor depends on how much of the colon is inflamed and how severe the attack is.

In more severe cases when the symptoms recur more frequently or when the colon becomes very seriously damaged by the inflammation the doctor may decide it is necessary to remove the colon. The remaining bowel may be attached to the anus by an ileoanal anastomosis. In some cases, the bowel is brought to the surface of the abdomen where a permanent opening is made, called an ileostomy. However, thankfully the majority of patients do not require surgery.

The aim of reflexology is to stimulate organ secretion to aid normal digestion, and to assist in the normal healing process. Reflexology helps the immune system and inflammation.

Areas to work

M/R. Work all intestinal areas, with special pressure applied to the rectum and anal reflexes. Also work all the brain area as the vagus nerve aids the movement of the bowels.

A/A. Adrenal glands are for any inflammation; this strong anti-inflammatory aids natural healing.

P/Hs. SI-3 and 4 help intestinal colic or constipation. Also LI-4 has an antispasmodic effect on the intestines.

Warning! LI-4 can be used only providing the person is not pregnant, as it is an empirical point to promote delivery during labour.

P/LL. ST-35 and 37 are very good for intestinal fluctuations, and ST-36 to strengthen the body.

P/AS. Work the large intestine, small intestine, rectum and anus points.

P/AA. Apex of antitragus is for ulcerative colitis, and centre of superior concha for abdominal pain or distension.

P/OM. Sympathetic nervous system is for intestinal spasms.

P/TCM. Sanjiao is for all abdominal problems; as the vagus nerve is contacted at this point it helps all the abdominal viscera as far as the splenic flexure.

P/HF. For constipation work the Chengjiang point (CV-24) on the lower lip.

Vaginismus

Symptoms

Any painful spasm of the muscles of the vagina, which may occur when there is contact with the vagina when intercourse is attempted. This may be psychological, in which case many factors need to be addressed. A medical reason, such as inflammation or tenderness, can also be the cause.

Areas to work

M/R. The aim is to relax the client. A good general treatment will aid and assist the whole body.

A/A. Work the groin lymphatics in case of any inflammation. Also work the spinal areas as the pelvic and pudendal nerve that arises from the sacral plexus, S2–S4, serves the perineum, the urethral sphincter and the clitoris.

P/Hs. LI-4 has a marvellous antispasmodic effect on the uterus.

P/LL. BL-60 will aid if there is any swelling of the vulva.

   Warning! LI-4 and BL-60 can be used only providing the person is not pregnant, as they are empirical points to promote delivery during labour.

P/AA. Centre of ear is very good if there is any neurosis.

P/OM. Endocrine point for all urogenital problems.

P/TCM. Shenmen for pain relief.

Vertigo

Symptoms

This may be caused by a disorder of the inner ear. The three semi-circular canals are responsible for maintaining our balance, and many things can cause this intricate mechanism to go awry. There is often a sense of tilting or reeling; infections can cause this, as in the case of Ménière's disorder, or labyrinthitis. There may be nausea or vomiting, and in some cases also tinnitus. Certain drugs are also responsible for causing side-effects of vertigo.

Areas to work

M/R. Work the brain area for the VIIIth cranial nerve, and ear areas, to ensure that fluid levels are balanced.

A/A. All relaxation techniques. Make sure you advise the patient to move slowly when changing position. Also work the cervical area.

P/Hs. PE-6 helps any nausea. TB-1 and 2 help ear problems and tinnitus.

P/LL. B-67 is a good point for vertigo.

   Note. Do not use this point in the latter stages of pregnancy.

P/AS. Midpoint of rim is useful in Ménière's syndrome.

Vomiting

Symptoms

Any unexplained vomiting should always be investigated. Reflexology will often help; treatment will also help motion sickness, and morning sickness in pregnancy. The hands are by far the best place to work for this unpleasant physical discomfort.

Areas to work

M/R. The aim is to calm the nerve centre in the brain that triggers off vomiting; this is the medulla oblongata, so working all the brain areas of the hands or feet will help.
A/A. Work the ear reflex to ensure there is no imbalance there.
P/Hs. PE-6 helps any nausea. Scratch the back of the hands as this also aids in alleviating any nausea. This is also especially helpful for treating morning sickness or motion sickness.

Whiplash injury

Symptoms

This should always be investigated in case there is any damage to the ligaments or cervical nerve roots. If the neck is immobilized by a support collar then reflexology treatment can help. Work as for neck problems and torticollis.

Wrist disorders

Symptoms

This covers carpal tunnel syndrome; for working *see* RSI and Sports injuries, pages 332 and 339.

Xerostomia

Symptoms

This is dry mouth, a very upsetting problem that can create a lot of stress; it is evident in patients with severe rheumatoid arthritis. This disorder can be made worse by some medications. The patient can have sore lips and the area of skin around the mouth becomes very inflamed and painful. Salivation is under the control of the parasympathetic nervous system. Sympathetic stimuli may arise in response to some stress, resulting in a dry mouth. Extreme stress over a period may change the salivary enzymes.

Areas to work

A/A. Work directly on the mouth reflex of the hands and ears. Work also all the brain area as the cranial nerves, the facial nerve (VII) and the glossopharyngeal nerve (IX) are responsible for stimulating salivation.
P/LL. ST-45 aids digestion.
P/AA. The apex of tragus is the thirst point; drinking water will aid the moisture of the mouth.
P/HF. The Chengjiang point (CV-24) on the lip is useful for a dry mouth.

Yawning

Areas to work

This is a reflex action that may be caused by tiredness or boredom; it has also been linked to indigestion.
M/R. A general treatment rejuvenates.

Note. Many of the case histories in this book show that stress may be the underlying cause of many physical disorders, creating adverse functioning of the body as a whole. For instance, stress often affects hormone levels, which may in turn create changes to the body's internal environment. Skin rashes on the feet are often external manifestations of internal disorder. Many of the patients mentioned had at some time consulted their doctors about skin complaints but had not subsequently obtained much relief. Although most of them had initially turned to reflexology for other reasons, their skin irritations were also cleared up as a result of the treatment. This shows how reflexology embraces the whole person, not just a single disorder, and that a holistic approach to treatment must be adopted at all times. (*See* chapter 9.)

9   Disorders of the skin: a practical application of reflexology

Reflexology is not only for the mind and body but also a must for the skin; it is a wonderful natural treatment that has shown to be effective with many skin conditions. Many skin problems that are common and troublesome in teenagers can also be helped. A relaxed state can help improve even the most chronic skin disorder. Many times the patient is not aware that a certain amount of relief can be achieved with self-help treatment. By addressing lifestyle and eating patterns, the patient gains a greater understanding of the not so obvious causes and problems. Reflexology helps to reduce any high stress levels thus aiding the patient to cope with everyday problems that may arise. A full treatment gives total relaxation and adjusts the inner equilibrium to balance the positive and negative forces of the body. A practitioner of reflexology should look on the therapy as an overseer to promote and conserve health in patients, thus helping to guide them through the healing procedure, giving them support and understanding.

No one medication is suitable for all skin problems. The use of topical steroids is now quite common. However, its value in routine long-term use may be questionable as many are known to have side-effects. We know that many sufferers respond to treatment but this does not necessarily alleviate all the problems.

Reflexology helps in a subtle way, with a very similar but less invasive action; stimulation to the adrenal glands induces the release of natural anti-inflammatory corticosteroids, reducing any inflammation. It helps to improve the circulation in general so that all the living cells get a fresh supply of oxygen and nutrients. Elimination is improved by the transport of excretory matter (matter arising from the end products of the chemical activities of the body) from the tissues. Many such substances diffuse into the lymphatic and capillary system and are then carried off in the plasma; this in turn reaches the kidneys and is finally removed and excreted as waste. However, any delay in the removal of this toxic matter from the system because of sluggish elimination causes many skin disorders to manifest.

Any elimination of any accumulated toxins from the system may affect the emotions. Often deep-seated problems may surface such as anger, agitation and hidden anxieties; these emotional discharges are as necessary as are the physical manifestations. It is most important that the holistic practitioner is aware of this and allows the space each patient needs.

The body energy flow is maximized during a reflexology treatment, ensuring improvement in health and harmony of the body in general. This energy, known as Qi to the Chinese, circulates in channels under the skin. Reflexology theory, like TCM theory, states that stimulation to a specific area on the skin will bring about a response which affects the functioning of the corresponding organs, but a reflexologist unlike an acupuncturist uses a non-invasive pressure or palpation on reflex points. Stimulation to the adrenal gland point would help release the powerful anti-inflammatory properties, which will calm the most persistent itching and relieve any tendency to wheeziness. This helps the bronchiolus to relax by opening up the air passageways, getting rid of congestion and any tendency to breathlessness, and calms the mucous membrane of the nasopharynx and aids the elimination of mucus.

Many patients are amazed at how the essential moisturising factor of the skin seems to be improved with regular treatments and it appears to advance the whole natural process of skin shedding and skin renewal; perhaps it is the stimulation to cells within the stratum germinativum that helps in this exfoliating process. The health of the skin depends on the healthy and efficient functioning of the whole organism and there is an intimate connection between the skin and the workings of the internal organs. All the eliminating organs, such as the skin, lungs, large colon and the kidneys, will try to get rid of waste but if they are not functioning properly they cannot eliminate these bodily processes quickly enough.

Anatomy and physiology

The integument is a marvellous covering of the body parts and a protector of the organs, enveloping the whole body, ie the skin, comprising the epidermis and the dermis, and all the appendages such as hairs, nails, sweat, sebaceous glands and mammary glands.

The skin also plays its role in helping to maintain the body temperature. Secretion is one of the skin's most important functions, the two secretions being sebum, a natural lubricant that also protects with its antibacterial action, and perspiration, produced by 2.5 million sweat glands. There are two types of sweat glands, known as apocrine and eccrine. Apocrine sweat glands are in abundance in the hairy parts of our body, in the axilla and the external genitalia. They are also found around the areola, the nipple of the breast and the eyelids. The apocrine glands are governed by the sympathetic nervous system; they discharge cellular matter as well as fluid. Eccrine sweat is a slightly acid and watery fluid that contains and excretes a certain amount of urea, one of the chief waste products of the body. This waste product is synthesized in the liver and discharged from the body in urine, which is carried to the kidneys in the blood. If the kidney function is slightly defective this product will then pass out through the skin; if the person has a skin disorder, this action is inhibited. The health of the skin depends on the healthy and efficient functioning of the whole organism; there is an intimate connection between the skin and the workings of the internal organs. All the eliminating organs such as the skin, lungs, large colon and the kidneys, will try to get rid of waste but if they are not functioning properly they cannot eliminate these bodily products quickly enough. If the sweat glands become blocked owing to debris and excess sweat, it can cause an intensely irritating rash, such as prickly heat. Sweating in the correct way is essential; hyperhidrosis and hypohidrosis are both disorders that can irritate the skin. The pH of the skin is most important; just like the pH of the body fluids, all must be maintained at a level of neutrality.

Reflexology has the most extraordinary effect on all secretions of the body, improving or normalizing the functioning of all glands and membranes, calming the blood vessels that may be dilated, which can cause erythema. Perhaps reflexology can delay the second stage, the formation of vesicles or papules that can thicken and become scaly. Thus, in the case of skin disorders, such as eczema, reflexology seems to help in the healing process, acting as an emollient and softening and soothing the skin if it is dry, hard or cracked. Reflexology will stimulate the whole circulation so that it functions more efficiently.

The skin is more than an inert excretory envelope enclosing the body. It is a vital and energetic organ. The health of the skin is essential to the general health of the body. The skin weighs about one-sixth of the total body weight and also holds at least one-quarter of the body's blood supply in the third layer, the subcutaneous tissue (hypodermis), which is rich in blood vessels. The blood vessels supply the skin, and their capillaries react either by dilating or by constricting in response to heat, cold or stimulation.

The skin provides a wonderful medium to work on as it is so rich in free nerve endings and we know there are even more pressure receptors within the dermis that respond to firmer pressure. These are the many corpuscles, which are small structures, usually microscopic in size, known as mechanoreceptors. There are a variety of tactile end organs that are responsive to low amplitude cutaneous displacement. These lie in the deeper portions of the germinative layers of the skin. These encapsulated structures are believed to be involved in impulse transduction; it is within these areas of the skin that the reflexologist will make a connection.

An experienced reflexologist will apply stimulation to the sensory nerve endings; some of those in the upper layer of the epidermis, such as the exteroceptors, are pressure receptors that respond to stimuli such as pain and touch. We know that stimulation of these may produce a reflex action. The recipient is aware of this stimulation but interpretation depends on the connections in the brain or the spinal cord. The many tactile corpuscles include Meissner's corpuscles and the Ruffini corpuscles, both of which are abundant in the fingertips, palms of the hands and the plantar surfaces of the feet and respond to even the most delicate of touch, therefore are ideal for hand and foot reflexology. Deeper within the dermis are those receptors that respond to a more penetrating pressure such as the Pacinian corpuscles; these lie in little groups in the dermal papillae. These corpuscles and the Ruffini corpuscles are found around the joint capsules, tendons and tendon sheaths; since they are receptive to a firmer pressure and any movement there is a need for stretching and relaxation procedures. However, patients with damaged skin on the feet cannot be worked on at this depth. In such cases a practitioner may use the hands or the ears. In the case of someone terminally ill the competent practitioner will know which pressure is suitable to use.

All receptors detect changes and then trigger impulses in the sensory nervous system, which may either send their messages to the brain, or they may synapse in the spinal cord, which then transmits responses to all parts of the body. Simple reflex arcs produce reflex actions, which then in turn stimulate the organs to function more efficiently.

Disorders

The skin problems that a reflexologist may come into contact with include: eczema, dermatitis, psoriasis, acne, urticaria, seborrhoea, shingles, erythema and ringworm.

Eczema

The word 'eczema' is taken from the Greek *Ek Zeein*, meaning to boil, seethe, or anything thrown off or out by an internal reaction. All of these definitions imply excess heat or excess turmoil within. Eczema and many other skin disorders often manifest because of poor function and activity in the internal organs. Any malfunction within is often displayed by the large amounts of toxic waste that the skin will try to eliminate when it cannot be excreted by other means. As a result of an imbalance, we may see a variety of skin disorders ranging from occasional pimples or pustules to chronic eczema. Eczema is a disorder that is often exacerbated by stress-related problems. In many cases it is just another attempt by the body to throw off the accumulated toxins from the system, which have amassed owing to the changes in the internal environment, passing these out through the skin. We know that stress can play a large part in these many skin diseases because stress can inhibit many functions of the body. A reflexologist sees these disorders as neither solely allergic in origin nor mainly as an inherited tendency, as these conditions have so many variable causes in the way they often appear and a proficient practitioner will embrace the total holistic concept.

According to TCM theory, the skin is related to the lungs, and it is amazing to see how many sufferers of eczema also have asthma or breathing problems. Stimulation to the adrenal glands reflex point would help release powerful anti-inflammatory properties, which will calm the most persistent itching, relieve any tendency to wheeziness, help the bronchiolus to relax by opening up the air passageways, and get rid of congestion and any tendency to breathlessness, calm the mucous membrane of the nasopharynx and aid the elimination of mucus.

Constipation

Constipation is another well-known problem that may cause skin eruptions. If the bowels do not eliminate in the correct manner some toxic waste is released through the skin in the form of minor eruptions. A malfunction of the hormones or the sebaceous glands can cause acne. Autoimmune disorders may affect the skin, as in the case of lupus erythematosus. In these instances we see the skin acting as a gateway through which the body eliminates lots of waste products. Many internal disorders resulting in skin eruptions are often brought about or exacerbated by incorrect eating habits or allergies to certain foods. If foods contain additives, these can often be the underlying culprits. So we see that skin disorders can be exacerbated by incorrect eating habits which cause an internal imbalance.

Dermatitis

The skin is very susceptible to outside influences; it may come into contact with many irritating substances, such as household products that may contain harsh chemicals, often causing dermatitis (inflammation of the skin). In panic, patients often apply substances or salves to the skin and this may force the problem deeper. It is imperative that the offending substance is found so that it can be tackled at its source.

Analysis and treatment

Skin assessment is one of our foremost tasks when we first apply our skills during foot or hand analysis. We need to check for any abnormality such as: skin colour, pallor or cyanosis, skin texture, skin temperature and humidity. During the normal ageing process the skin becomes thinner and loses some of its suppleness but it is necessary to examine the elasticity of the skin. This needs to be observed closely to see if there is a condition of anhidrosis which may be due to poor peripheral circulation. One of the main aggravations we often find with the skin is a fissure or slight defect in the skin of which the patient is often unaware. This could prove to be a site for entry of bacteria which can be exchanged quite easily by personal contact or touch. It is of the utmost importance that the practitioner ensures the highest standards of hygiene when handling any area that has a break in it to prevent infection or cross infection. A reflexology practitioner must adopt best and safe practice at all times. Also, it is crucial to note if there are any signs of circulatory problems such as swelling, blanching, varicose eczema or any other pigmentation that may be present. If there is any severe skin problem on the hands or feet we first have to establish if it may be an allergic disorder, such as contact dermatitis, which may be caused by a multitude of substances to which the skin is sensitive. Even sweaty feet can release chemicals from dyes in shoes or by a reaction to washing powders, when traces may be left in footwear. These skin eruptions can vary from slight redness to severe inflammation. It is so much better for the patient to try reflexology first, prior to the use of any prescribed corticosteroid creams. Reflexology improves the general elasticity of the skin because it stimulates the whole blood transport system, oxygen, nutrients and other necessary chemical messengers, such as hormones, overall circulation improves which then improves the general tone and quality of the skin.

We must also inspect nails for fungi or viral infections. These can easily be transmitted by touch and it is imperative that the practitioner safeguards themselves from cross infection. The most common examples are caused by the tinea group, which include tinea pedis (athlete's foot) and tinea unguium (ringworm of the nails). These may be caused by direct or indirect contact with other people or contaminated articles that may contain recently shed infected skin cells. Ringworm, a tiny organism, flourishes in moist, warm areas making the skin become very itchy and flaky. Usually it affects the top layer of the epidermis and it is when shedding takes place that infection can be spread. Thus, it is imperative for the practitioner to maintain a very high standard of hygiene at all times: ensuring each patient has their own towel, sweeping the area before and after each treatment session and washing one's own hands.

Diet should also be looked at, as this is often the reason that the person's defence system is low. All processed foods should be eliminated, restrict foods that have hidden sugars, any words ending in 'ose' indicates a sugar, ie lactose, sucrose etc. One should also be aware of sugar substitutes, as they do not contain any nutritional benefits whatsoever, they are artificially refined carbohydrates and there is no need for them in the diet.

Often eczema sufferers have a totally congested and acidic system. This is shown by the colour of their skin, which may have a grey tinge or poor colour. You may find the colon area on the feet or hands puffy and inflamed; this may be due to a deficient diet often high in either hidden sugars, dairy products or processed foods. The ingestion of known irritants such as tomatoes, oranges, green peppers, cucumber, potatoes, mushrooms, condiments, spices and curries, also excess tea and coffee, can play a part in causing more aggravation to the existing problem.

When patients come for reflexology they are often unsure as to whether they will get a response or not. They are therefore amazed at how the essential moisturising factor of the skin seems to be improved with regular reflexology treatments. Treatment appears to advance the whole natural process of skin shedding and skin renewal; it is the stimulation to cells within the stratum germinativum that helps in this exfoliating process. Stimulation also seems to help its secretory functions. The two main excretory substances are sweat and sebum (*see below*).

Reflexology also brings about a profound sense of well-being and complete relaxation, thus reducing any stress, which is often very evident in people suffering with a skin complaint. A reflexologist will aim to help regulate the general homeostasis of the body. As the kidneys play such a vital role in regulating the composition of the internal environment, extra stimulation on this reflex point is very important. The kidney reflex needs to be worked several ways to ensure proper activity within the organ. The internal environment of the body is kept within narrow but normal limits by feedback mechanisms; many systems or organs of the body are involved. The hypothalamus regulates many hormonal functions. The lungs improve the gaseous exchange within the alveolus helping the intake of oxygen and expulsion of carbon dioxide which is by diffusion. The liver balances the blood glucose concentrations maintaining the correct levels. The role of the skin is in making sure that the body temperature does not deviate too much beyond accepted limits. Reflexology has a wonderful way of helping balance all the above systems of the body and all secretory functions. Secretion is one of the skin's most important functions. Sebum, a natural lubricant from the sebaceous glands, keeps the epidermis supple and helps to reduce any tendency to dryness; it also protects with its antibacterial action and antiseptic properties. Perspiration contains some sodium chloride, small quantities of urea and lactic acid; it is secreted from the sudorific glands. These two main substances together create what is known as the 'acid mantle', with a pH between 4.5 and 6; this helps protect the skin from any growth of organisms. It is essential that the correct balance is maintained. The pH of the skin is most important, just like the pH of the body fluids, all of which must be maintained at a neutral pH level.

The sweat glands are governed by the sympathetic nervous system. Often when there is excess stress or an emotional overload, activity within the glands increases and they discharge cellular matter as well as fluid. This is shown when there are sweat spots on the feet or hands; these often arise when there has been any overload on the emotions or there is undue stress. Eccrine sweat is a slightly acid and watery fluid which contains and excretes a certain amount of urea, one of the chief waste products of the body. Excess tension in the body can exacerbate this natural process. If the liver or renal function is slightly defective, this waste product will then try to pass out through the skin. If the person has a skin disorder, this action can be inhibited further causing internal imbalances. It is vital that the sympathetic nerves are calmed down and the hormones of the endocrine system are stimulated, as both are involved in the regulatory mechanism. Thus, in the case of skin disorders, such as eczema, reflexology seems to help in the healing process with an action similar to an emollient softening and soothing the skin if it is dry, hard or cracked.

Usually, at the first treatment session, I suggest a fast for 2 to 3 days (see chapter 11, page 385) with lots of water to flush through the toxins. However, I instruct patients to do this only if they confirm that their GP is in agreement and they are able to have a quiet couple of days. Then a restricted diet for about 2 weeks is recommended. The diet should consist of lots of raw salads or lightly cooked vegetables; dressings can be made with olive oil and lemon. Quantity does not matter, individuals should let hunger be their guide. They must ensure, however, that they do not have any mucus-building foods during this period, then a bland diet together with reflexology sessions should follow until all eruptions have completely healed and disappeared.

It is important to check first to see whether there are any stomach problems; flatulence or acid regurgitation is often a sign that there may be an allergy or a lactose intolerance, and dairy products could be making the problem worse. Reflexology is a marvellous way to detoxify the body; working on the liver reflex will help to eliminate any excess heat in the body and help normalize and balance its function.

Energy in the body takes many forms; chemical energy, electrical energy and heat energy from muscle contraction. This energy flow is maximized during a reflexology treatment, ensuring improvement in health and harmony of the body in general.

Chinese philosophy

In the early human embryo there are three germ layers that are formed as a result of mitosis. The outer layer is known as the ectoderm; this forms the nerves and the skin and its other appendages, which have a close connection to the other two germ layers: the mesoderm and the endoderm. The mesoderm forms the majority of the skeletal system and the musculature, the circulatory system, the excretory and most of the reproductive system. The endoderm forms all the other various internal organs, their linings and tracts in the course of their growth. According to

Chinese philosophy there are connections or points from the inner to the outer cellular layer of the human embryo: the ectoderm forms a line to a particular organ, so we see all organs having a line of association from the skin, ie their own meridian. The 12 organs are clearly associated to the 12 limb meridians. The brain, nerves, sense organs, endocrine glands and reproductive system can all be contacted and successfully treated through the other meridians. So stimulation of the cutaneous area would have a repercussion on the associated organ and this intimate connection should prevail throughout life. This same idea is fundamental to the understanding of reflexology, in which the very act of stimulating the sensory nerves produces some form of functional activity.

Urticaria

Usually patients with acute urticaria, where the attack has no connection with any digestive derangement or any other causal factor (other than a possible relationship with stress), have been suffering over a period of time and have been given antihistamine drugs by their GP. But these are often found to be restricting because of their extreme sedative effect and their effect on the patient's general co-ordination. Also they limit the ability to drive and do other daily activities. A reflexology treatment seems to have a similar effect to these drugs but without any side-effects. Stimulation has a direct sedative effect on the brain area; it calms the patient, who is often alarmed by the uncomfortable swellings and irritation. A reflexology treatment will also reduce redness and irritation in the eyes and nose, thus reducing sneezing and any watery discharge. Reflexology, by its very nature, will bring about deep inner tranquillity and aids in diminishing any feeling of stress. It does not remove the stress, but it helps the patient in their reaction to it.

Hydrotherapy

The therapeutic use of water has been known for centuries. Water is something that many sufferers of skin conditions do not ingest enough. It is essential that an adequate intake of fluids is maintained as it is crucial to flush through toxins. Hydrotherapy baths are very popular, but there are contraindications to their use in many skin problems. I have found that utilizing water by external application on the reflex points, if correctly applied, does not cause further impairment to damaged skin and is very effective in reducing inflammation and subduing pain and discomfort. First, apply a short sharp spray of the entire area with cold water, then a direct jet so that the force or pressure of water then makes contact with each of the reflex points involved; all the organs concerned with homeostasis (*see below*) need to be stimulated. Finally, a good surge of water over the whole foot or hand is most beneficial.

Just as in a general reflexology treatment, we can contact all of the reflex points associated with homeostasis by using water, starting with the hypothalamus reflex, on the great toe or thumb. Then the liver area is worked, mainly on the right foot or hand; applying slightly less force on this zone for at least 4 minutes helps to detoxify the body. Stimulation of this reflex seems to help neutralize the body's natural toxins, which are produced by microbes within. Then direct the stream on to the pancreas. These two reflexes together aid in the metabolism of carbohydrates, to maintain normal blood glucose levels. Apply a short sharp, but forceful, burst for 30 seconds on the left foot or hand reflex of the pancreas. The kidneys are the next reflex as they are of vital importance in adjusting the body fluids; by harmonizing and balancing this organ we stimulate this marvellous filtering and waste disposal system. It is essential to give both kidney reflex points a good direct surge as it is involved in the acidity and alkalinity of the body and regulation of water balance. Another reflex that must be given extra attention is the spleen; this stimulates the production of lymphocytes and antibodies and is responsible for the quality and quantity of the blood in the general circulation, all of which feeds the skin. In TCM the spleen and the kidneys have a very close relationship of mutual nourishment and mutual support. The spleen can function only when the right type of energy is produced from the food we eat.

Direct the jet on the adrenal glands reflex for 6 minutes to stimulate their powerful anti-inflammatory properties. This point is ideal for any allergic conditions, any rheumatic problems or bacterial infections. If the ears are not affected by the eczema you can contact this point on the top of the lower eminence of the tragus, a very potent point. The solar plexus points on both feet or hands relate to the coeliac plexus of the sympathetic ganglia and its radiating nerve fibres. In TCM this reflex is the Kidney point KI-1 known as the 'Bubbling Spring'; stimulation to this point has a remarkable effect on the body in general. It is used in any conditions where there is an Excess pattern, as it reduces heat, which is often present in any inflammatory disorders.

Finally observe whether there are any reflex points that still appear slightly red or puffy, and apply the spray of water to these areas. It is essential that the force should never be more than the patient is comfortable with. The use of water is advantageous for all those reflex points concerned and the whole system is balanced and generally stimulated. Over a period of time healing takes place and new skin is formed, then allowing you to work and apply pressure and palpation in the correct way directly on the area, often within a very short space of time. To summarize, a practitioner of reflexology should look on this therapy as an overseer to promote and conserve health in all patients.

Skin care routine

Hygiene of the feet is of the utmost importance, as fungal infections can be very contagious. Many people now go to aerobics or exercise classes; these are often undertaken in bare feet. If you then shower or use any changing room where many people congregate, this is the most likely time when you could contract a fungal infection. Families that share shower facilities, often use the same bath mats and towels, and if anyone in the household has any foot disorder it is imperative that everyone keeps their own personal towels or bath mats. Fungal infections can affect all the toes, especially in between the lateral three toes. They can also spread to the plantar and dorsal aspect of the foot if not treated correctly.

First-aid tips

Shoes or trainers that do not allow the feet to breathe exacerbate foot disorders. Fungal infections proliferate in moist dark places, and shoes such as trainers or heavy boots, or rubber wellingtons encourage this problem. The client should be advised to try not to wear synthetic materials, and to try to wear open shoes that allow the skin to breathe.

For hands and nails people should use their own nailbrush and towels. If they visit the beauty salon they should take their own nail utensils; those in the salon may not have been sterilized properly. Hygiene is also relevant in the use of foot spas. There are many products on the market. However, tea tree oil is antifungal, antibacterial and antiviral, and this used daily in a footbath helps to ensure that problems are nipped in the bud before they can become rampant. Tea tree oil applied directly to the area will help clear up most problems. If there is excess moistness and the skin is white and pulpy, then it needs to be dried up, using an antifungal powder. Tea tree cream is recommended for all fungal problems, if there is soreness or irritation. Tea tree hand wash also helps in preventing you, the practitioner, from catching other fungal infections.

10 Stress

What is stress?

Stress is not a disease: it cannot be caught. The word 'stress' is taken from a Middle English word *stresse*, which is short for distress.

Stress is a physical, chemical or psychological factor, or a combination of factors, that may arise and pose a threat to the overall homeostasis of the internal environment of the body. Such factors could include worry, injury, infection or disease, which will then act on the body which produces a defensive response. In fact it is anything that is a threat to our mental or physical well-being.

Stress is a part of everyday living and no two people respond to stress in the same way. Virtually everyone has to cope with stress at one time or another; how we respond is the key question. The body adjusts to normal homeostatic changes during stress. It is only in the case of extreme stress there may be a problem. Being overcompetitive at work or in everyday situations, at home or in our leisure pursuits, may make you more at risk of becoming stressed and then developing a related disorder. We cannot cure stress, get rid of stress or even alleviate stress but what we can do is to manage it correctly; this helps us to cope with the pressures that life puts upon all of us, so that our health and general performance are less affected.

Stress is increasingly common and people vary in the amount of stress they can tolerate. 'Stress disorder' is now a common diagnosis in the medical profession. There are many 'stress-related' symptoms such as high blood pressure, increased heart rate and poor digestion, which can be caused by long arduous working hours and continually driving on the body. This stimulates the action of the adrenal glands. Disease, worry and emotional stress can lead to many so-called psychosomatic disorders, which can cause physical symptoms. Extreme stress, for example wounds from accidents and operations, can cause great changes in the body, even circulatory collapse. This is where Western medicine can be so beneficial. However, stress can also be a prime factor in causing many other physical diseases such as stomach ulcers, duodenal ulcers, migraines, eczema, heart attacks and even cancer; the list is long. The medical profession often treat parts of the body. We as holistic healers know that the parts get better if the whole is well. So one can see the need to tackle and identify a stress-related disorder holistically. One only has to read the many case histories in this manual to see that stress is a common cause of many problems.

Physiology of stress

There are two ways that the body may respond to stress: fight or flight. A stressful situation causes sympathetic nervous impulses to flood the hypothalamus; these nervous impulses then travel to the adrenal glands via the sympathetic nerves. The adrenal medulla is the only endocrine gland to have a rich nerve supply. Nervous stimulation of this causes the release of adrenaline and noradrenaline; these prepare the body for immediate action. While this is very helpful in emergency situations, too much of this stimulation may result in anxieties developing. Clinically, this is how anxiety, nervousness and tension are caused as the balance between certain chemicals in the brain and body is disrupted.

Adrenaline and noradrenaline are released in response to any short burst of activity or stress; the body is then prepared for fight or flight. This alarm reaction can often get us out of a dangerous situation, as the immediate response is mobilization and some physical activity. Adrenaline and noradrenaline act on all the tissues throughout the body. This effect of nervous stimulation is helpful in an emergency, since it helps to divert blood to areas where it is needed most. There is an increased breakdown of glycogen in the liver, increasing cardiac output, dilatation takes place in the bronchioles, blood pressure increases, as tone is raised in the walls of all larger blood vessels. The pupils dilate, increasing alertness. Activity is increased in the sweat glands in anticipation of production of more heat from the boost in physical activity. There is a decrease in the peristaltic action within the alimentary canal; digestion is slow when the body is very active.

If there is such a shock to the nervous system and no activity takes place, then the blood pressure may fall rapidly and the person is liable to faint. Increased activity of the fight or flight system over a period of time (eg the workaholic or someone constantly verbally berating you so that you are angry and tense) without any physical activity can lead to the many harmful stress-related disorders developing. Adrenal stimulation over a long period will deplete the body's systems, so the organs do not function as efficiently as they should. These stresses are first felt in the heart and blood vessels; hence elevated blood pressure is a response to stress. Frequently also the adrenaline produced in response to this stress is not dissipated properly owing to insufficient physical activity. Exercise helps excess adrenaline to be burnt off. Constant stress can even change the balance of hormones in the body. Medication can help the problem of stress but it will not cure it until you remove the stress factor.

Stress as a cause of illness

The pace and pressures of modern-day living are tremendous. Stressful lifestyle is quite common. If there is a continual force on the body's internal mechanisms, many other physical conditions and disorders may arise such as pain in the neck and in the lower back, cystitis, dermatitis, diarrhoea, eczema, urticaria, ulcers, heartburn, indigestion, irritable bowel syndrome, migraine, repeated sore throats, stomach and duodenal ulcers, sleep disorders and palpitations, to name but a few. Healing cannot take place, regardless of what medication is given, unless the offending problem is addressed. Many people realize that tranquillizers are only a crutch and these can cause many other serious problems, as there are often unwanted drug-induced effects. Most people now realize that relaxation is a must and should be part of their everyday lives.

Stress in women can completely upset their hormonal cycle; the right balance between oestrogen and progesterone is essential. Imbalance of hormones is thought to create premenstrual syndrome (PMS) including symptoms of water retention, anger, depression, fatigue, irritability and tension, tender and enlarged breasts, and headaches. If the correct balance of these hormones is maintained there is a comparatively trouble-free cycle.

Persistent anxiety is harmful to the physical body. Reflexology can help people to relax, thereby balancing the whole biological system on which health depends.

Stress shows the way our physical and mental system respond; our emotions and temperament often change under stress. Many situations such as shock, fear, loneliness, even surprise, can cause the heart rate to speed up, while blood pressure may rise, and we perspire more. Most stress produces a defensive response; this can be physical and emotional trauma or ill-health or disease, which is taken from an old French word '*desaise*', '*des*' like 'dis' being a prefix that forms the opposite of the word, and '*aise*' meaning comfort, hence dis-ease – we are not comfortable with something. Being at ease is a state of being relaxed without worry or anxiety.

Stress can lead to disease or distress quite quickly if we do not recognize its onset or we are unaware of its causes. Road rage is a phenomenon that has reared its ugly head; it is due to stress, irrational anger and increased irritability over traffic problems and delays. The person loses all common sense, and there is immediate wild uncontrollable anger that may last only a few moments, but in that time something dreadful may happen, like a physical attack on the person whom they felt had caused the problem. The deep breathing exercises below (page 375) will always help in any emergency, when anger may overcome reason. Relaxation techniques should be practised whenever possible. Tolerance is also a keyword, and making sure that sufficient time is left so that you can get from A to B.

Chronic stress can also be caused by long-term emotional problems. These may be due to pressure or difficulties in everyday life, such as working with a manager who harasses or does not support the person. This can cause biochemical changes in the body, which may play a part in many occurrences of frequent headaches or neck pain or lower back problems. The old adage 'You are a pain in the neck' or 'You are a pain in the backside' has a lot of truth in it. Indirectly this may contribute to high blood pressure, digestive disorders, anxiety and depression.

Depression is often a term used to cover a range of emotional states. It can be a passing phase, or it can become a burden and life can become a problem. There is often a feeling of inner emptiness and despair. This state is often caused by bereavement or break-up of a relationship, and the person feels unable to move on. (*See* case history under Depression in chapter 8, page 275.) Everyone feels sad at some time or another, and even the most successful people may harbour fears or doubts and suffer anxiety at times. (*See* plate 13 of a person suffering from anxiety.) However, understanding our psychological distresses is part of the healing process. For relaxation or relief of stress, many of us reach for another alcoholic drink or smoke too many cigarettes, or drink too much coffee. All of these are stimulants and bring about only artificial relief. If depressed we may require antidepressants or tranquillizers. The widespread use of these drugs is questionable. It is much better to try an alternative way to cope.

Physical and mental indicators of stress

The different physical manifestations that may arise from stress include the following:

- You are hot and sweaty in your body.
- You are aware of your heart beating and palpitations, and you get butterflies in your stomach.
- You feel breathless, with a lump in the throat, and have rapid, shallow breathing.
- Your mouth feels dry.
- Diarrhoea, constipation, flatulence are just part of your every-day life and you suffer from indigestion or nausea.
- You suffer general muscle tenseness, particularly of the jaws, and you grind your teeth.
- Often you find you have your fists clenched, you hunch your shoulders and suffer general aches and pains in your muscles. You may also suffer night cramps.
- You are very restless, you are hyperactive and cannot sit still; you bite your nails and you find yourself finger drumming, or foot tapping, and your hands shake.
- You often feel tired, fatigued, lethargic, totally exhausted.
- You may have sleeping difficulties.
- You may feel faint and suffer frequent headaches, or frequent illnesses such as colds and upset stomach.
- You may be sweaty, especially on the palms and upper lip, with a hot flushed feeling all over.
- You have cold hands and feet.
- There may be a frequent desire to urinate.
- It is quite possible that you overeat, or suffer loss of appetite.
- There is an increase in your cigarette smoking, or in your alcohol consumption.
- There is a loss of interest in sex.
- There is an urgency in everything you do.

The different mental manifestations include the following:

- You feel distressed and often worried and upset; you may be tearful, often deflated, with a feeling of helplessness and hopelessness, or hysterical.
- You may be withdrawn, feeling unable to cope, anxious, depressed.
- You feel very impatient and you are easily irritated and aggravated. You are often angry, hostile and aggressive.

- You feel frustrated, bored, inadequate, guilty, rejected, neglected, insecure and very, very vulnerable.
- There is a loss of interest in self-appearance, in your own health, in the right diet; you have low self-esteem and no interest in other people.
- You feel you are doing too many things at once. You are rushed and you jump from one task to another, often failing to finish any task before moving on to the next. Because you feel you have so much to do you end up not knowing where to start, so you do nothing.
- You have difficulty in thinking clearly or concentrating and making decisions.
- You are often forgetful. There is a lack of creativity and you feel irrational. In general you feel you are non-productive and inefficient.
- You are prone to making silly mistakes and having accidents; you spill or drop things.
- You are hypercritical, often inflexible and unreasonable; you overreact to most situations.

The role of reflexology in stress

Reflexology is the most wonderful stress buster. By definition it is a science based upon the principle that there are reflex areas in the hands, feet and ears that correspond to all the internal organs of the body. Reflexology deals with internal energies if these become blocked because of stress factors such as death of a loved one, marital breakdown, losing your job, moving home, monetary problems, pressures at home or at work, all of which may create a block in the energy flow.

Reflexology may not be the first remedy a person thinks of, but it is the most natural non-invasive holistic therapy, and is a means of relieving many of the stress-related symptoms and balancing the internal energies. With reflexology a person is more able to cope. There is a general change in temperament, and the person has much more interest in all situations at home and work or in recreational pursuits. Energy levels improve. All the senses are more relaxed and there is less feeling of nervousness or panic. A more positive attitude follows, with less negative imagination and emotional sensitivity such as tearfulness. The hormones become balanced and the metabolic rate is stabilized as the thyroid function is facilitated. Even though this gland has its own internal control system, the hormones produced must be kept within narrow limits as the slightest disorder can easily upset their function.

Relaxation is the key to good health. A good well-balanced diet should also be maintained, with less of the addictive stimulants, like caffeine, or nicotine from smoking, and comfort foods containing sugar, like chocolate, cakes and fizzy drinks. A gentle regular exercise programme should be upheld. Together these factors will combat stress. Relaxation can be anything that will release built-up tension and anxiety, from sport to whole-body relaxation like reflexology, which not only helps balance the mind and body but can generate energy as well.

Reflexologists will use their skills in assessing what a patient needs. As the treatment commences, and the patient begins to relax and totally unwind, a unique experience evolves. Tranquillity and relaxation, together with the reflexology and soothing music, create a powerful ambience to calm the inner emotions, and help to refresh the mind. The head relaxes, the eyes close, and the shoulders release their tension so the neck and head start the relaxation process. During a treatment many relaxation techniques are used. There is a focus on breathing allowing the patient's body to feel it is sinking into the treatment couch. These techniques help release muscular tension to bring about a state of complete calmness. Stimulation to the brain reflexes helps to release serotonin, which is a natural tranquillizer and mood enhancer. This substance is present in many tissues of the body and in the hypothalamus and basal ganglia of the brain, and is believed to affect behaviour; it also plays a part in the biochemical mechanism of sleep, thus helping sleep patterns. It acts as a neurotransmitter (see chapter 2, page 45).

I often feel that reflexology should be referred to as nature's tranquillizer as it helps to alleviate many stress-related disorders such as anger, anxiety, depression, hypertension, insomnia and irritability. Overall harmony and well-being are achieved and stress responses are more under control. People sleep naturally and more soundly, and wake up fresh and relaxed and full of energy without the use of any other aids. It is a very effective method of reducing and helping in the prevention of disorders developing. It is also remarkably effective in alleviating many problems that people would normally go to their GP for. Patients should, however, realize that it usually takes a series of treatment sessions to bring about total relief. People who have reflexology develop an holistic approach because they become aware of the factors that cause the stress responses. This gives a much broader perspective to plan for any future stressful occasions that may arise.

Encourage all patients to pause and ask themselves how often they relax. Often their only relaxation is sitting in front of the television after work and this is insufficient. They should be encouraged to look around; there are enough yoga relaxation classes, sports halls, dance classes, books and tapes on relaxation. It takes practice to become a cool, calm and collected person, but relaxation is a prerequisite to good health. Remember that 80 per cent of the ailments common to most of us are caused by tension or stress.

Simple stress management techniques

1 Mental relaxation

The aim of this is to produce a relaxed state of mind. Ideally the person needs privacy and quiet surroundings, but with practice it can be used anywhere. This should always be combined with deep breathing. A visualization is used as follows.

In your imagination try to visualize your own ideal stress-free situation and then concentrate on this image for 3 or 4 minutes. It may help if you consciously try to discard any problems from your mind first – you might, for example, visualize an open window through which all your problems are passing, to be replaced by an image that gives you a sense of peace and well-being. Imagine being stretched out on a beach, with the water lapping at your toes. Or imagine floating on a cloud.

2 Simple breathing exercises

These are essential as most people when tense or agitated tend to breathe shallowly, often using only the upper part of their lungs. This often provides the body with insufficient oxygen.

Good deep breathing from the abdomen uses the lungs to their full capacity. This should be done whenever there is a feeling of stress or anxiety. One should always inhale through the nose, not the mouth; patients can be advised to put their hands on the abdomen to ensure that they are using it. (The chest should barely rise.) Then very, very slowly they should exhale, again feeling the abdomen.

Another good tip is to put the arms in front of the body on a support at about shoulder level, while doing the deep breathing exercise. This enables the diaphragm and rib cage to relax.

There are many variations, but the following exercise is one of the simplest. The person should ideally lie flat on the floor but it can also be practised sitting in a comfortable position.

Breathe in through the nose, slowly and deeply, for three counts, hold for three counts, then breathe out slowly through the mouth for three counts.

Continue like this, maintaining a steady rhythm, for 3 or 4 minutes.

As you breathe, particularly when holding the breath, make sure your muscles are relaxed. Then repeat, this time holding a finger over one nostril so that it is blocked; then change over and hold the other nostril.

3 Progressive muscular relaxation

The aim of this is to work through each of the main groups of muscles in the body, first tensing and then relaxing. The person should lie on their back, on the floor with their arms by their sides, and feet uncrossed. The following is a reflexology technique.

Rotate your wrist, then first with your fingers tense, hold for 5 seconds and then relax. Allow the sense of relaxation to travel up the arms and into the shoulders. Clasp your hands together and hold for a few minutes. All these simple exercises will relax the neck and calm the mind.

Starting now with the toes and feet, tense and hold for a few seconds, then slowly relax. Breathe deeply. Repeat this with the toes, wriggling them this time. Then move to the ankles, stretching them and then relaxing. Repeat with the calf muscles, then the thighs and buttocks, clenching them tightly then relaxing them.

Now arch the back gently and relax it. Next pull your stomach in and hold to the count of three, then push out. The arms and shoulders should be flat on the floor. Now take the elbows out to the side at right angles from the body; this allows the scapular to lie completely flat. The face muscles now need working. Accentuate a grin, and do this several times to relax the face muscles. For the mouth, suck in the cheeks then puff them out, and slap them to make a popping sound – this exercises the mouth, nose, eyes and forehead.

Finish with the deep breathing exercise given above.

Self-help exercises with another person

These stress-dissolving exercises can be performed in the home or in the workplace; they help to relieve tight and fixed muscles. There is no need to remove any clothes. (*See* plates 36–8 for massage sequence.)

1 Support the person's shoulder with the hand opposite to the one you are going to work with. Use the heel of your hand and apply a circular movement over the whole area of the shoulder and upper back.

2 Work the other shoulder, making sure the person's chest is supported as this shoulder and the scapular area are massaged.

3 Both hands can be placed on the shoulder and, using the thumbs, apply small circular movements over the whole area, right up to the nape of the neck. Gentle pressure is the secret. This contacts vital parts on the hairline, to release stress and tension.

4 Finish the shoulders by gripping and releasing, and gently squeeze to relax the area; this eases tension. The shoulders usually relax considerably.

5 Now support the head and work with one hand. Points on the face, head and neck (see chapter 7, page 227) can be worked using thumb and fingers, with slight rotation on all points. By moving the fingers and thumb apart, you can stretch the skin away from the midline of the neck. Repeat but this time draw the skin towards the midline of the neck; this procedure relaxes the neck area. Pick up the tissue and relax it.

6 Lean on the recipient's shoulders with your forearms; this applies gentle pressure and encourages them to relax their shoulders even more.

11   Natural nutrition

What is nutrition?

Nutrition is the process of supplying the body with all the essential nutrients in adequate amounts to maintain efficient functioning. Hippocrates said: 'Let food be your medicine and your medicine be your food.' There has always been a study of food in relation to the physiological processes of the body. Nutritional imbalance can cause many problems. These may range from mild to chronic.

The body needs food for growth, repair of the tissues and energy production. The science of nutrition includes studying the role of different diets in maintaining health. Essential nutrients include carbohydrates, proteins, certain fats, vital minerals and water. These are known as the macronutrients. The one element that is often forgotten is water, which is important both inside and out. The micronutrients are the vitamins and the trace minerals required by the body in small amounts and these are also vital to sustain life. There are 13 major vitamins: A, C, D, E, K and the 8 B-complex vitamins. These are essential constituents of the diet; therefore we must rely upon dietary sources to produce them. These substances are required daily for normal development and healthy growth. Most people obtain sufficient quantities of these from natural sources in a normal varied diet.

The term 'diet' is taken from the Greek word '*diaita*' meaning 'a way of living, life, food'. A good diet means a balanced diet, containing all the natural nutrients in the right quantities, to provide for the daily functioning of the body without depleting or increasing the body stores of nutrients. On such a diet, a person would maintain their body-weight and their overall health would be good.

A balanced diet means adapting good dietary habits. We should eat a variety of foods that help to keep the system as alkaline as possible. (This does not mean 100 per cent alkaline because this would not be sensible or healthy.) The body functions better when all the fluids are balanced. Nutritional evidence tells us that sound health is determined by a balanced alkaline and generally acid-free body, whereas ill-health is often associated with an extremely acidic body. Good dietary advice is that we should avoid excess coffee, tea, salt and sugar as these have an adverse effect upon our mineral balance.

It is only comparatively recently that more people have become aware that diet may play a part in their disorder, that it may be partly caused by their overconsuming certain types of foods or eating foods to which they may be hypersensitive.

Components of a good diet

A good dietary routine should include the following: fresh green leaf vegetables, fresh raw fruit, salads, whole-grain products, plenty of pulses, fish, poultry and minimal amounts of meat; these all help to maintain the alkalinity of the body. Fresh foods are generally rich in vitamins and minerals. These form the necessary major food components, together with dietary fibre, which is the indigestible part of any plant. The intake of these foods will help to protect against many of the colon disorders and other health problems. A balanced diet should contain, on average, 20 per cent protein, 20 per cent fats and 60 per cent carbohydrates.

Macronutrients are the major food components required by the body. Dietary deficiencies of these can lead to illness. They include:

- Carbohydrates – an energy source. Obtained from plants, cereals, sugar and vegetables
- Proteins – for growth and repair of tissue, obtained from dairy and meat products, cereals and pulses
- Fats – an energy form, but needed in lesser quantities, obtained from animal products (saturated) and oils (unsaturated); the latter supplies the essential fatty acids, which cannot be synthesized by the body.

Proteins

These are essential to the body, as they help form the structure of muscles, tissues and organs. We obtain our proteins from the food we eat. We need only a small quantity daily to stay healthy. Excess proteins not required by the body are converted into carbohydrate and stored to be used later as an energy source.

Two types of proteins can be obtained from the diet:

- Complete proteins – these provide a correct balance of the necessary eight amino acids, which are the building blocks of the body; the foods that supply this are of animal origin, such as: meat, poultry, seafood and dairy products

- Incomplete proteins – these are provided in foods such as wholegrain cereals, peas, seeds, nuts and beans. They do not individually supply all the essential amino acids, but can be combined to do so (eg seeds with pulses).

Amino acids are a group of chemical compounds that form the basic structural units of all proteins. Amino acids are formed in the digestive system as the final breakdown product of proteins. There are 20 different amino acids; 12 of these can be made by the body, but the remaining 8 need to come from dietary sources. Amino acids cannot be stored by the body; those not used immediately for protein formation are deaminated in the liver. Absence of protein in the diet can lead to many disorders.

Carbohydrates

These are a group of compounds composed of carbon, hydrogen and oxygen. They supply the body with its main source of energy. Carbohydrates fall into two groups:

- Available carbohydrates – these are the simple starches and sugars metabolized in the body for energy requirements, for cell metabolism, muscular growth and activity and the functioning of all organs
- Unavailable carbohydrates – these are cellulose and demi-cellulose, which make up the bulk of dietary fibre and cannot be broken down by the human digestive system; they have the capacity to hold water, thus adding bulk to the faeces facilitating bowel movement.

Carbohydrates are an important source of energy. They are manufactured by plants and obtained by man and animals by dietary intake. They are broken down in the body into the simple sugar glucose, which can then take part in the energy producing process. Excess carbohydrates are stored in muscles and the liver in the form of glycogen, which may be rapidly turned into glucose when needed. Glucose is the major fuel for the brain.

There are three hormones involved in carbohydrate metabolism. These are:

- Insulin – a protein hormone produced by the beta cells of the islets of Langerhans, within the pancreas
- Glucagon – produced by the alpha cells of the islets of Langerhans, also within the pancreas
- Adrenaline – from the adrenal glands.

These substances all work together to maintain the correct amounts of glucose in the body and control carbohydrate metabolism. Too much sugar is a prime factor in many disorders. Excess of this substance leads to obesity, and to heart disorders, diabetes, hypertension, gall stones and tooth decay. Excess sugar can also exhaust the adrenal glands. We should cut down on all hidden sugar products, such as many tinned foods, drinks and all confectionery, and choose foods such as potatoes (especially eating them with their skins on), plenty of pasta or brown rice but not too many cereals, which tend to raise body acidity and often contain sugar.

Fats and oils

Fat is one of the three main constituents of food and is the principal form in which energy is stored in the body. Fat is stored in adipose tissue. This thick layer of connective tissue is formed around the kidneys and in the buttocks; it also forms a layer under the skin and acts as an insulating layer, and an energy source. Fat is stored only when food is consumed in excess of requirements.

Fats are nutrients that provide the body with its most concentrated form of energy. Some dietary fats are sources of fat-soluble vitamins such as A, D, E and K. There are three types of dietary fat:

- Saturated fats – found in dairy products and meat (excess of these tends to raise blood cholesterol levels)
- Monosaturated fats – found in olive oil and avocados
- Polyunsaturated fats – found in fish and vegetable oils (these tend to lower blood cholesterol levels).

Fats are broken down by the digestive system and absorbed in the intestines as fatty acids and glycerine (glycerol). Fat is also conveyed to the lymphatic system and enters the circulation via the thoracic duct.

The fat content of our diet should be low, even though fat provides us with energy. Fat is necessary in the diet to provide an adequate supply of what is known as the fatty acids. These help in the absorption of the fat-soluble vitamins (A, D, E and K). These fatty acids are found in nuts, seeds and cold-pressed oils, and we need these every day to maintain our cholesterol levels. A deficiency can produce dry skin, water retention, lack of energy, skin disorders, allergies and a sluggish metabolism.

We should use monounsaturated or polyunsaturated fats and vegetable oils as these help in reducing high levels of cholesterol.

We all consume too much fat, the largest part often being saturated fats, and excess consumption of these tends to raise blood cholesterol levels. Cholesterol and its esters (an acid-derived compound) are important constituents of all cell membranes and are precursors of bile salts. Cholesterol in the right quantities aids in the general metabolism of carbohydrates; it also helps to produce some of the steroid hormones synthesized by the adrenal cortex, including powerful anti-inflammatory steroids and androgens (sex hormones). Cholesterol is made naturally in most tissues of the body, except the brain. However, the right balance of cholesterol and other blood fats is essential. The correct levels are also of great importance. The blood concentration is normally around 3.6–7.8mmol/l. Elevated levels may lead to atheroma, degeneration of the walls of the arteries owing to a build-up of fatty plaque, which may limit blood circulation. Abnormalities in blood levels also often play a part in coronary heart disease, peripheral vascular disorders and strokes. In order to lower the levels of cholesterol, specific foods will aid the balance. For instance, onions and garlic have amazing properties; they seem to act like a vasodilator and are thought to have a cleansing action on the blood, lowering blood pressure. Apples taken daily are also beneficial, as the pectin is thought to decrease fat absorption and lower cholesterol levels. Patients who suspect that they are at risk from high blood cholesterol should get their levels measured before commencing on any restrictive diet.

Fibre

This is considered to be helpful in the prevention of many of our Western diseases such as: appendicitis, diabetes, bowel disorders and obesity. It is often referred to as roughage and is the part of food that cannot be digested and absorbed to produce energy.

The main products that contain fibre are fruit, root vegetables, nuts and wholemeal cereals. These are called high fibre foods and are very necessary and beneficial in the diet. If you have a high fibre diet it is rare to have a bowel problem.

Water and minerals

Macrominerals

These include the following:

- Calcium – this is obtained from dairy products, green leafy vegetables, nuts, seeds, lentils, soya bean products and hard water.

Calcium is a metallic element, essential for normal development and functioning of the body. It is a very important constituent of bones and teeth. It also aids the nervous system, helps the heart to beat regularly, and also helps to alleviate insomnia.

- Magnesium (known as the antistress mineral) – this is obtained from green vegetables, apples, grapefruits, lemons, corn, almonds, seeds, milk, fish, wholegrain cereals and hard water. Magnesium is a metallic element, essential for the proper functioning of muscle and nerve tissue (muscle cramps are a sign of deficiency). It also aids the bones and teeth, prevents calcium deposits in the kidneys and gall bladder and promotes a healthy cardiovascular system; it is a very essential mineral for all metabolic processes.

- Sodium – this is contained in most foods; it is controlled by the kidneys. Sodium is an essential mineral element that controls the volume of extracellular fluid, thus maintaining the acid–base balance. This is related to maintaining the correct level of fluid balance for normal blood pressure. Also, as it maintains the electrical potential of the nervous system, it has a necessary role in the proper functioning and maintenance of nerves and muscles. It also helps in heat prostration or sunstroke.

- Potassium – this is obtained from oranges, bananas, potatoes, mint leaves, green vegetables and wholegrain cereals. Potassium is a mineral element. It helps to make up the intracellular fluid together with sodium, thus helping to maintain the electrical potential of the nervous system, also normalizing heart rhythms. It also aids muscle function, assists in the correct working of the heart, and aids in maintaining blood glucose levels; it is present in all cells.

Water

The water content of the body in humans by weight is approximately 73 per cent of the lean body mass. Blood plasma is composed mainly of water (90 to 95 per cent).

The water we drink contains various other substances. Hard water contains an appreciable concentration of calcium or magnesium salts. Soft water contains much smaller amounts of calcium and magnesium. Spring water contains an appreciable amount of calcium and magnesium, and also smaller amounts of other minerals: sodium, potassium, fluoride, chloride, nitrate, sulphate, and larger amounts of bicarbonate, making it alkaline.

Nitrate and sulphate are simple chemical compounds. The former is a substance found in nature, the latter is one of the inorganic salts needed by the body. Bicarbonate is an alkali. In solution it has a neutral pH, showing its balance of acidity and alkalinity. A daily intake of water, tap or bottled, is so very essential to life. Six to eight glasses every day are often recommended.

Water is nature's diuretic, increasing the urine output, often helping to dilute the concentration of substances with less likelihood of any stone formation. The skin texture improves because it is one of the constituents of blood and tissue fluids. The digestion improves as well. Water also plays a role in maintaining the body temperature.

Water has been part of many therapeutic treatments over hundreds of years. Hydrotherapy is treatment with water internally and externally (*see* chapter 9, page 364).

Additives

Anything that has a long shelf life will probably contain an additive to preserve it. Substances that are added to food during processing include emulsifiers, flavourings, colourings, thickeners, curing agents, antioxidants, bacterial inhibitors, yeast, mould and, in small amounts, some vitamins and minerals. This highlights the need to eat food as near to its natural state as possible to ensure that not too many of these substances are taken in.

It is best to avoid eating white flour, white sugar, or other refined carbohydrates as these can cause a wide variety of harm to the body and do not contain any essential nutrients. Preserved, packaged or convenience foods are also often high in hidden sugars, and often these prepared foods are low in fibre. It is necessary that we should take in sufficient fibre as this has a direct beneficial effect on the gut (*see above*).

A healthy lifestyle

Diet

Diet is a very complex subject. It includes not only the nature of food that is eaten, but also how it is eaten, the season that the food is produced in, and the regularity of meal times, which should be adhered to so that the body has a natural rhythm and flow of energy at regular times throughout the day. Eating at the wrong times can affect the body so you are often unable to digest food properly.

Some good advice about diet includes the following. It is always wise to:

- Eat a breakfast
- Do not overeat
- Do not eat too fast
- Do not eat on the move
- Do eat regularly
- Do eat in the right conditions (not in an emotional state)
- Do not go for long periods without food, unless you are fasting, and then you need to rest.

Certain natural foods will aid the body. Certain foods also have some healing benefits. Some foods such as prunes, celery, fennel and leeks can help in elimination. Some substances, like salt, can be harmful in excess.

The right nutritional diet aids weight loss, and is healthy and effective. There are many nutritional books on the market; these will give more in-depth advice. The references that are made here will aid in any holistic healing programme in conjunction with reflexology.

Fasting

Fasting will help in the curative process as a whole. Ceasing to take food into a depleted system enables the body to start its cleansing process with more effective elimination; this helps toxins and impurities to be released. Reflexology helps with this process by unclogging tissues and aiding the removal of any congestion that causes a blockage in the energy pathways, also detoxifying and balancing the internal environment of the body that has been abused by faulty eating habits. Prolonged fasts can be weakening, so it is better to have a short fast of 2 days. It will achieve beneficial results and the person should have no misgivings about it. However, always check with the GP before recommending or undertaking any fast. Each patient must realize they play a part in the whole holistic curative process. The effects are usually so rewarding that the person often cannot believe that slight attention to diet plus reflexology and exercise can bring this wonderful feeling of well-being, new health and renewed vitality. A fruit-only diet is nature's finest natural eliminator. The value of fresh fruit in helping to overcome any congestion and many problems, such as arthritis, rheumatism, catarrh and constipation to name but a few, is quite amazing. Together with reflexology this method of body cleansing and ridding the system of impurities helps to restore a depleted nervous system. Factors such as stress, worrying, fear, anger, nervous tension and overwork all cause deterioration of health in the body, often causing nerve enervation and exhaustion. This can mitigate against a swift recovery. Note, however, that if a person is very ill with any severe pain, or with a depleted system because they are frail or underweight, the daily diet should never be changed without consulting their GP.

Exercise

Patients should be encouraged to combine exercise and diet. By lowering their calorie intake they lose weight gradually, whereas crash diets are very bad for the system. Exercise is an essential part of healthy living; any repetitive or systematically varied activity will have a cumulative effect by improving, maintaining or restoring health. Regular activity helps improve bone density; a sedentary lifestyle with little or no exercise may lead to a reduction of calcium in the bones, and together with a poor diet in early years may lead to osteoporosis. All the weight-bearing exercises such as walking, jogging, running and simple exercises can help reduce calcium loss from our bones.

Nutritional knowledge is an aid to healing. As holistic practitioners it is a must to have an awareness of the nutritional requirements necessary for a healthier body. Many illnesses or disorders are made worse by the wrong types of food, such as overrefined products, and by the chemicals that are added at every stage from the growing seed to the final product. Some of these chemicals can build up in the system at an alarming rate and cause excess toxins or allergic reactions.

What is an allergy?

The word 'allergy' is derived from two Greek words: '*all(o)*' and '*erg*' meaning 'altered reaction'.

Many people present themselves to a practitioner on the first visit with vague symptoms such as extreme tiredness, fatigue in the mornings (but feeling better by midday), irritability and depression; these may be due to a food intolerance. The person also complains of fluid retention and weight gain; this is often linked to hormonal imbalance but can also be associated with food. Food allergies may also cause mood swings, with the person often craving the very food they should not be eating.

As a holistic practitioner the reflexologist will remedy allergies by including all these factors, as well as consideration to diet and lifestyle. A reflexologist would treat the immune system with extra stimulation to the liver, adrenal glands and digestive system: the liver specifically to detoxify, the adrenal glands to stimulate the naturally occurring glucocorticosteroids, which have a very powerful anti-inflammatory effect, and the digestive system because with any allergy the stomach produces excess acid. A general treatment would improve the function of the immune system, thereby improving the circulation, and this would stimulate the body to produce antibodies calming the immune system's response to whatever antigen is causing the hyper-sensitivity or allergy.

It is no good just giving a treatment; attention must also be paid to the cause. By elimination of specific foods you will find which foods are the main culprits. Food allergies are initiated by ingestion of certain specific foods. Known irritants include: peanuts, some soft berries, dried fruits, shellfish, coffee, tea, milk products, eggs, chicken, alcohol, oranges, tomatoes, wheat, oats, barley, rye, corn, rice, potatoes, onions and sweet corn. Symptoms may include diarrhoea, vomiting and skin rashes, aches and pains in the joints, constipation, abdominal bloating, flatulence, pre-menstrual problems and muddled thinking. These can take place immediately after ingestion or up to several hours later. These ingested allergens are often a trigger in cases of asthma, hay fever, eczema, urticaria and migraine.

If any patient complains of intestinal discomfort in any way, such as constipation, diarrhoea, abdominal bloating or extreme flatulence, one should suspect gluten intolerance or a wheat allergy. Gluten may be the problem; it is a protein that is present in wheat, barley, rye and oats. By looking at dietary habits a practitioner can often help to alleviate the problem. Reflexology will calm the whole system down.

Disorders where diet and reflexology work together

Bowel disorders.   An apple a day does keep the doctor away; the pectin in apples encourages natural growth of intestinal flora and can aid in most intestinal disorders. Broccoli is high in calcium and chromium (a necessary microelement in carbohydrate metabolism) and is a must for healthy bowels and plays an important role in a healthy intestine. Bananas aid in cases of diarrhoea; the dietary fibre soaks up fluid, which prevents excess fluid loss, and helps safeguard against loss of vital potassium. Garlic is nature's antibiotic for most problems. Also honey is excellent for enabling fluid to be utilized from the tissue, rather than giving other fluid replacements, plus it has an antibacterial effect. Reflexology aids in all bowel problems: it has a normalizing action on bowel function (*see* relevant sections of chapter 8).

High cholesterol. Pectin in apples aids in helping lower cholesterol levels. Most people have a cholesterol level of around 5:1. A ratio above this is not advisable as there is a danger of cardiovascular disorders manifesting. Patients in doubt about their cholesterol levels should consult their medical practitioner.

Common cold. Zinc tablets aid sore throats and help to lessen many of the symptoms better than many other patent medicines. Eggs and wheatgerm are good sources of zinc. Citrus fruits and green-leafed vegetables supply lots of Vitamin C to fight colds.

Cystitis. This is inflammation of the inner lining of the bladder. This inflammatory process of the mucosa and the submucosa of the bladder is often due to the bacteria known as *Escherichia coli*. Many women suffer from this disorder, sometimes with only mild discomfort, sometimes extreme pain. Many people seek their medical practitioner's help immediately for antibiotic drugs. They do not realize that, while they may get relief, often settling the infection and killing the bacteria within 24 hours, one of the main disadvantages is that continued use of antibiotics over a period of time can destroy the friendly bacteria as well. This then sets up a cycle of cystitis – antibiotics – cystitis. We can use many natural products to help if we have an attack. The use of live yoghurt is beneficial. It is also necessary to increase water intake, and the use of sodium bicarbonate can make the urine more alkaline. It is important to pay attention to personal hygiene. It is essential to avoid wearing synthetic clothing as it inhibits airflow to this region of the body. Cystitis can return time and again. Regular changes in a person's diet can help this problem and break the cycle of misery that this disorder brings.

As holistic practitioners, the aromatherapist and reflexologist may suggest the use of tea tree, sandalwood or bergamot to aid the problem. This alone is not enough, as the diet must be made more alkaline quickly because the patient's system is overloaded with toxins. This is where reflexology can help. Stimulation to the liver reflex will aid in detoxifying the body; together with this, working the kidney and adrenal reflexes and the groin lymphatics will help reduce inflammation and reduce pain. Drinking beetroot juice, cranberry juice or spinach juice, together with copious amounts of water, will alleviate an attack. A change in dietary habits is most essential. All the refined products must be avoided, less coffee and tea consumed, and condiments should also be restricted, as should pickles, spices and sauces. If a person smokes this can also aggravate the problem.

It was thought at one time that it was necessary to make the system more acidic so that it was hostile to germs. However, it has been found that cranberry products (which are alkaline) taken over a period of time help to keep the *E. coli* bacteria from adhering to the tissue of the bladder wall. Reflexology will help to reduce any inflammation by applying extra stimulation on the adrenal reflex; this will alleviate the burning heat and pain and control the overall mineral balance. Stimulation needs to be applied to the groin lymphatic reflex and the spleen to increase antibody production to fight the infection.

High blood pressure (hypertension).   This has often been linked to the wrong diet and lifestyle. A reduction of all animal fats (except oily fish) in the diet is essential; the intake of salt and all other stimulants such as tea, coffee and alcohol, should be drastically reduced or withdrawn immediately from the diet. Taking onions and garlic is thought to benefit greatly anyone who suffers with high blood pressure, as it is thought these act as neutralizers of toxins, and also vasodilators, widening the blood vessels. High stress levels are often thought to elevate blood pressure levels. Gentle to moderate exercise is one of the most important ways of maintaining a good circulation and may help in the reduction or decrease in high blood pressure. The use of exercises that induce relaxation is thought to have a beneficial effect. Many doctors now feel that hypertension should be treated by nutritional means and relaxation techniques, whenever possible, rather than resorting to medication. The level of blood pressure can fluctuate daily, so it is imperative that more than one reading is taken. (Just the thought that your medical practitioner is going to take your blood pressure, is enough to elevate it.) A good reading should be 120/80, but it is usual to have an increase in this measurement as you age. The rule of thumb often used is to take the systolic blood pressure, an average reading of a 100, plus your age if over the age of 50 years old, giving you a reading of 150/80 (to get the average for an older age group). However, Dr Michael Colgan of the Institute of Optimum Nutrition, felt this was too high and was a cause for concern. His feelings were that, with the right nutritional supplement programme, the blood pressure readings should remain the same 125/85 at any age, with a good resting pulse rate of 65 beats per minute.

Reflexology is a marvellous way to calm and relax a person. It will strengthen the cardiovascular function and regulate metabolism. Because of these effects blood pressure is lowered. Together with the right diet and exercise this should achieve a healthy stress-free body.

Prostate problems. According to many articles now written, not only zinc aids this problem, but also several portions of tomatoes (rich in Vitamin C) taken daily helps to protect against prostate cancer.

Respiratory disorders. An age-old remedy has been to take boiled onions for coughs and colds; this aids the lungs and the upper respiratory tract.

Nutrition is one of the first basic steps to a healthier body. We are what we eat and drink, and even the smallest change can bring about the most amazing benefits. Outlined in this chapter are the basic ideas of choosing the right foods for general well-being and vitality. A person does not have to go without; it is a matter more of getting the combinations and balance right. Diet and reflexology make you feel good both inside and out, improving energy levels and the functioning of the eliminating organs, and stimulating the general metabolism of the body. Also the importance of water in the diet cannot be stressed enough – at least six to eight glasses daily should be taken.

12   The reflexology practice

The public are now aware of complementary therapies as they perceive the need to have a fit and healthy lifestyle. This is made available to them in many ways. You can set up a practice through existing beauty salons, health centres, health farms, leisure centres, or simply work from home. To capitalize on this growth area it is essential to use as many marketing skills as possible, and ensure that you promote yourself extensively.

It is imperative that the surroundings are conducive to relaxation; this is the first step in setting up your practice, regardless of whether it is a salon or a clinic in a fine building, with all the right staff. A lot of thought needs to be put into setting up the treatment room. Salon owners or managers, or complementary practitioners working from home, all need a well-run business regardless of size. This all adds to your professionalism. Overall management is down to you.

Setting up a practice

There are various factors that you need to know about when setting up a practice:

- Treatment room – it is imperative to find suitable space or premises with a serene and tranquil ambience. This can be a building or part of an existing practice, or even a room in your own home if it is suitable. There must be reasonable access to toilet and hand-washing facilities. Heating must be satisfactory, with adequate ventilation.
- Equipment – suitable equipment to work on includes a treatment couch or reclining chair.
- Insurance – third party indemnity is necessary; this covers a person not named on the insurance agreement but who will be protected by the insurance if there is an accident on the premises. Professional indemnity covers you against any litigation arising in the case of accidents during or connected with treatment.

- First aid – qualifications in or knowledge of first aid is most important if someone is suddenly taken ill (*see* Appendix II, page 416). A first-aid box is necessary in the case of minor injuries.
- Safety – a fire extinguisher is advisable but not compulsory in all premises.
- Administration – recording of daily affairs, appointments, treatments and financial accounts is essential. Accounts should include a record of debits and credits and all receipts. Tax laws can be complex and an accountant can often advise you to claim for the correct current amounts and percentages of purchases. Many expenses are subject to tax relief. You need to be aware of PAYE, which is the system by which income tax is deducted from wages of someone you may employ, and the self-assessment system, and VAT liability.
- Certification – display all professional qualifications with pride; also display current insurance certificate and membership of any established professional body.

Planning the business

Professional image is of the utmost importance, not only in your uniform or outfits, but also in your business or appointment cards, your stationery, and your premises.

To get started in your practice you need to promote yourself; if people do not know that you have a service to offer they cannot take advantage of this facility.

You can put out some printed leaflets locally; the response rate is not usually that good, usually 2 per cent of output, but it can inform your local community that you have a practice in reflexology to offer. If you get a 2 per cent response from people who recommend you to their family and friends that is ultimately a much greater percentage response. Patient referrals are the best form of advertising.

Advertising in local newspapers, or your local directories, is also a possibility. It is a good idea to contact your local paper and offer a free treatment to someone who covers health issues for the paper's editorial department as you are setting up in practice; in return you may get a free mention in the editorial pages.

Invite a few acquaintances, asking them to bring a friend, and give a short talk and demonstration. Leave some leaflets around explaining and outlining the treatment procedure. You can repeat this by asking anyone if they would like to do the same in their home, asking them to invite a minimum number of guests to make it worthwhile. In turn you can offer a free treatment to the host. Contact your local groups, the WI, the sports centre, or leisure centre; all are possible outlets or places that may like a presentation, while giving you the chance to improve your profile. Speaking engagements offer you the opportunity to explain to others about your practice and the facilities that you offer.

Business terminology

Most leading banks will offer services to help you set up your own business. It is not easy to set up any type of business, no matter how small. Planning is the keyword, and most business packs address all stages that you need to cover, from your original idea to the marketing plan. This includes knowing your market and how to promote yourself. The usual pack includes details on formulating a business plan, legal and tax obligations, even staffing and recruitment advice.

There are many organizations offering courses of interest to people who wish to start their own business. For any further information about starting up in business, go to your nearest Job Centre where they will also give you expert advice on contracts of employment. Each town usually has a local Training and Enterprise Council, and an Enterprise Agency if you require any more information.

Bookkeeping

While you are in business it is essential that you keep a detailed account of the amounts of money received or paid out on every transaction that takes place. This is the law, and also the details of your financial transactions enable the correct amount of income tax to be collected, and VAT if relevant.

Some of the terms you may meet in business administration are as follows:

- Net profit – this is the amount of profit after payments like income tax have been deducted.
- Cash flow – this is the movement of money to and from the business.
- A balance sheet – this is a clear statement showing how much money has come into a business, or goods that you have purchased that are of value and can be sold to pay a debt; these are your assets. How much money is paid out of the business is

your outgoings; these go to cover debts that must be paid and are your liabilities.

- Petty cash – this refers to an amount of money specifically kept ready for making small payments for everyday purchases.
- Petty cash book – this is a book that is kept to record the date and amounts paid out from the petty cash.
- Standing order – this usually refers to an order to pay a set amount from your bank account each month or each year.
- Direct debit – these are usually requested by the person who requires the payment for a regular service or for goods supplied on a regular basis. For this you sign an agreement or mandate with your banking details on, which sanctions the request, so that the person can instruct your bank to deduct from your account the required amount of money. This is very useful if the amounts fluctuate as it saves you a lot of time and trouble.
- Lease – this is a written agreement made according to law, which enables you to have the use of premises for a set period of time, for which you are charged rent.
- Rent – this is an amount of money you may pay for the use of premises; this may be a room or a set space within another business, or a building.
- Franchise – this is the authorization by a producer of goods or someone who already conducts a successful business in a tried and tested way, given to you to carry on a type of business in a particular area, for which you pay a fee. A formal agreement is usually signed. Check with your local bank to see whether they have a franchise guide.
- Contract – this is a document or signed agreement on which terms and conditions are written. (One should never enter into or sign a contract until it has been read from beginning to end and you are entirely sure that you can fulfil all the conditions as stated.)
- Licence – this is an official document that shows you have permission to do something; this is often given and in return you make a fixed payment for this official permission.
- Accountant – this is a person who keeps or examines the money accounts of your business, and will recommend appropriate legal ramifications. A chartered accountant is a certified public accountant, a person who has undertaken and passed specified official examinations and has full professional recognition.
- PAYE – this is pay as you earn, a system by which income tax is deducted from your wages prior to you being paid.
- National Insurance – this is a system of insurance run by the government to which every employed or self-employed person makes set regular contributions; there are various classes of

payment. This money is used to benefit those less able to support themselves because of age or illness.

- Tax – this is a sum of money paid in accordance with the law to the government in proportion to income earned, property, or goods purchased. It includes:

    Income tax – a sum of money charged on one's income, that is, money that is received regularly for work, or interest received on investments. Your local Inland Revenue office are always pleased to give any other information that you may require.

    Value added tax – often known as VAT. If a company or business has a turnover greater than a set amount (the amount at the time of going to press is £46,000), a sum of money or tax is levied by the government for most of the business transactions over and above this set amount. The business has to register for VAT and charge it. VAT is currently standing at 17.5 per cent; this must be charged on all products and services sold, and it is similarly paid on all goods or services purchased from VAT-registered companies. It is imperative that a very detailed account of all negotiations is recorded. The VAT tax period is every 3 months, when it is necessary to fill in the appropriate forms, known as VAT returns. These record the amounts, and should the VAT exceed a certain level a sum must be paid to HM Customs and Excise. However, if this amount is far less than this level it can be reclaimed from HM Customs and Excise.

- Self-employed – this means you are earning money from your own business and are not being paid a wage by an employer; your tax and National Insurance contributions are usually calculated on your profits.

- Employer – this means you pay a person a wage to carry out required tasks or activities. They are a paid worker and you, the employer, have certain obligations. You are required to collect a proportion of the wage of an employee on behalf of the Inland Revenue.

- Employee – this means you are a paid worker; for this you receive an amount of money known as wages.

Creating the correct atmosphere and suitable accessories

The following tips are good basic guidelines to get you going.

1 Make sure your treatment room is fresh and crisp. You do not need to spend a fortune, but it should be clean and airy.

2 Flowers or plants are good window-dressing aids; have a fresh display weekly.

3 Make sure the temperature is even (not too hot or too cold).

4 There should be an abundance of clean towels, one for each patient.

5 Antiseptic or wet wipes should be provided for freshening the feet or hands; also you may need to wipe your hands if you sneeze or blow your nose.

6 A tissue roll saves changing the pillows after each client.

7 Use a vaporizer or burn oils in a container; fragant oils are relaxing and soothing, which is all part of the therapeutic technique.

8 Play some soft music, but remember it should only be background sound. This also relaxes the client and can be quite uplifting.

9 A fan is a good investment; if the weather is too hot it is refreshing to walk into a fresh cool room. The other advantage is that if it is noisy outside you can close the window to keep noise to the minimum and still remain cool.

10 Finally, your image is most important, especially if you work from home. Remember, a patient may arrive on the wrong day, or they may turn up earlier than expected. Always leave sufficient time to prepare yourself, if you try try fit housework in between clients.

11 All utensils should be at hand, including talcum powder or corn silk powder, and cream to complete the treatment with a nice relaxing foot and leg massage, or a hand and arm massage.

Working from home

Regardless of where you work from, home or local premises, you may need a licence to trade, as there may be some small clause in your property deed that has a restriction. You need also to check to see whether there are any local bylaws that may limit certain activities. Nuisance regulations may cover excess parking in a built-up area. Always contact your local Planning Office for further advice. There are many advantages to working at home: there are no travel costs, overheads are cut to the minimum, and many tax deductions are available. If in doubt, it is always advisable to have a business solicitor.

Regulations

There may be local bylaws, or special rules laid down by some local authorities or local councils governing massage treatments.

Often a licence is required to practise. Some councils insist on this for reflexology. It is your responsibility to check to see whether you require such a licence prior to setting up in business. Your Local County Council Trading Standards Department will give you advice on whether you need a licence for reflexology. Each county may have different rulings. This licence is usually required prior to giving chiropody treatment, massage of any body part, and in certain cases reflexology to any member of the public. If so, you will be requested to submit details of qualifications and any staff you may employ. References are often requested from two professional persons who know you and are prepared to give a testimonial of your character. Often an inspection of the premises is required, and occasionally there may even be a police check to ensure that you are of good character. Once you are approved by your authority a registration fee is charged and you pay an annual fee for this licence. However, you may get requests for periodic inspections.

Each country has its own laws governing the practice of some complementary therapies. It is each person's responsibility to check for any legislation that may impede their work.

Each town or county in the UK usually has the following:

- A Health and Safety Executive
- HM Collector of Taxes
- HM Customs and Excise
- A Trading Standards Office
- A Department of Social Security (DSS), of which there are two agencies usually: the Benefits Agency, dealing with income support, sickness benefit and pensions, and the Contributions Agency, dealing with National Insurance contributions
- A Job Centre, where job opportunities are advertised, and advice is given on training and counselling services; some opportunities are available for the self-employed
- An Environmental Health Service, where advice is given on all health and safety regulations pertaining to premises, and also information that you may need regarding legislation and hygiene measures.

The general law of the land detailed below applies to England, Wales and Scotland. Other countries have their own legislation.

Criminal law discourages any harmful behaviour to the community as a whole, and this includes deliberate fraud, sharp practice and the use of unsafe appliances. In England, Wales and Scotland the courts can order compensation for personal injury, loss or damage to those who have suffered because of the actions or omissions of someone who may be negligent. Negligence is a failure of duty to care, for instance the duty of the practitioner to care properly, to accepted professional standards, for the patient.

Statutory law covers both criminal and civil law. A library will have detailed information on the various Acts of Parliament; those listed below are an abridged version of the most relevant ones.

Health and Safety at Work Act 1974

These are regulations laid down by law to ensure the rights of the employee and the employer. It is the employer's responsibility to provide a safe and healthy workplace. They cover:

1 Correct safety procedures (fire exits)
2 Health and safety policy to which all staff must have access
3 Regular training sessions in all aspects of safety procedures
4 Any equipment that is used, which must be deemed safe and must be regularly serviced.

Employees should adhere to the above and follow all safety procedures as laid down by their employers. Any equipment that may appear faulty in any way should immediately be reported.

Fire Precautions Act 1971

This covers the duty for all employees to be trained in emergency fire procedures. These may include the following instructions:

1 Knowledge of all fire exits
2 Assembly point in the case of evacuation
3 Use of stairs rather than lifts
4 Closing all windows and doors, if possible, before leaving the premises
5 Not bothering about belongings
6 Types of equipment to be available on the premises

Electricity at Work Act 1990

This covers the duty to ensure that all electrical equipment is regularly checked and dated. For instance, all exposed wires should always be reported and use of the equipment must be discontinued. A qualified electrician should visit annually to check plugs and wiring.

Trades Description Act 1968, 1972

This makes it a criminal offence to describe goods falsely, whether written or spoken. This is applicable to many different kinds of description, including services.

Ethics

This is a general set of moral rules and codes of conduct that a professional practitioner should abide by. Some ethical guidelines are as follows:

- Always conform to accepted standards of moral values and rules of conduct.
- Maintain professional confidentiality regarding patients' case histories and other individuals at all times. This is of the utmost importance when dealing with more than one family member or their close friends and work colleagues.
- Refrain from criticizing or finding fault in the work of a fellow practitioner or any member of the medical profession.
- If a patient is having current treatment for the same condition elsewhere, encourage the patient to ask the medical or health care practitioner if they have any objections to the patient receiving treatment.
- Never recommend that a patient discontinues any drugs he or she may be taking; that decision must be taken by the patient and general practitioner.
- Never offer cures for specific conditions.
- Confine treatment to your own particular therapy; do not offer advice such as taking patent medications or other nutrients unless qualified to do so.
- Observe rules of conduct and standards as indicated by your governing body.
- When you accept a patient into your care you are obligated to give the most fitting treatment of which you are capable.
- Observe 'good and safe practice' at all times.

Professionalism

There is no quick way of learning how to be a professional person; this is attained over a period of time. However, there are some guidelines.

Give your patient your wholehearted attention; forget about the previous patient's problems, and refer only to the present patient's personal problems and their dilemmas.

Encourage your patients to discuss their interests, leisure activities, pastimes and other pursuits of relaxation, as they all play a significant role in the well-being of each individual.

Always wear some covering or other professional uniform. This protects your clothes and your professional image. White coats can put some patients off and make them a little apprehensive; a neutral colour is just as good.

Always make a point of washing your hands so that your patient is aware that you have done so, especially after blowing your nose, or if you change the limb or ear you are treating. It is good to talk, but do not gossip. Remember, the patient should be kept quiet. One should not enter into discussion on unethical topics.

Never get involved emotionally with your patient; this is unprofessional. Your behaviour and skill show your qualities of professionalism and high standards.

Making an introductory presentation to an audience

The following section provides some guidelines to help you to prepare for a presentation to a group of people. This can be two or three or even 1,000 people. Adhere to the following and you should have no problems.

Essential preparatory stages

The work on a presentation can be broken down into a number of stages:

1 Establishing your objectives
2 Analysing your 'audience'
3 Making a preliminary plan
4 Organizing your material
5 Thinking about your manner and technique
6 Practice and rehearsal
7 Timing.

Establishing your objectives

What are you aiming to do in your presentation? It seems a very obvious question but often we are so concerned with what we are going to say that we lose sight of why we are saying it. You need to think about both short-term and long-term objectives and tailor your presentation accordingly. You also need to think realistically about what you can achieve in the time available and what you can expect from your audience. You need to whet their appetite quite quickly, so it is best to keep your talk quite short.

Analysing your 'audience'

What you say, and how you say it, should be tailored to suit the people to whom you are trying to communicate. This means thinking about their knowledge of the therapy. For example, a good presentation can go very wrong if you use oversophisticated methods with a very unsophisticated group. Analysing your 'audience' helps you to determine who to expect, which age group, whether it will be females only or a mixed group, and so on. This enables you to adapt the following:

- Your general approach and style
- The level of your presentation
- How much jargon, technical vocabulary, etc to include or omit
- How much supporting material to use, for example evidence, statistics, visual aids.

Making a preliminary plan

It is a good idea at this stage to make notes as a starting point to structuring your presentation. This includes the main ideas and concepts you want to put across and the general history of reflexology. Include a few case histories, and a brief demonstration. Then take questions from the floor. Before you commence, consider the following points. First, know your history, and have a few dates ready to show that it is an age-old therapy, with refined techniques. Think of the facts you want to use as examples, for instance a description of simple nerve pathways. Decide the emphasis you want to make, for instance reflexology as a natural non-invasive therapy. Consider other material you might use – statistics, evidence, etc, and possibly two or three case histories. Suitable material that might be appropriate for visual aids, for example, would be charts copied on to transparencies, or a photograph of a person's foot showing hallux valgus. (This marked lateral deviation invariably indicates neck problems or shoulder problems.)

Organizing the material

Even experienced speakers find it best to make notations of their ideas initially as they occur to them and to then sort them into some structure. A common device also is to sort the points into four categories:

1 What you must include – use only points that are necessary and essential.
2 What you should include – do not fabricate but only state true facts; remember, reflexology is not a panacea to all ills, only 90 per cent of them; give an outline of research to date.
3 What you could include – remember, certain points may become irrelevant if you follow a speaker who has spoken on a similar theme.
4 Organize your material.

The simplest way of constructing your presentation will be to think about the following:

- The opening
- The main body of the presentation
- The conclusion.

The opening is clearly essential and critical to get the group's attention and make them immediately interested. You must also introduce your purpose and the main ideas you wish to put across. There are several options open to you here:

- Direct statements – you may begin your opening sentence with a phrase such as 'I'm going to talk about' or 'My presentation is about'. With a direct statement you always appear to be plain speaking.
- Indirect statement – the alternative is to start with a sentence like 'You may be wondering why I am speaking to you all this evening.' With an indirect statement, however, you may often be meandering and the talk may appear drawn out.
- True to life examples or comparisons – case histories can be used to exemplify the treatment process.
- Using quotations – you may wish to add historical interest by including statements such as 'Fitzgerald said . . .'
- Statistics – for instance, you may wish to make a comparison on price; by stating 'The current cost of a treatment session is . . .' and also quoting what it would cost for hairdressing or the cinema makes reflexology more desirable.

Remember not to overdo the introductory stage; it should take up no more than 5 per cent of your overall time.

The main body of the presentation should develop your ideas; here it is important to retain your audience's attention and ensure that they are understanding your points. Visual aids may help, though not necessarily if they are too involved and not well prepared (*see* Visual aids, page 408). It will probably be important to give examples, comparisons and supporting evidence or be able to illustrate a point with a 'story'. It is also worth bearing in mind that the ideas you want to be remembered may need to be repeated, possibly two or three times, and that this will be most effective when you present them each time in a slightly different way.

The conclusion needs careful thought so that it is fairly brief and concise while still rounding off the presentation smoothly. Summaries are useful and are a systematic way of concluding.

Thinking about manner and technique

Your main aim is to enlist the group's attention and interest. Again, analysis of your audience helps to determine the most appropriate style of delivery. Most people find that they develop a personal style with experience, but some feedback is essential in order to assess and improve performance.

Practice and rehearsal

Important presentations are definitely improved by practice and rehearsal before the event. This is not always possible, but where time allows a 'run-through' with a friend or partner is a great confidence builder and it also helps you to master the timing. A willing and helpful observer can also be an effective way of getting some feedback.

When full rehearsal is impossible, make sure you know exactly how you are going to begin and end your presentation. You need to ask yourself a few questions regarding your audience.

- Why are they attending this presentation or meeting?
- Are they used to listening to presentations?
- How many will there be? (So how far can you encourage participation?)
- Do they expect you to be formal or informal?
- What is their knowledge of the subject? Is it general or limited? Remember to make sure you know what level of technical or non-technical vocabulary to use to help their understanding.
- How open-minded are the audience and willing to accept the

theme of the presentation? Be aware of atmosphere and be prepared to give another demonstration if needed. Or ask 'Are there any questions so far?'

Timing

Any occasion must have timetables so that the arrangement of stated events can happen. This ensures that everyone who is booked to speak does so in their allotted time, thus allowing for the time of arrival and departure to be strictly adhered to, if a venue is reserved for a particular time.

Ten tips for effective speaking

1 Public speaking is a performance. It is important that you know how to use your voice, face and body to make yourself effective. Most speakers could improve their delivery. Note that the best preparation can be simply wiped out by poor presentation. Keeping it short and concise is the most effective way. Reflexology is not a subject that you can cover in 5 minutes. It is said that most listeners' attention will drop after 15 minutes and usually reaches saturation point after 30 minutes, unless it is a lecture. Where appropriate it is often useful to say at the start something to the effect that you intend to keep the presentation short to allow more time for questions. Remember, most speakers are more interesting when answering questions than when lecturing.

2 Your general manner is most important. Try to be as natural as possible; make sure you relax (*see* page 411) and that you smile. Look directly at individuals and then traverse your audience. It is essential that you like and show enthusiasm for your subject; if you do not feel positive then the audience will not be able to. Your most important and interesting points should be at the beginning when you have the most attention. Limit yourself to four or five main points, getting to the point fairly quickly. Begin with opinions with which the audience will usually agree; this increases your credibility and the audience's confidence so they will be prepared to listen to the rest. Show that what you are saying is relevant or will benefit the listener and always state the opposite point of view, as a heavily biased presentation is usually badly received. Show that you are aware of, and have considered, all other arguments.

3 Remember that the listener often finds it harder than the reader to take in a message. This is because they cannot take it in at their own pace, so it is advisable to keep the structure simple and the sentences short. It is important to repeat at least twice the concepts you wish particularly to strike home and be remembered. You must find ways to repeat yourself that are interesting and different – paraphrasing, giving examples, citing authoritative references, quoting, giving statistics and summarizing. You can say the same thing over and over in different ways.

4 Posture is most important as it adds to your presence; also it enables you to move or gesture with ease. In general, try to avoid looking stiff and making overexaggerated movements. Always stand unless your audience consists of less than 10 people. Stand with your feet slightly apart and keep the weight of the body on the balls of your feet. This enables you to move around without any stumbling, and it makes you appear more relaxed. Relax your arms, letting them hang quite loosely at your sides or put them behind your back. Traverse your audience as eye contact is a powerful persuasive tool. Each person listening to you needs to feel included and it is a good technique to move your eyes across the audience while speaking. If you are sitting remember you must still look around your audience and address them directly.

5 Too many unnecessary gestures can be offputting, and do not fiddle with your notes, chalk or pen, coins or your hair. If you are an inexperienced speaker or the audience is small, it is probably better that you keep gesticulations to the minimum. With a large audience, the non-verbal impact of gesture, or moving towards the audience, can be vital to compel the attention. It is a useful tool to express any meaning.

6 Voice production, quality and force of sound are particular to each individual person. When used effectively, the human voice can express every kind of feeling. If used correctly it can be powerful, holding people's attention immediately. It can be a great aid to clarify the meaning of something. Inflection and modulation of tone are important, as is varying the volume level depending on the size of the area you are speaking in; if there is no variation in your voice it can be boring to listen to. Speak clearly, concisely, slowly and to the point. If you feel nervous then deliberately slow down, pausing occasionally to allow time for the audience to take in some of the finer details. Use your natural voice; do not try to speak with an affected tone. Use straight-forward language, avoiding sentences with a complicated

structure. If the hall is large use a microphone rather than straining or raising your voice too high. If you are worried about your voice, form all the vowels, and give some additional attention to the consonants at the beginning and at the ends of words.

7 Do not overemphasize points inappropriately; tell the audience what is important by the way you say it, using your voice to show the importance of the meaning. If you dry up, try summarizing key facts. Think of your presentation as a conversation with the audience – speak to the people in front of you. Talk to them, never at them. Even when preparing the talk, try and think of it as a discussion with people you know. Capture their attention by using some humour, or short anecdotes. Avoid meaningless words or phrases. The beginning and the last sentences are the most crucial; they must be clear, resounding and striking. Many good speakers actually write these out and learn them even when the rest of the presentation is left entirely in note form. This always results in a far more effective and natural presentation.

8 Some mannerisms can be irritating, and may be distracting. They can also make you appear nervous. Try to avoid verbal mannerisms such as repeating the same word many times (like 'you know', mutters such as 'um' or 'er', 'something or other', 'and so forth', 'all that sort of thing' and so on). Also avoid phrases like 'I could go on and on, but', or 'I will have to leave it at that for now'. These phrases are not necessary and can be quite irritating to the audience. Do not constantly clear your throat, and always have some water handy. Behaviour mannerisms can be equally offputting; for instance, men should not put their hands in their pockets and rattle change. Do not walk around too much, unless you are making a point.

9 It is good to have notes, but do not try to read them word for word. When written material is spoken aloud it can sound too highly organized. Use headings for each part of your presentation. Do not try to conceal your notes, hold them at waist level to avoid dropping the eyes too far, glancing up from time to time, so that you do not break contact with the audience too much.

10 Timing is important. If you have been given 30 minutes, keep to it. Make sure you can see the time easily; if you cannot see a clock, put a watch on the table or somewhere convenient, or get someone to give you a 10-minute time-check. Mark time checkpoints in your notes. If you digress, do not rush in order to cover everything else in the time; it is better to omit the less vital points. Always adjust your presentation to suit the audience reaction. When you say 'Finally', make sure that it is final.

Handling questions from the audience

Taking questions from the floor can be more nerve-racking than making the presentation. However, it is an excellent way of making contact with an audience and meeting their needs more thoroughly. It gives your listeners a chance to participate, especially if you are worried about the level of interest or of comprehension, and questions can give you some valuable guidance. They give you feedback, but remember that if indifferently handled then questions can diminish a good speech. However, well-handled questions can improve the content immensely.

Decide at what stage you wish to take questions. Some people feel comfortable about being interrupted and allow questions to be asked at any stage. If this is so, tell the audience at the outset. Sometimes, it may be appropriate to generate questions after each section to help understanding. Again, make it clear how you wish to operate as you may wish to deliver your speech in its entirety before handling any questions. Again, say so at the beginning.

Make sure that everyone knows what the question is. It is a good idea to repeat it as it may have been inaudible or badly phrased and this is particularly important if you have a large audience so that everyone is aware before you answer. By repeating the question clearly, this also gives you a little more thinking time. Ask yourself, Why is the question being asked? Do I understand the question? Has the rest of the audience understood? If it is a technical question from a professional audience, translate any jargon for the benefit of the rest of the audience and take advantage by passing it back to the person to answer, saying, 'You are the professional, what would you do?'; you may be able to use the question to advantage in reinforcing one of your points. Be wary of allowing a single questioner to dominate the proceedings, especially if she or he has a particular axe to grind. Keep to the point, and be short but not abrupt. Be friendly, and firm but fair. Avoid ever being aggressive or personal. If the questioner is aggressive, then try to keep composed but look directly at the person when speaking. With sarcastic questions, do not be drawn but try to take a light-hearted approach or throw them back to the audience for their comments. Always acknowledge a good question, whether it is good in its own right or because it helps you make your point.

Do not let the questions digress too much. If irrelevant issues are being raised, then tactfully indicate that you would prefer to stick to the subjects covered in your talk. Unless the answer is simple, always think before responding on another theme. Be sure that the questioner is satisfied. This makes sense, builds up goodwill and gives you more credibility with the audience. Look over the audience's heads or drop your gaze while reflecting. Be clear about what your personal views are. Do not fix your gaze constantly on the questioner when replying, but look at the beginning of a row and at the end. Do not forget those in between; by traversing the audience you involve the members in the answer.

If the question is on policy, or is 'sensitive', state your position and say something like 'I am not able to go into any detail on that at the moment unfortunately'. Whenever dealing with areas of policy, there are three courses of action:

1 You can agree; there is little difficulty in this.
2 If in doubt and you don't know the answer, do not bluff. It is much better to admit the fact. If you ought to know the answer then offer to find out; you can advise them at a later juncture or in writing. Alternatively, you could try throwing the question back to the questioner or to the audience in general, saying, 'This is an excellent question, would anyone like to answer it?' For anyone who is totally sceptical or doubtful, you should aim to stress the common ground between you, and appealing to reason should suffice.
3 You can openly disagree. You must, however, try to make the audience appreciate your point of view by providing some evidence and examples. If this fails and you feel it is important to persevere, open up a further dialogue and aim to explore the questioner's views and feelings. Counter-questioning can be a useful strategy for handling objections and helps to get you off the defensive, although it should not be overused. Always reserve yourself the right to offer to answer a personal question individually after the session has finished.

Summarize by involving the whole group wherever practicable, and giving a short general account.

Visual aids

This is apparatus that can be used to enhance even the smallest presentation; for larger presentations it is essential. We absorb information mainly through two of our five senses in the following proportions: hearing makes up 10 per cent, while sight makes up 80 per cent, with taste, touch and smell making up the remainder. In reflexology we use four of the five senses, the latter two being as important as the former two. Audiences are often almost entirely dependent on hearing to get the message of a talk. Therefore, the visual aid is a vital additional tool for the speaker, helping to make points clear to facilitate and augment the retention levels of the listeners.

Seeing something is also helpful to reinforce learning and remembering. The advantage in using a visual aid to reinforce, supplement or clarify a message is that the audience is more likely to remember what it has seen as well as heard. If there is something to look at it also adds a certain amount of interest and variety to a presentation.

Visual aids are also time savers; just one picture can be worth its weight in gold, and certain points can be emphasized more strongly. Some may be difficult to convey verbally. If you have a lot of material, then visual aids can be used to pull out or summarize key issues. Boards or overhead projector slides can be designed to take the audience step by step along a line of thought, building up their understanding gradually. Good, attractive visual aids can help to maintain interest; audiences like them and they can be self-prepared using fibre- or felt-tipped pens, Letraset or adhesive coloured plastic. Transparencies can also be made from photocopied material provided the detail is clear.

There are disadvantages, however. Good visual aids need time and care to prepare, and some may require special materials and skills that you do not have. Many businesses or copy shops have the facility to produce colour transparencies, however. Too much visual material can be distracting. Being reliant on 'technology' also has its disadvantages and can be problematical, with bulbs blowing or machines breaking down. Always set up and check electrics in good time; preferably check equipment operation in advance to avoid embarrassment. Also make sure you have a spare bulb.

The following are the most commonly used visual aids:

- Good old-fashioned chalk and blackboard – this is perhaps the most versatile. Or you can use the white board and felt-tipped pens.
- Overhead projector (OHP) – this projects a transparency on to a wall or screen behind the speaker. Transparent acetates are used, either in single sheets or fixed in a cardboard frame or surround, and sometimes on a roll attached to the machine on the glass top. The advantages of OHPs are that they can be used in a room that is dark and the speaker can still face the

audience. Nevertheless, skilful use still takes a little practice and the machine should always be switched off when the visual aid is no longer being referred to, as the noise from the equipment, and the visual aid itself, can be distracting.

- Projectors – this apparatus enables you to project film or pictures on to a surface. A carousel of slides is helpful. These can be worked through quickly to give an overall view or at more length to give a detailed discussion of specific photographs, ensuring that the details are large enough to be clearly seen.
- Foot or hand charts, and other posters – these should illustrate what you are describing, and they attract and arouse attention.
- Demonstrations – these are useful if you can get somebody to act as a model. They help you explain or show how a reflexology movement is made, how you obtain a response to an area that you may have palpated on and you know may be out of balance, and other points. This is more advantageous than anything else to get your message across. You can also ask the model for comments and impressions.

In conclusion, we can see that visual aids are a powerful means of getting information across. But thought must be given to how they can be made to work for you, because they certainly can also work against you. This means careful planning, preparing and rehearsing, always bearing the type of audience in mind. Above all, remember that they are just a support to aid communication, not a complete explanation in themselves. They will not always make your point, but they will help you to confirm it.

Notes

Good notes should contain: the first sentence, the last sentence, and key words. They should be written on cards. Use one side only, with one theme or idea per card. Each card should be numbered. Each card then can be put at the bottom as each separate theme or idea is completed. This allows flexibility if time is short, as less important themes or ideas can be missed if necessary. Cards are convenient as they can be held quite easily at waist level.

Checking

Always make sure of the name of the place where you are expected, and exactly where it is. Check how you can get there.

Check also how big the venue is, and where you will be in relation to the audience. Ask questions such as: Will you be on a stage or rostrum? What is the seating arrangement for the audience and for you? On the day, make sure you arrive in plenty of time; it is better to be too early than late.

Check arrangements for equipment: are you providing it, or is it being provided? Are the technical details thought through, for example the distance the electrical equipment is from the sockets? Check that it works and that you know how to use it. On the day, ensure that there are no trailing wires to trip over. Check the layout of the room, move the chairs and move tables or equipment if you want to. Ask people to move if you feel it will help the layout. Finally, check that any aids you may need, like papers, pens or board cleaners, are all to hand.

A final checklist is as follows:

- Have you got your visual aids?
- Have you got your notes?
- Have you got a watch or clock you can see?
- Do you feel you are dressed appropriately and comfortably?
- Have you had time to rest beforehand?
- Have you had some fresh air?
- Have you had too much to drink (alcohol)?
- Have you got something to drink (water)?
- Have you planned to arrive in time to look at the room?

Having checked all these objectives, probably some of them several times, you should have allayed a whole range of very real fears about what could go wrong. Regardless of how many times you may speak, there is always the chance that something unforeseen may happen. These thoughts can plague you and sometimes they will not go away; this psychological response needs to be addressed by calming yourself down, as there are certain things that are out of your hands. Use the relaxation techniques below to help allay any unnecessary anxieties. These are techniques you may often suggest for others but rarely use yourself.

Nerves

Most people feel nervous before any sort of presentation, even an informal one. In fact sometimes this can be an advantage, as the adrenaline can help prepare you, but equally it can leave you dry mouthed and panicking. So it is most important to make allowances for your own nerves. Frequently it is the most informal of speeches, such as a presentation to a retiring member of staff, a short speech at a wedding, the acceptance of a gift, or a simple vote of thanks, that is the most nerve-racking. Nevertheless, as stated, a degree of nervousness provides energy and zest, which, if correctly focused, can provide the drive to make a presentation more effective.

Relaxation techniques

To calm yourself, either do deep breathing or rest with your eyes closed, maybe with pads of moist cotton wool over the eyes; this feels wonderful for a few quiet minutes. A quiet walk taking in the fresh air is also most beneficial. Clenching and unclenching your fists, or shaking your hands and arms briskly or running on the spot as you might do on a cold day, all help release tension. Drop your chin to your chest to stretch out your tight neck and shoulder muscles.

Just prior to speaking try to relax, using whatever method above suits you best. Try to drop your shoulders so that you relax your neck muscles, and clench and unclench your hands again and again to relax them. If your mouth feels dry then have a drink of water or suck a sweet. Unless your audience consists of less than 10 people, stand to give your talk as this helps your breathing and your voice.

Last of all, just remind yourself that this is not actually a matter of life and death; you have probably chosen to do this, and think how good you will feel when it is all over. A useful point to bear in mind is that you are not the only nervous person in the room. The audience also is, at the least, apprehensive. They are often apprehensive on your behalf, because, even in situations where they might be hostile or in disagreement with what you have to say, they none the less will want you to say it effectively. As you warm up and become more confident they will feel more relaxed about your presentation and listen more intently to what you are saying. They may argue with you but that may be one of the responses that tells you that you are starting to get your message across.

Key points for designing handouts

A good way to ensure that your audience remembers the main points of your talk is to provide handouts. Here are some pointers:

- Decide what your audience may need from the handout. The simple way is to take the observations from giving a presentation, in terms of what they must know, should know, or could know.

- Know your audience as it helps to have some idea of their previous level of knowledge or educational background.
- Always use a clear and simple style. Try to write as you talk, using short sentences. If in doubt, put a full stop and start a new sentence and keep to short paragraphs. Use diagrams or illustrations and examples only if necessary to make your meaning clear.
- Decide on the layout as the finished product must be pleasant to look at. Use both lower and upper case writing, as this gives impact. Leave a space clear all round the page and enclose it in a frame. Leave plenty of space between paragraphs or sections. Avoid too much underlining or the use of too many capitals or different fonts for emphasis as this can be visually confusing. Use boxes to emphasize key points.
- Decide on the method of duplicating copies. The final decision may depend on quantity, as one method may be cheaper than the other, if required in large quantities.

APPENDIX I

Statutory support systems

You will be able to obtain advice about help and welfare services from your local advice centre, where invariably there is also information on local services available. Each country or state has their own rules and regulations; check with your local health information bureau. These lists provide information on support available in the UK. They often indicate a wide variety of groups that exist to give expert help when needed. If your local centre does not produce a list, then compile your own to aid and support your client. The following are the types of information that may be needed:

Addictions

Alcoholics Anonymous – these often operate a 24-hour helpline.
Drugs Advisory Service – the aim is to provide the necessary support for substance users and their relatives and friends. This entails counselling, so an appointment is compulsory.
Emergency Drug Line – sometimes there is a 24-hour helpline.
Gamblers Anonymous – these often offer self-help groups to support the person and family.
Most doctors operate a 'quit smoking' session.

Age

Local voluntary wardens are listed.
Day centres provide services for retired residents.
Most towns have an Age Concern number to contact.

Children

Child guidance services include: babies in need, advice for sexually assaulted children, antibullying childline (often this is a freephone number).

General health

For cases of bereavement, cot death, miscarriage and cancer, most towns have local support groups or helplines; these offer practical advice, friendship and understanding.
The Samaritans operate a 24-hour helpline.

Miscellaneous

There are very long lists to cover every eventuality, from marriage guidance centres, to local charities and religious organizations.

These types of lists are often similar from one town to the next and they usually include addresses and telephone numbers. In a time of crisis most people are unsure where to turn. Because we are holistic practitioners we often become more involved in the family problems. During your time in practice it is beneficial if you are able to offer support and advice, so keep a list to hand. I have had parents wrongly accused of child abuse. I have also had parents extremely upset because their teenager is taking drugs. I also treat many elderly people, who are often lonely and need a little bit of advice and compassion. A practitioner often acts as a counsellor and the greatest skill is to offer sympathetic listening and understanding, which paves the way to self-help so that they can deal with their own personal relationships, and any occupational or social problems.

APPENDIX II

First aid in the treatment room

First aid is treatment on the occurrence of an injury or sudden illness, using whatever means that are available to you at the time; this may take place prior to a medical practitioner arriving. We advise all students before commencing in practice to attend a basic 'first aid at work' course. The purpose of first aid is:

- To preserve life
- To prevent the person's condition worsening
- To promote recovery.

The following is just a guide for emergencies. If a patient becomes unwell or falls down on your premises it is your responsibility to ensure their safety.

- Remain calm – assess the situation and diagnose what is wrong.
- The principles of diagnosis – these are the same as we always use with patients.
- History – if the patient is conscious, ask what happened.
- Symptoms – ask the patient about any pain or sensations he or she may feel.
- Signs – look at the colour of the patient's face; is the breathing shallow or are they sweating? Use your senses. Smell, look, listen and assess.

The main conditions you may come into contact with are listed below.

The following heart attack conditions are the result of reduction of the blood supply to the muscular wall of the heart causing lack of oxygen to the heart muscle.

Angina pectoris
This is often described by the sufferer as severe indigestion. It is a strangling, constrictive pain extending to the left shoulder and arm, and sometimes pain is felt in the throat. This pain is due to insufficient oxygenated blood reaching the heart muscle.

Coronary obstruction
In this condition, again excruciating pain is felt in the chest, often following the same course as the above. In both conditions, the patient would complain of pain in the chest, anything from mild to severe. This pain can be such as to make them stop in their tracks or feel giddy, and lean against something for support or even fall to the ground. The breath is short and the pulse is weak. Nausea and dizziness and sweating are common. Their skin is often ashen and their lips are blue.

Emergency treatment.   Do not move the patient unnecessarily. Loosen tight clothing and call for medical aid immediately. In the mean time, leave the person in a half-sitting position, with head and shoulders supported and knees bent, propped up against a wall if possible. If unconscious and breathing place the patient in the recovery position so the airway is unobstructed.

Cardiac arrest

In this condition, the pumping action of the heart stops suddenly, with total loss of consciousness; there is no pulse, and no breathing. A person who is still breathing is not suffering from cardiac arrest.

Emergency treatment. If breathing fails, try to start the patient breathing as follows. Pinch the nose and tilt the head back while supporting under the neck. Make sure there is no obstruction in the mouth. Put your lips around the mouth and blow at least 10 times and then check to see whether the person is breathing. If not, repeat. Call an ambulance as soon as possible. Cardiac compression should not be done unless you are a qualified first aider and have a knowledge of the correct procedures.

Epileptic fit

Do not move or restrain the person unless there is any danger that they may hurt themselves more. Do not attempt to put anything in the person's mouth or try to open the mouth in any way. When the attack is over, place the person in the recovery position. On recovery, encourage the person to rest for a while. It can take up to 15 minutes for the person to regain consciousness completely.

Fainting

This follows a temporary reduction to the blood supply to the brain. This has been known to happen during a treatment of reflexology. It may be because the patient has remained in one position too long, or the room is overheated and there is insufficient ventilation, or the stimulation was too strong, or the patient is apprehensive and unsure. The person may also have been excessively fatigued on arrival, and they stood up too quickly after treatment. Finally, diabetics are sometimes prone to fainting (*see below*). Elderly people need to remain resting for a few minutes after treatment. Some drugs can also cause episodes of fainting. Always watch the patient for any signs of change of colour in the face. Sudden pallor often indicates a problem.

Emergency treatment.   Sit the client down on the floor and put the head between the knees. Get the person to breathe deeply, loosening all tight clothing. If the patient becomes unconscious but is still breathing, elevate the legs above chest level. If the patient does not regain consciousness, check for any breathing, and if this is absent continue resuscitation as above (*see* Cardiac arrest). Then put the patient in the recovery position and send for aid.

Hypoglycaemia

This condition usually occurs in insulin-dependent diabetics, who may have a low level of glucose in the blood. This is a serious condition because the brain must receive sufficient glucose or it could lead to an impairment of certain functions. The problem may arise from too much insulin, too much exercise, or insufficient food intake. The person may appear drunk and incoherent, they may even be sweating profusely, and have a pallor to their skin. Their breathing is shallow and they have no odour on their breath.

Emergency treatment. If conscious, give the person something sweet to drink or eat (containing glucose or honey – or the person may be carrying glucose/dextrose tablets). If there is an improvement this is an indication that the insulin dose is possibly too high, so the medical practitioner should be contacted so that the insulin dosage can be reviewed. If the patient becomes unconscious put in the recovery position, put a glucose tablet in the mouth (or rub honey, if available, around the gums), and call for medical help immediately.

Note. Never apply too hard a pressure when treating diabetics with reflexology. If unconscious, check to see if the person has a bracelet indicating that he or she is diabetic.

Hyperglycaemia

This is excess glucose in the blood and insufficient insulin in the blood. This can simply be due to an inadequately controlled diet (eg excessive intake of carbohydrates and sugars). Usually the patient is aware that there is a problem.

Emergency treatment. If the person feels unwell, treat as for fainting. Suggest the patient sees the medical practitioner as soon as possible.

Nosebleeds

This can be an annoying problem; the patient may simply have blown their nose too hard, or possibly bent down and knocked their nose on some edge of furniture. If there is any profuse flow of blood from the nose, keep the head forward. Working SP-1 on the great toe helps to stem blood flow from the nose.

Note. Do not let the person raise their head as blood may be swallowed or inhaled, causing vomiting, or affecting the breathing.

Emergency treatment. Loosen all tight clothing, and pinch the soft part of the nose, do not encourage the person to speak. Let the blood trickle down, and mop it up as much as possible. Release the pressure after at least 10 minutes; if the bleeding has not stopped continue for another 10 minutes. If there is still a constant stream of blood after 30 minutes seek medical help immediately.

Bleeding varicose veins
These are veins that are varicosed (swollen) and superficial; they are vulnerable to any slight knock on a chair leg or piece of furniture, and can bleed profusely. If blood flow is not controlled immediately the condition can be fatal.

Note. Before giving reflexology treatment always remove your watch and ensure your nails are well trimmed. Do not leave wires trailing or have loose rugs whereby a person can easily trip up.

Emergency treatment. Apply pressure to the area, and elevate the leg immediately. Treat as for shock, and call for medical help at once.

Shock of any kind
If the patient becomes unconscious but is still breathing, elevate the legs above chest level. If the person does not regain consciousness check for breathing. If this is absent, follow the resuscitation procedure above (*see* Cardiac arrest). Call an ambulance as soon as possible.

Soft Tissue Injuries/Sprains and Strains
Apply the RICE routine: rest, ice, compression and elevation. This will help to alleviate any immediate discomfort such as pain and tenderness around a joint.

Cramp
When cramp occurs in foot muscles, apply something cold to the plantar area of the foot and gently push the foot towards the body. For leg muscles, push the leg gently towards the body whilst elevating it slightly. For hand muscles, straighten all the fingers very firmly but gently. Gently massage all the affected muscles.

APPENDIX III

Complementary therapies that may assist reflexology

Acupressure. Traditional Chinese system of healing through pressure on certain areas using the thumb and finger and other parts of the hand; the pressure points are the same as in acupuncture.

Acupuncture. Traditional Chinese system of healing through needles being placed at certain points which lie along channels called 'meridians'. The theory is that this method stops pain and cures organ imbalances.

Alexander Technique. Originated by Frederick Mathias Alexander. A technique of improving health through correcting posture.

Aromatherapy. A method of treating illness with concentrated plant-based oils, known as essential oils; these can be applied either by massage or by aromatic baths and steam inhalations.

Bach Flower Remedies. Originated by Edward Bach (1880–1936). It used homeopathic-type preparations made from plants and wild flowers, spring water and alcohol. These tinctures are given according to the person's attitude and emotional outlook.

Bates' Method. Originated by Dr William H Bates (1860–1931). A method of eye treatment through exercises to improve vision.

Biochemic Tissue Salts. Originated by Dr W H Schuessler (1821–98). Remedies consisting of mineral salts. A correct balance of minerals must be maintained to help everyday ailments.

Chiropractic. Originated by David Daniel Palmer (1845–1913). A technique of treating disorders through manipulation. Its theory is that skeletal displacement and soft tissue trauma may cause malfunction and irritation of nerves and muscles, causing disorders of the body. McTimoney chiropractic uses a much gentler manipulation than the original method.

Counselling. In this the person talks to someone trained in sympathetic listening skills. The patient is enabled to unburden himself or herself to help with the problem.

Herbal Medicine. In general use by many people. Plant-based remedies have powerful healing properties to restore health.

Homeopathy. Natural remedies to boost the body's own healing process. Based on the Samuel Hahnemann (1755–1843) principle of treating a disorder using minute doses of a substance that in large quantities produce symptoms similar to the disease.

Iridology. Used as a very useful diagnostic tool, the theory is that the organs of the body are laid out on the iris; through observation disorders are often noted prior to manifestation in the physical body.

Massage. Practised in early Egyptian times and also in ancient Greece (3000 BC). Hippocrates was known as the 'Father of Medicine'; he stated that an oiled massage daily would improve your health.

Naturopathy. Treatment is aimed at helping your body to heal itself through natural means. Changing the diet, breathing exercises, gentle physical exercise, hot/cold baths, massage, and manipulation are all part of the natural healing process.

Osteopathy. A therapy relying on manipulative techniques, especially of the spine. The theory is that many diseases are caused or exacerbated by displacement of bones.

Shiatsu. Pressure on vital points. Practitioners also use many other parts of the body to apply pressure on tsubo (points on the meridians).

Tai Chi. Dating back to the 11th century. Another holistic therapy using a series of slow, continuous moves that are thought to achieve balance of Yin and Yang. It combines a meditation-like mental focusing with breathing and correct body alignment through motion.

Yoga. (Indian origins). A system of spiritual and mental and physical training to enhance the body, through mind control.

APPENDIX IV

Astrology and health

Astrology can be a valuable guide in helping in the diagnosis of imbalances. There are 12 divisions or signs of the zodiac. The following are general descriptions of their characteristics (note that they apply both to the individual's sun sign (the sign the sun is in at birth) and to their rising sign (the sign on the horizon at birth)).

Aries (the ram)

These individuals are usually pale skinned, tall and thickset, and often quite athletic and energetic. Females may be equally striking, often with long flowing hair. They may develop lung problems, which could lead to asthma. Their weak spots are the head-related areas, eyes, ears, maxillary area, jaw and teeth.

Taurus (the bull)

These individuals are generally sturdy, and often of medium height, with strong muscular legs. Males often have a moustache or beard. Females have a good head of hair that is well kept. Their weak spots are the mandible, jaw and lower teeth, throat area and thyroid gland. The kidneys could also be weak. Diabetes could be a problem, as they have a sweet tooth. Basically, however, they are very healthy.

Gemini (the twins)

Male Geminis are usually compact and dapper, while females are very trim and fashionable; both sexes often look younger than they are. Their weak spots are the upper appendicular skeleton, hands, arms and shoulders. There could be a weakness in the respiratory tract. As the nerves govern this sign, any of the autonomic nervous system may suffer. Irritable bowel syndrome and skin disorders are often evident.

Cancer (the crab)

These individuals tend to be well built and often appear top heavy; they often have small hands and feet. Their weak spots are the digestive system and thoracic area, lungs, and breasts in the female. They often have a negative attitude to life. But they are kind-hearted, honest and reliable, with very good business skills.

Leo (the lion)

These individuals often have a full head of hair and are well built. They are very proud people and like to look good. They love excesses of food and drink, and are gourmets. Their weak areas are the spinal column and the heart and the reproductive organs.

Virgo (the virgin)

These individuals tend to be slim with a good head of hair, and possessing a strong jaw; they are very photogenic. They are also neat in appearance. Their weak spots are that they are prone to allergies such as hayfever, asthma or eczema. They are often plagued by the nervous system, which could affect their bowels, causing irritable bowel syndrome or colitis.

Libra (the scales)

These people are tall or medium in height. They are charmers, with well-balanced features. A typical individual likes company and calm surroundings. Their weak spots are the urinary tract, bladder and kidneys. The liver or the pancreas could also be weak, which could cause diabetes, and the lumbar area could be a trouble spot. They need to drink plenty of water and keep to a good diet, otherwise they could become overweight.

Scorpio (the scorpion)

These people are generally well built and often aloof and unsmiling. Their weak spots are the lower lumbar area and reproductive tract, and sometimes the legs.

Sagittarius (the archer/centaur)

These individuals tend to be tall and well built, and very strong and physical. They are usually non-aggressive and popular, but very outspoken. Their weak spots are the thighs and hips.

Capricorn (the sea goat)

The Capricorn male is often well built and stocky, while the female is usually much more slender. Both are quiet and dignified in their manner. Their weak spots are the legs and knees; they may suffer from depression.

Aquarius (the water carrier)

These are generally tall and slim people; they are very fair minded. They may suffer with weaknesses in the ankles, with strains and sprains and even breaks; often other leg problems can develop, such as Achilles tendon strain.

Pisces (the fishes)

These individuals are usually tall with broad shoulders. They always take whatever opportunities come their way. Their weaknesses are the feet, and they suffer greatly when they are stressed; this can lead to problems developing in the glandular system.

The figure shows how the areas of the foot correspond to the signs of the zodiac.

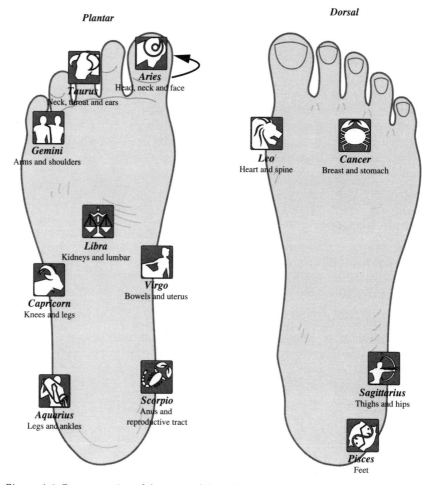

Figure A.1 Representation of the signs of the zodiac on the foot

APPENDIX V

Some questions that students may be asked in an examination

1 Why is it necessary to position the patient correctly?

Suggested answer. It enhances the effects of the treatment. Patients find it easier to relax. Cushions are there to support them; these are placed behind the head and under the knees. A loose covering over patients ensures they are warm, or if they are female and wearing a skirt they do not feel uncomfortable with their legs slightly apart. Clothing is loosened so that they do not feel restricted in any way.

2 What do you understand by contraindications?

Suggested Answer. These are any factors in a patient's condition that make it unwise to pursue a particular line of treatment.

3 What are the main four contraindications to reflexology?

Suggested answer. Patients should not be treated if they have severe fungi or viral infections of the feet; varicose veins that are very distended; complications such as thrombosis, phlebitis, history of miscarriages, they are pregnant and unused to reflexology; on strong medication such as IVF or drugs that cause changes to a system as in some heart problems. (In infectious illness, always wait until the acute stage has passed and there is no fear of cross infection.)

4 Name four abnormalities of the feet that can affect that reflex zone.

Suggested answer. Any of these: pes planus, spine problems, hallux valgus, shoulder and neck problems, hammer toe, mallet toe, corns, calloused areas, problems within the zone, such as eye or ear disorders. (In leg shortening, observe the ankle point as it could indicate lower back problems.)

5 What professional and ethical considerations must a reflexologist observe?

Suggested answer. (Refer to code of conduct.)

6 If a patient had a urinary problem what would you look for?

Suggested answer. A puffy or raised red area on the medial side of the foot, striations on the heel near the rectum point, and a very red colour in the pelvic area on the base of the heel.

7 Name the direct areas you would work for a bladder problem and the areas of assistance.

Suggested answer. Bladder, ureter and kidneys. The area of assistance is the lower spine for all the pelvic nerves, pelvic or groin lymphatics, reproductive areas and the spleen.

8(a) What is the definition of first aid?
 (b) What is the purpose of first aid?

Suggested answer. (a) Procedures used in an emergency. (b) To preserve life, to try to prevent the condition becoming worse, and to aid or to promote recovery of the person.

9 If a person fainted what procedures would you follow?

Suggested answer. Symptoms/signs are usually a slow weak pulse, and the person is pale and clammy often because of a brief temporary reduction in the flow of the blood to the brain. This could be due to a nervous reaction, an emotional upset, lack of food, overtiredness, or could also be due to a long period of inactivity. The aim is to position the fainted patient so that gravity helps the flow of blood to the brain. Raise the legs and maintain an open airway; loosen clothing; keep the patient cool; fan them or open a window. Always check to see if they had sustained an injury when falling.

10 What is the meaning of referred pain?

Suggested answer. This is pain that is experienced in a part of the body quite distant from its point of origin. This effect is brought about by the many sensory nerves around the body that share a common nerve pathway; each pathway arises from the spinal cord. Pain can be caused by irritation of a nerve, injury or inflammation of a nerve. (Pain in the left arm may be related to heart disorders. Pain in the leg or foot may be due to irritation of the sciatic nerve. This can be confusing to the patient as it often occurs when there is movement on the other side of the body, such as when they get in and out of a car or flexion of the foot while driving. Pain in between the shoulder blades, followed by feeling sick or vomiting after meals or coffee, is often due to embedding of a gall stone in a duct, causing biliary colic. In appendicitis, pain is first felt quite high above or around the navel area. This can move around, but if it is appendicitis it moves down into a lower area on the right side of the abdomen. This is very evident in phantom limb pain. This is because impulses from the remaining portion of the limb are interpreted by the brain as having come from that limb.)

APPENDIX VI
Useful addresses

United Kingdom

Crane School of Reflexology
135 Collins Meadow
Harlow
Essex CM19 4EJ
International and countrywide courses.
Tel 44 (0) 1279 421682
Fax 44 (0) 1279 441304

For a list of training establishments contact
any of the following:

Association of Reflexologists
23 Old Gloucester Street
London WC1N 3XX
Tel/Fax 0990 673320

The British Council of Complementary
Medicine
PO Box 194
London SE16 1QZ
Tel 0171 237 5165
Fax 0171 237 5175

British Complementary Medicine Asociation
249 Fosse Road South
Leicester
LE3 1AE

British Reflexology Association
Monks Orchard
Whitbourne
Worcester WR6 5RB

Guild of Complementary Practitioners
Liddle House
Liddle Close
Finchampstead
Berkshire RG40 4NS

The Institute for Complementary
Medicine
Unit 15, Taverns Quay
Commercial Centre
Rope Street
London SE16 1TX
Tel 0171 237 5165
Fax 0171 237 5175

International Institute of Reflexology
32 Priory Road
Portbury
Bristol BS20 9TH

International Therapy Examination
Council Limited
James House
Oakelbrook Mill
Newent
Gloucester
Tel 44(0) 1531 821875
Fax 44(0) 1531 822425

Reflexologists' Society
249 Fosse Road South
Leicester
LE3 1AE9PG

Scottish Institute for Reflexology
57 Horsley Dale
South Shields
Tyne & Wear
NE34 6LA

Rest of the world

Austria

Academy of Reflexology Austria
Achsengraben 12
Pregarten, A-4230

RWO-Shur Health Institute Intl
Geyrstrasse 80
6020 Innsbruck

Australia

Reflexology Association of Australia
National Enquiries
PO Box 366
Cammeray, NSW 2062
New South Wales
Tel (047) 214752
Fax (02) 9631 3287

PO Box 349
Morningside 4170
Queensland
Tel (07) 3229 3203

PO Box 624
Rosney Park, 7018
Tasmania
Tel (03) 6239 9669

27 Collins Street
Brighton, 3095
Victoria
Tel (03) 9899 4760
Fax (03) 9593 2221

PO Box 1032
Leederville, 6901
Western Australia
Tel (09) 388 2941

Belgium

Europese Akademie Voor
Complementaire Gezondheidszorg
Weg naar As 267
Genk 3600

National Vevrbond Der Begische
Reflexolgen
t.a.v. Achterlee 183
2460 Lichtaart

Canada

Reflexology Association of Canada (RAC)
Box 110
Brussels
Ontario
N0G 1HO

Reflexology Association of British
Columbia
214–3707 Hember Place
North Vancouver
BC V7G 2JY

China

China Reflexology Association
PO Box 2002
Beijing 100026
Tel/Fax 86 1 5068309

Denmark

Forenede Danske Zoneterapeuter
(Danish Reflexology Association)
FDZ Secretariat
Chr. Winthersvej 13
DK-6000 Kolding
Tel 45 7550 1250
Fax 45 7550 7447
Email fdz@.fdz dk
Web http:/www,fdz dk

Finland

Finnish Association of Natural Therapies
Pilspan
Kylantle
01730 Vantaa

France

Institute Yung
22 Rue Caumartin
75009 Paris

Germany

Fortbildungszentrun Fur Komplexe
Reflexzonetherapie
D-6232 Bad Soden

Deutscher Reflexologen Verband
Lloyd G Wells Strasse–15
Berlin 14163

Greece

Hellenic Association of Reflexologists
Alkionis 85
Paleo Falivo
Athens 17562

Hong Kong

Rwo-Shr Health Institute International
Room 192 Java Commercial Centre
128 Java Road
North Point

Ireland

Irish Reflexologists' Institute
3 Blackglen Court
Lamb's Cross
Sandyfd
Dublin
Tel 01 2952238
Secretary
4 Ruskin Park
Lisburn
Co Antrim

Israel

Israeli Reflexology Association
Mordechai 38
Kriat Tivon 36023

Israeli Reflexology Association
PO Box 39220
Tel Aviv 61391

Italy

Federatzione Italiana Di Reflessologia
del Piede
Via Rinaldini N10 Bis
Vestone
(Bresica) 25078

Federatzione Italiana Di Reflessologia
del Piede
Via F. Sforza, 48
20122 Milano
Tel/Fax 39 2 58303814

Japan

Reflexology Association of Japan
Akasaka TS Building, 5-1-36
Akasaka
Minato-ky
Tokyo 107

Malaysia

RWO-Shur Health Institute Intl
1–11 Wiayah Shopping Centre
Jalan Campbell 50100
Kuala Lumpar

Netherlands

Bond van Europese Reflexologen
AFD Nederland
PO Box 9009
Amsterdam NH 1006 AA

Vereniging Van Nederlands Reflexzone
Therapeuten
Noorderhaven 37A
Groningen 9712 VH

Reflexology in Europe Network
R. van Brederodestraat 24
1471 Kwadijk

New Zealand

New Zealand Institute of Reflexologists
PO Box 67 083
Mt Edan
Auckland

New Zealand Reflexology Association
PO Box 31 084
Auckland 9

Paraguay

Asociación de Reflajoterapist de Paraguay
C/O Gotthoid
Diaz de Solis 2546

Russia

I M Sechenov
Moscow Medical Academy
Department of Complementary Medicine
B, Pirogovskaja
2/6 Moscow 119881
Tel 7 095 246 99676
Fax 7 095 248 0214

South Africa

South African Reflexology Society
PO Box 201858
Durban North 4016

South African Reflexology Society
PO Box 1780
New Germany 3620
Kwazulu, Natal

Sweden

Axeisons Gymnastiska Institut
Box 6745/Gastrickegatan 10–12
11382 Stockholm

Switzerland

Association Suisse D'Etude de la
Réflexologie
2001 Neuchâtel
Casa Postale 126

United States of America

American Reflexology
Certification Board
P.O. Box 620607
Littleton CO 80162
Tel 303 933 6921
Fax 303 904 0460

Foot Reflex Awareness Association
PO Box 7622
Mission Hills
CA 91346

Reflexology Association of California
PO Box 641156
Los Angeles
CA 90064

Associated Reflexologists of Colorado
7043 West Colfax Avenue
Denver
CO 80215

Reflexology Organization of Wisconsin
904 Gail Place
Ft Atkinson, W1 53538

Iowa Assoc of Reflexologists
1315 Hammond Avenue
Waterloo
IA 50702

Maine Council of Reflexologists
PO Box 969
Jefferson
ME 04348

Reflexology of Minnesota
PO Box 662
Hinkly
MN 55037

Missouri State Reflex Association
12817 East 47th
17 Grove
Independence
MO 64055

Reflexology Association of America
4012 S. Rainbow Boulevard
Box K585
Las Vegas
Nevada 89103–2059

Nevada Reflexology Organization
836 Monika
Las Vegas
Nevada 89119

Reflexology Research Project
PO Box 35820
Albuquerque
NM 87176

North Dakota Reflexology Association
PO Box 411
Lisbon
ND 58054–0411
New York State Reflex Association
1492 Sweeney Street
North Tonawanda
NY 14120

Florida Association of Reflex
1270 Bently Way
Odessa
FL 33556

Ohio Association of Reflexologists
313 S Fifth Street
Tipp City
OH 45371

State of Oregon Reflex Association
2291 Jubilant Avenue
Medford
Oregon 97504

Pennsylvania Reflexology Association
1900 Emerson Street
Philadelphia
PA 19152

ICR Board of directors

International Council of Reflexologists
PO Box 621963
Littleton
CO 80162
USA
Fax 303 904 0460

January 1st 1997–December 31st 1998

Bill Flocco, President
606 East Magnolia B
Burbank CA 91501
USA

Russel McAllister, Vice President
PO Box 1032
Bondi Junction 2022
NSW
Australia

Christine Issel, Secretary
4311 Stockton Blvd
Sacramento
CA 95820
USA

Eugine Dietriech, Treasurer
384 Alper Street
Richmond Hill
Ontario
L4C 2Z4
Canada

Barbara Mosier, Administration Assistant
11129 W. Tulane
Littleton
CO 80127
USA

Hang Xiongwen, Director
PO Box 2002
Beijing 100026
China

Derthe Krogsgard, Director
Selgade 34-porten
1307 København K
Denmark

Beryl Crane, Director
135 Collins Meadow
Harlow
Essex CM19 4EJ
Great Britain

Sandy Rodgers, Past President
PO Box 290
Sunshine 3020
Victoria
Australia

Glossary

Acupressure A non-invasive treatment of healing and relieving pains using differing forms of pressure with fingers or thumbs on strategic points, which originated in China.

Acupuncture A traditional Chinese system of healing and inducing anaesthesia by inserting needles at strategic points.

Allergen Any type of substance that can cause an allergy, for example: pollen, animal fur or feathers, dust, house mites, moulds and fungi, some foods. Some additives used in processed foods can cause gastrointestinal discomforts. Chemicals in household products and in cosmetics can cause skin allergies.

Anterior The front of.

Antibodies Proteins produced in the body to destroy foreign invading bacteria or toxins (antigens).

Anticonvulsant A medication that can be used to prevent epileptic fits.

Antigens Any substance that may cause an antibody reaction by the immune system.

Anti-inflammatory Any substance that can reduce inflammation (often refers to a type of medication).

Autonomic nervous system The branch of the nervous system that usually works totally independently of our will and consciousness and is responsible for the vital functioning of some of our internal organs.

Beta blocker Medication that is used to calm the sympathetic nervous system down, thus slowing the heart rate and reducing blood pressure; often used in heart conditions.

Biomechanics The structure and movement of the locomotor system.

Borborygmus The noises made by the intestines; this is caused by the movement of gas and fluids, and this often increases during reflexology treatment.

Brachial plexus The complex array of nerves that arise from the cervical spine and supply everything from the fingers, hands, forearms and certain parts of the shoulder girdle.

Bronchodilator Any substance or force that causes widening of the airways, achieved by relaxing the smooth muscle of the bronchi and their principal branches.

Cancers Tumours that are malignant.

Chorionic gonadotrophin A hormone produced in the placenta during pregnancy and excreted in urine.

Contraindication An indication that a particular treatment may be unsuitable because of specific factors in a patient's condition.

Diabetes mellitus A disorder with complex causation, in which there is a disruption of carbohydrate metabolism because of a lack of, or resistance to, the pancreatic hormone insulin. There are two types: insulin-dependent and non-insulin-dependent.

Differential diagnosis In reflexology, a diagnosis in which the aim is not to ascertain the nature of the disease, but to diagnose an imbalance that may be caused by many other factors. In orthodox medicine, a diagnosis that distinguishes between two or more conditions with similar signs/symptoms.

Dorsal The back surface.

Dorsiflexion Moving the foot or toes so that they are flexed towards the body.

Dorsum The back of the hand or the top surface of the foot.

Dyspnoea Any laboured breathing, often evident in asthma, emphysema, and other lung or heart disease.

Eminence A rounded protuberance.

Emollients A substance that has a softening or soothing effect on the skin.

Epilepsy A disorder characterized by an abrupt loss of consciousness and possible convulsions.

Evert To turn outwards.

Fungus Micro-organism producing spores. Some types feed on the protein keratin, which is found in the skin, the hair and the nails.

Gamete The mature sex cells: the ovum in the female, and the spermatozoon of the male.

Gastrocnemius A large double muscle forming the bulk of the calf, ending below; in the Achilles tendon.

Gonadotrophins Hormones synthesized and released by the pituitary gland, and acting on the gonads.

Gonads The testes or ovaries of the male and female reproductive tract; they produce the gametes.

Hallux rigidus Stiffness or rigidity of the great toe; this can be due to trauma.

Hallux valgus An outward displacement of the great toe; a bunion is the swelling of the joint between the first metatarsal bone and the toe.

Hammer toe A condition usually affecting the middle joint of the second toe, which becomes bent. It is often due to incorrect footwear. If all the toes are so affected then it is referred to as 'claw foot'.

Homeostasis The maintenance of physiological stability (eg blood pressure, blood glucose, body temperature, and the acid–base balance) in the body.

Hormones Substances released into the blood that have an influence on the performance of other organs and tissues.

Hyper An excess of something.

Hypo A deficiency of something.

Hypothenar The padded tissue or protuberance at the base of the little finger.

Intrinsic muscles Those muscles situated within an organ.

Invert To turn inwards.

IVF (in-vitro fertilization) Fertilization of the ovum outside the body.

Kinetics The study of all aspects of motion and the forces affecting motion.

Ligament Bands of connective tissue that join bones together.

Lisfranc's joint line Line of amputation of the foot through the tarsometatarsal joint, discovered by Jacques Lisfranc, a surgeon in Paris, France (1790–1847). In reflexology it is used as a guide line from the distal edge of the medial cuneiform bone to the proximal end of the fifth metatarsal notch, as it follows the representation on the foot of the base of the rib cage.

Lumbago Severe pain or restriction in the lower back.

Mallet toe A condition where the distal phalanx of the toe cannot be extended.

Meissner's corpuscles Corpuscles sensitive to touch that are abundant in the fingertips and the pads of the toes.

Menopause Cessation of the menstrual cycle and release of egg cells from the ovaries. This occurs in women aged between their mid thirties to their mid fifties.

Meridian In TCM theory a channel through which Qi flows in the body; an imaginary line connecting the acupoints of an organ system.

Metacarpals The five bones of the hand that form the metacarpus.

Metatarsal The five bones of the foot that form the metatarsus.

Metatarsophalangeal The metatarsals and the phalanges, the toe bones.

Musculature The muscles of a region.

Musculoskeletal Both the muscular and skeletal systems together.

Mycosis Any disorder caused by a fungi.

Myelogram An X-ray of the central canal of the spinal cord, involving the injection of a dye into it.

Occiput The area at the back of the head joining it to the neck.

Oedema Any excess accumulation of fluid beneath the skin or in any body part.

Pacinian corpuscles Pressure receptors found in the skin, consisting of minute sensory nerve endings. They are very responsive to pressure.

Palmar The anterior surface of the hand, extending from the base of the fingers to the wrist.

Palpitations An irregular or more forceful beat of the heart, often felt in times of stress.

Paraesthesia Sensations of burning or pricking, usually of the areas served by the peripheral nerves.

Pes cavus A condition of claw foot, in which the instep of the foot is extremely arched.

Pes planus An abnormality of the arch, in which it drops almost to touch the ground.

Pes valgus A condition in which the foot is displaced and twisted outwards (*see* talipes).

Pes varus A condition in which the foot is displaced and twisted inwards.

Phlebitis General inflammation of a vein.

Phobias Any unreasonable fear of objects or certain situations.

Placenta The temporary organ that grows with the embryo and supplies it with nutrients and oxygen; it is expelled in the latter stages of labour as the afterbirth.

Plantar The sole of the foot.

Plantarflexion A downward movement away from the body.

Posterior The back of.

Proprioceptors Sensory nerve endings that respond to internal stimuli.

Psoriasis A skin disorder that sometimes has a hereditary link, in which there are red raised eruptions, usually appearing on the elbows and knees.

Pulmonary Pertaining to the lungs.

Qi or Chi A Chinese term, often translated as life energy, or vital force; a basic principle of TCM theory and Chinese thought; within the body it flows through meridians, and imbalances in it eventually manifest as illness (*see* Yin and Yang).

Sanjiao The Triple Burner/Heater/Warmer meridian in TCM, so named as it regulates the balance between the upper, middle and lower portions of the body.

Schizophrenia A mental disorder in which there is a progressive disintegration of normal mental functioning.

Seminal vesicles Paired organs secreting the liquid element of semen; they are usually referred to as male accessory sex glands.

Systemic Pertaining to the circulation of the body, as opposed to the circulation of the lungs.

Talipes A condition also called club foot; there are several forms.

Tarsal Relating to any one of the seven bones that form the tarsus (the bones of the ankle).

Tendon Tough cords composed of fibrous tissue attaching the end of a muscle to a bone.

Thenar The palm of the hand; the thenar eminence is the padded tissue or protuberance at the base of the thumb.

Thrombosis A blood clot formed within the blood vessels or the heart.

Tinea pedis A condition, sometimes referred to as athlete's foot, which is a very contagious infection often predominant in the webs of the third to fifth toes.

Tinnitus Any noise within the ear; it may be caused by some structural damage to the auditory pathway, or by some drugs, but usually the cause is unknown.

Vascular Pertaining to blood vessels, or supplied with blood vessels.

Vasoconstriction Narrowing of blood vessels.

Vasodilation Dilation and relaxation of blood vessels.

Venous system The system of veins in the body.

Verruca A highly infectious benign growth, usually on the plantar aspect of the foot, but sometimes on the hands.

Vulva The fleshy areas of tissue in the female sex organs surrounding the entrance to the vagina and urethra.

Yang The male, strong, positive, and active principle in TCM.

Yin The female, soft, negative, inactive principle in TCM.

Index